Symbols Summary

 MW01070675

gf = g

 GF Lines or Facility; o
No chance of cross-contamination

 Gluten Testing is performed

 Gluten-Free based on review of ingredient label
(as no GF list was provided)

 Procedures to Mitigate Cross-Contamination are in place,
although there are shared facilities or equipment

 Cross-Contamination is possible; or, Made with "gluten-free ingredients" (with no mention of overall status by the company)

No Icon. The company reported that the product is gluten-free
but provided no further context.

For the full key, see page 21 >>

Quick Reference Table of Contents

BAKING AISLE cont'd

**CANNED &
PACKAGED GOODS**

CONDIMENTS cont'd

SNACKS & CONVENIENCE FOODS

Baby Food & Formula

Frozen Foods

Meat

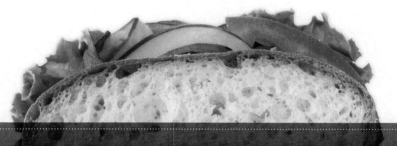

WE'RE BRINGING
SANDWICH BACK

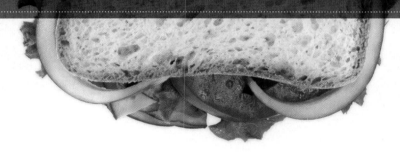

All of Udi's gluten-free breads are crafted by hand and baked for great taste. So pile the fixings high and enjoy. **The sandwich is back.**

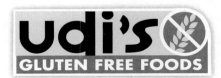

Fresh GF News

Free & Delivered Weekly to your email inbox

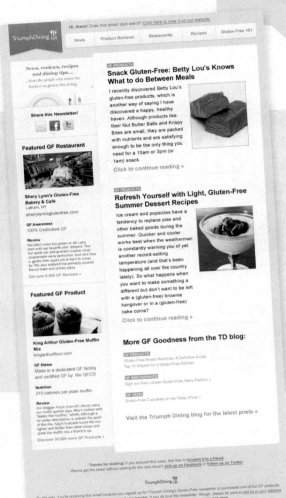

- All the Latest GF News

- GF Product Reviews

- GF Recipes

- GF Restaurants

And, check out the all-new feature, "GF 101: A Gluten-Free Guide for Beginners."

Sign up for free at

www.triumphdining.com

We will never rent or sell your information. The newsletter is always free.
Unsubscribe at anytime with the click of a mouse.

The gluten-free world is changing from one of frustrations and restrictions to one of choices and adventures. We at Triumph have been around since the height of the frustrations and restrictions—since before gluten-free beer and when Mr. Ritt's was the only GF bakery (long before you could get fresh GF baked goods at mainstream grocery stores).

And now, look where we are: We have gluten-free flour mixes that are sold at huge supermarkets like Safeway, Kroger, and Publix. We have six brands of gluten-free beer and 27 brands of gluten-free cereal. We have over 30,000 gluten-free products in this guide—somehow, I don't think you need all of them to make tonight's dinner.

The gluten-free world is expanding fast—and my hope is that this guide makes it easier for you to find all of the options that are now available to us. We've listed more products from an increasing spectrum of sources—regional stores, national mega-chains, major national brands and small, dedicated facilities with wide distribution.

However, despite the improved climate for gluten-free, we still have to exercise caution when making our grocery purchases. When we were editing the lists provided to us by brands and stores to make this guide, we did catch a few mistakes. The workers composing these lists at the food manufacturing companies are human, just like all of us. We have to be careful to avoid pitfalls and read labels carefully, even if we're told a product is gluten-free.

In the past, we've also found brands with quirks that could easily trip up a gluten-free shopper, like the brand with gluten-free teriyaki sauce but NON-gluten-free teriyaki marinade. These things can be dangerous—especially when the bottles are hard to tell apart. It's easy to confuse the two. I, for one, certainly would not expect the sauce to be safe while the marinade was not.

So that's the thing about expectations. We have to balance them with an open mind, so that we don't end up missing extraordinary opportunities to integrate new foods into our daily diets. But we also need to hang on to our expectations, to some extent, because they keep us healthy. For example, I'll read a label for teriyaki sauce much more closely than I'll read a label for, say, canned vegetables, because I expect that the teriyaki sauce is likely to have gluten in it.

New developments in gluten-free have changed the way we shop, but they haven't eliminated the challenge. Still, very few products are labeled "gluten-free," and still, no one is really quite sure if their definition of "gluten-free" is the same as the next person's. The FDA hasn't regulated this definition yet (even though it's more than two years overdue), so many companies hesitate to confirm that their products are gluten-free, even if you ask. Other companies gladly share the gluten-free status of their products, but only when asked.

So then our challenge becomes: How do we ask companies about 40,000 products? (That is, after all, the number of products sold in the average American grocery store.) The answer is this guide. It narrows down the grocery aisles to the products you'll want to inquire about more deeply; it enumerates your many options while saving you the time and effort required to sift through all of the products at the store. We want to help you eat well while saving time and money, anywhere you shop.

So please—if there's any way we can better serve you, if we can make your trip to the grocery store even easier, please let me know. Write to me at any time—I read each email personally, and I take your feedback to heart. We're always looking for ways to improve this guide and to make it more useful for you.

Happy gluten-free shopping, cooking, and eating,

Ross Cohen
President
Triumph Dining
ross@triumphdining.com

GENERAL TIPS FOR GROCERY SHOPPING

Everyone knows how to grocery shop—we've all been doing it most of our adult lives. The interesting thing is that each person approaches shopping slightly differently. Some people spend hours methodically comparing prices in search of the best deal, and others race through the store as quickly as possible so they can move on to other things. There's no right or wrong way to shop, but what follows are a few basic tips and ideas to help make your gluten-free shopping trips a little more successful—no matter what your personal shopping style is.

Choosing a Grocery Store

Some grocery stores are simply better for the gluten-free shopper than others. Generally, I prefer to do my shopping in stores that cater to gluten-free clientele in some way—it makes my shopping easier, and I prefer to support the businesses that focus on my needs.

A store's focus on gluten-free customers can manifest itself in several ways:

1. Grouping gluten-free goods in one section, like Kroger does;

2. Stocking an extensive selection of gluten-free products—many smaller, specialty stores like Martindale's in Springfield, PA, Against the Grain in Salt Lake City, UT, and Gluten-Free Trading Company in Milwaukee, WI pride themselves on carrying hundreds or thousands of specialty gluten-free items;

3. Labeling gluten-free foods—either in the grocery aisle like Whole Foods, or on packaging itself; Wegman's in New York marks their gluten-free private label foods with a little "G";

4. Publishing a list of gluten-free items that can be found in their stores, like the Trader Joe's chains do.

Stores that fit into these categories will tend to have more options for gluten-free customers, resulting in a better shopping experience. Try to frequent these types of stores when you can.

But, we understand that not everyone lives near a Trader Joe's, or can afford to buy all their groceries from premium and specialty stores. That's why this guide is designed to help you find gluten-free options in any grocery store—whether or not it specifically caters to gluten-free customers.

COMMON PITFALLS TO AVOID

One ongoing concern for people on the gluten-free diet is cross-contamination. It can happen anywhere, there's no way to know whether it's happened to a product, and it's rarely ever flagged for us. Also, the Food Allergen Labeling and Consumer Protection Act does not set specific standards for using cross-contamination advisory statements or require manufacturers to identify the possibility of inadvertent cross-contamination. (See the next chapter for a more in-depth discussion of the FALCPA.)

And, concerns about cross-contamination extend beyond grocery store shelves, to bulk bins, deli/meat counters, and the prepared foods sections.

Bulk Bins

Bulk bins are largely left unattended by grocery store personnel. There's often no way to tell that other customers haven't inadvertently shared serving scoops across products, potentially contaminating anything that otherwise would have been gluten-free. And, there's no indication whether products rotate through the bins or, if they do, whether the bins are thoroughly cleaned before transitions. In other words, the bin that holds a seemingly gluten-free product today could have been full of wheat flour last week. For these reasons, we recommend avoiding bulk bins and buying packaged items, instead.

The Deli Counter

Deli counters and prepared food sections present a different challenge. Here, store personnel directly handle food products meant for your consumption. The easiest way to navigate these challenges is to think of the deli counter and prepared food section as "mini restaurants." (For more information about issues to consider in gluten-free restaurant dining, please refer to *The Essential Gluten-Free Restaurant Guide*, also available from Triumph Dining.)

Before you make a purchase, you need to understand both the ingredients in the food and the preparation methods used to create it. There are many issues to consider in making a decision about these foods. Some examples include: Do gluten-containing meats go in the deli slicer?

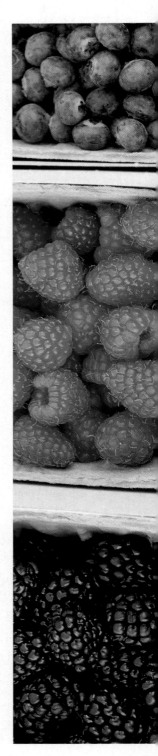

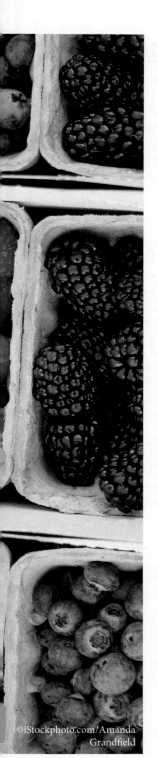

What, if any, precautions are taken in the prep area to avoid cross-contamination? Are there ingredient labels on the prepared foods? How accurate are those labels?

Often, however, it's challenging to interface with the employees who prepared these foods. At some grocery stores we've seen, the prepared foods are made off-site or by an early morning crew that's long since cleared out by the time the typical person shops, making it hard to get questions answered about dish contents and preparation methods. For these reasons, we recommend frequenting deli counters and prepared food sections only when you've done due diligence to confirm that the products you're purchasing truly are gluten-free.

Selecting Your Groceries

Despite a restricted diet, there are still many wonderful foods for gluten-free shoppers to choose from. When given a choice, I prefer to support the companies that cater to the needs of gluten-free customers. Some of these companies produce specialty products for the gluten-free market. Others have dedicated manufacturing lines and/or carefully test their products for gluten. Please consider buying their products and calling or writing in to let them know you appreciate their efforts. The more we support these businesses, the more products we'll have to choose from in the future.

Consider Your Information Source

When thinking about which products to purchase and evaluating information available to you, please keep in mind that primary source information, like ingredient statements on packages and manufacturer statements, is always better and more reliable than secondary source information, like postings on message boards and compilation lists (this guide included). Think of it like a game of telephone—the more people who handle information before you receive it, or the older that information gets, the greater chance there is of it having inaccuracies or other problems.

Always Read Labels

The goal of this guide is to drastically cut your label-reading time, but the reality is that no product obviates the

©iStockphoto.com/Amanda Grandfield

need for label-reading entirely. Product formulations can change without notice, companies can make mistakes on their gluten-free lists, and people compiling information can make mistakes as well. That's why you need to read labels every time you make a purchase, and regularly contact the company to confirm the gluten-free status of the products you consume.

Never Make Assumptions

When contacting companies, please keep in mind that the FDA has yet to issue a rule defining the term "gluten-free." Meanwhile, there's a lot of conflicting information on the gluten-free diet, even among dieticians, support groups and the many other experts in the field. Some believe that blue cheese is gluten-free; others do not. And the emerging question about the suitability of oats in the gluten-free diet adds even more confusion. So, don't expect a company to guess what your definition of gluten-free is. Always ask questions to make sure you understand what they mean when they say "gluten-free."

Where to Find More Information

This guide pre-supposes that you are familiar with the gluten-free diet. But for those just starting out, there are some excellent resources available to help you understand the gluten-free diet and to make informed choices. For example, there are a host of helpful resources available from local and national support groups, widely available books and online materials. Doctors and nutritionists are also an excellent source of information. In short, please be proactive about educating yourself. When it comes to the gluten-free diet, the educated shopper really is the only healthy shopper!

Gluten Free Oats?

Ask your doctor to see if "gluten-free" oats may be right for you. Recent research suggests that moderate consumption of oats can be safe for most Celiacs. However, there's a catch . . . it's only pure, uncontaminated oats.

In contrast, normal oats and oat products, like the ones found at your local grocer, are usually cross-contaminated with wheat during harvest, transport, or processing. Consequently, they are unsafe for the gluten-free diet.

However, pure, uncontaminated oats are available. They have to be specially grown and processed to avoid cross-contamination, so they are harder to find and more expensive than traditional oats. But if you're hankering for oatmeal-raisin cookies or a crunchy bowl of granola, you may finally have a safe option!

BOB'S RED MILL
(800) 553-2258

CREAM HILL ESTATES
(866) 727-3628

GLUTEN FREE OATS
(888) 941-9922

Effective January 1, 2006, the Food Allergen Labeling and Consumer Protection Act of 2004 (FALCPA), set requirements for the labeling of eight major allergens on packaged foods. This is a quick overview of the elements of the FALCPA that are likely to be relevant to consumers on a gluten-free diet.[1]

Allergens Covered

The FALCPA covers eight major allergens that are credited with causing 90% of all food allergies. Those allergens include: milk, eggs, fish, crustacean shellfish, tree nuts, peanuts, soybeans and, most importantly, wheat. The FDA notes that, for the purposes of the FALCPA, wheat includes common wheat, durum wheat, club wheat, spelt, semolina, Einkorn, emmer, kamut and triticale.

Allergens Not Covered

It's important to note that the FALCPA does **not** cover barley or rye. Nor does it cover oats, which are likely to be cross-contaminated with wheat.

Labeling: What's Required

The FALCPA requires food manufacturers to identify allergens in ingredient lists in one of two ways:

1. In the ingredient listing, the common or usual name of the major food allergen must be followed in parentheses by the name of the food source from which the major allergen is derived. For example: "Enriched flour (wheat flour…)," or

2. Immediately following the ingredient listing, a "Contains" statement must indicate the name of the food source from which the major food allergen is derived. For example: "Contains: milk, wheat and eggs."

Allergens present in flavorings, coloring and additives must also be identified in one of the two ways listed above.

Labeling: What's Not Required

It is important to note that the FALCPA does not apply to major food allergens that are unintentionally added to food as a result of cross-contamination. Cross-contamination can result during the growing and harvesting of crops, or from the use of shared storage, transportation or production equipment.

---

[1] Please note this brief overview is not meant to be comprehensive, nor is it intended as medical or legal advice. If you have questions about food labeling laws or their impact on your dietary choices and decision making, please consult a legal professional, dietician or doctor, as appropriate.

The FALCPA also does not address the use of advisory labeling, including statements designed to identify the possibility of cross-contamination. The FALCPA does not require the use of such statements, nor does it specifically articulate standards of use for advisory statements.

Application

The FALCPA applies to all packaged foods sold in the U.S. that are regulated by the FDA and that are required to have ingredient statements.

It's important to note that the FALCPA does not apply to meat products, poultry products and egg products that fall under the authority of the USDA.

The Big Picture

What does this all mean for people following the gluten-free diet? There are three important limitations of the FALCPA to keep in mind:

- As far as gluten is concerned, the FALCPA does not cover it. The FALCPA covers wheat, but not rye, barley or other potentially troublesome grains.
- The FALCPA covers only products regulated by the FDA that require ingredient lists. For any product that does not require an ingredient list (such as raw fruits), or that falls outside the FDA's jurisdiction (such as meat, poultry and egg products that fall under the authority of the USDA), the FALCPA does not require manufacturers to identify major allergens.
- The FALCPA does not require manufacturers to identify the possibility of inadvertent cross-contamination, nor does it set specific standards for using advisory statements warning of potential cross-contamination.

The important thing to remember is that, despite improved labeling laws, hidden gluten in grocery items is still a very real possibility. Gluten can come from non-wheat sources, result from cross-contamination, or can occur in products not covered by the FALCPA. For those reasons, it's important to remain vigilant and carefully scrutinize the products you buy. It's not enough to just read labels; contacting manufacturers directly is often necessary.

What is Gluten-Free Anyway?

One final note on the FALCPA: The FALCPA required the FDA to issue a rule to define and permit the use of the term "gluten-free" on food labels by August 2008 (clearly, this ruling has been delayed by quite some time). We expect that ruling in the future, but when it comes, it will not require food companies to label gluten-free products as such. Rather, the FDA will establish a uniform standard definition of the term "gluten-free" to be used voluntarily by food manufacturers, likely after some period of notice to allow companies time to comply. For more information, please visit the FDA at www.fda.gov.

USING THIS PRODUCT LIST

Our goal is for this guide to make your shopping trips easier, safer, and full of choices. There are a few things you need to know about this guide's content and organization to help us fulfill that goal.

PRODUCTS FEATURED

Our guide covers over 30,000 products from hundreds of different brands. The products listed are likely to be found in typical American grocery stores like Wal-Mart, Meijer, Hy-Vee, etc. They include brand names, as well as private label brands from some of the larger grocery chains. In cases where the grocery chain's name is different from their private label brand, we've also put the chain's name in parentheses next to the private label brand name.

When "All" are Gluten-Free

Some brands publish a list enumerating each gluten-free item, while others chose to simply say all foods in a particular category are gluten-free. In the latter case, we list the brand name in the appropriate category and sub-category, followed by a description of the products covered and the word "All," where applicable. For example, if a company, let's call it "Brand X," tells us that all its cheeses are gluten-free, it will be listed under "Brand X," followed by "Cheeses (All)." Alternatively, sometimes the brand communicated that all of their products are gluten-free, in which case, they will be noted in the guide as "Brand X (All)," regardless of category.

"All BUT"

Sometimes, the brand communicated that all but a few of its products were gluten-free. In those cases, they're listed as "Brand X (All BUT . . .)." That qualifier will always appear with Brand X across all categories to cut down on the need to cross-reference multiple sub-categories as you shop.

PRODUCTS NOT FEATURED

You will not find many "boutique" gluten-free brands in this guide, unless they are likely to be found in typical grocery stores. This list is far from comprehensive; there are smaller brands and new items popping up all the time. Just because a product isn't listed in these pages doesn't mean it's not gluten-free. If there's something you're interested in that's not listed in this guide, call the company directly or let us know, and we'll look into adding it for the next edition.

We haven't listed some items that are generally accepted and widely known to be gluten-free. For example, plain dairy milk is not listed. However, we have listed

Navigation Tip

The Easy Reference Table of Contents on the inside front cover is a quick visual reference for the different categories and sub-categories. Or, use the index in the back, if you prefer.

flavored milk, sour cream and other items that contain ingredients (e.g., thickeners or other additives) that may be of concern to some shoppers. Of course, what is "generally accepted" and "widely known" to be gluten-free is subjective. So while one person may find an entire sub-category of items we cover in the guide to be obviously gluten-free, some will not. We try to be as inclusive as possible for the sake of the latter audience.

For the sake of simplicity, this guide only lists items on a company's gluten-free list. We have excluded items that were not reported to be gluten-free.

Finally, there are some brands missing from the product listings because they simply do not provide or maintain lists of their gluten-free products. Unfortunately, companies are not required to maintain or share their gluten-free lists, so not every company can be listed in this guide. See the opposite page for details on some major brands that don't maintain or share gluten-free lists.

GENERAL OVERVIEW OF ORGANIZATION

The product list is organized into a three tier system: first by category, then by subcategory, then by product name.

Organization by Category

The products listed in this guide are arranged like a typical grocery store. The list is organized first by master categories that align with aisles in a grocery store, like those for Dairy and Eggs, Snacks and Frozen Foods. Our hope is that organizing the guide by grocery aisle will make your trip through the store quicker—you can follow along in the guide as you shop through the store.

There are a few exceptions to the link between master category and grocery aisle: in some cases, our consumer research found it more helpful to organize items by general category as opposed to aisle. For example, while refrigerated

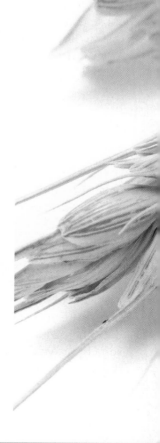

Why Can't I Find My Brand?

Some brands (including some private label store brands) don't provide gluten-free product lists, so you won't find them in our guide. Some brands cite reasons such as the high frequency with which ingredients change. Others are simply unwilling to claim a product is gluten-free until the FDA issues a final ruling on the definition of "gluten-free." Whatever their reasons, we can't force a company to share its gluten-free list.

On the bright side, several of these brands, while they don't provide complete lists, do have ways for you to investigate the gluten-free status of their products. **Sara Lee** brands, for example, have a "truth in labeling" policy, while **Supervalu**'s customer service will look up the status of its private label products (be sure to have the UPC code ready). Other stores, like **Trader Joe's** and **Whole Foods**, have full or partial gluten-free lists online or at their store locations.

"How can I find out the details about my brand's gluten-free products?"

We've compiled a list of the biggest, most popular stores and brands that don't offer traditional gluten-free lists. We've also investigated their reasons for not having a list, as well as the steps consumers need to take to get information about the gluten-free status of products. Just visit this page on our blog for more information:

www.triumphdining.com/blog/brands-without-gf-lists

"What are the chances that my store will ever have a gluten-free product list?"

The chances are a lot higher if you contact the brand and tell them you want it! On our blog, we've also included contact information for the brands and stores we've researched. Call or write to them today to let them know that you are a valuable customer and want to see an official gluten-free product list. If enough people ask, they'll deliver!

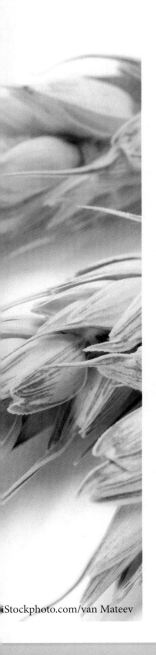

orange juice is often found in the Dairy and Eggs aisle, you'll find it listed here in the Beverages category.

Organization by Sub-Category

Each master category is further sub-divided by sub-categories that align with the particular types of food products found in the master category aisle. For example, sub-categories within the Snacks master category include: Chips, Cookies, Crackers, etc. Sub-categories are organized alphabetically within the master category.

Organization by Brand & Product

Within these subcategories, you'll find individual products listed alphabetically by brand name (in bold), then product name (not in bold). While we've done our best to organize the products into the "correct" category and sub-category, we hope you'll understand that it was a subjective process and there will be some variance.

Information on all items listed, except the items in gray (more about these later) is obtained directly from the brand, manufacturer or brand representative (we refer to these as the "company" for short). Occasionally, they also send along additional information, ranging from legal disclaimers to in-depth notes on manufacturing procedures.

In order to make this guide portable and convenient, it's not practical to reprint all of the notes provided by a company. But, there are a few exceptions. We know that you want to know which items may pose cross-contamination concerns and, conversely, when companies go the extra mile by having dedicated production lines or gluten testing, for example. Therefore, those and other relevant situations are marked with special symbols.

We'll discuss each symbol in-depth here, but don't worry, there's a cheat sheet on page 1 to jog your memory when you're actually at the store.

Placement of Symbols

If a symbol applies to all of a brand's listed products, we placed the symbol next to the brand name. If it only applies to a particular product, the symbol will appear next to that specific product. For example, if Brand X's entire line comes with a cross-contamination warning, the disclaimer icon will appear next to the Brand X name. If the warning only applies to its Chocolate Chip flavor, we place the symbol next to the Chocolate Chip flavor listing only.

Limitation of Symbols

Another thing to keep in mind is that any information, including disclaimers like cross-contamination warnings, are provided by companies at their discretion. Unfortunately, companies are not required by law to warn shoppers of cross-contamination, so just because a company does not have a cross-contamination warning does not necessarily mean it's not an issue! We sincerely hope that the FDA will resolve this confusion in the near future.

Symbols In-Depth

Reading Symbol

Some prominent brands do not maintain or share gluten-free lists. When you're gluten-free, your choices are, by definition, limited. The goal of this book is to open up more choices.

So, in cases where brands do not have a gluten-free list but DO have a policy of accurately labeling for gluten, no matter how small the amount, Triumph independently reviewed each product's ingredients (based solely on the product labeling) to determine which are gluten-free.

The information for these particular product listings did not come directly from the brand or manufacturer, as with the other products in this guide, so we have distinguished them with a special glasses symbol and gray text color.

Gluten Testing Symbol

This symbol indicates that a company has tested its ingredients, finished products, machinery and/or equipment, etc. for gluten.

Gluten-Free Processing Symbol

Here's another happy symbol: this symbol indicates that the company reports any of the following:

- They use gluten-free lines, equipment or facilities; or,
- Items are produced in a gluten-free environment; or,
- Cross-contamination is not an issue for whatever reason (be it because they have a dedicated facility, rigorous testing policies, etc.).

Cross Contamination/Shared Equipment Symbol RED

A company may get this symbol if it reports any of the following:

- Cross-contamination may be an issue; or,
- Their products are made on equipment, lines or in a plant that also process gluten-containing items; or,
- Their products are made with gluten-free ingredients, but they would not provide information on whether the manufacturing process is gluten-free.

So, does this symbol mean that you need to avoid these products entirely? The answer is complicated, I'm afraid. I don't like the answer any more than you're going to, but this is the world we live in and the hand the FDA has dealt us.

Some companies—too many, in my opinion—use language like the above bullet points in the hopes that it will cut down on litigation. In other words, they don't want to get sued. In these cases, it's not their Quality Control teams that are writing these disclaimers, but their legal teams.

So it's very possible that these products may be safe with little to no chance of cross-contamination, but the companies want to cover their legal bases by noting the chance, no matter how remote.

Unfortunately, there are also many cases where there may be a legitimate chance of cross-contamination. There's no surefire way to distinguish these "real" cross-contamination risks from an overzealous legal department. Trust me, we've tried!

Cross Contamination Symbol ORANGE

 Something felt wrong about lumping together companies that write "cross-contamination is a possibility" and those that state "cross contamination is a possibility but all our personnel are trained in handling allergenic materials, which are stored separately, and we sanitize and swab test shared machinery between each product run."

That's why this symbol covers companies that noted cross-contamination or shared equipment, like the RED cross-contamination scenario, but also informed us about counter measures they have in place. Such measures may include the following:

- Special handling and/or segregation of gluten-containing ingredients or products; or,
- Scheduling equipment and machinery so that gluten-containing items are processed at different times than gluten-free items; along with,
- Thorough cleaning/sanitization procedures between gluten-containing and gluten-free product batches; or,
- Their products are made with gluten-free ingredients, but they will not claim their product are gluten-free, though they do have processes in place to minimize cross-contamination (e.g., like the procedures above).

Of course, this is not an exhaustive list of the many different methods companies take to minimize cross-contamination. But, I think you get the picture!

Strange Bedfellow

So you probably have this symbols thing down by now. But, then you may see ⓘ and ♟ together. And you may rightly wonder, how can something be made on a dedicated gluten-free line or facility and still have a risk of cross-contamination symbol. Well, a possible scenario may be that they have four lines in a plant, and three are dedicated gluten-free, but the fourth is used for gluten-containing items. So, in this case, there is both a gluten-free line (♟) and non-gluten-free facility (ⓘ).

No Icon

When collecting gluten-free product lists, we always ask companies about cross-contamination. Not all companies, however, choose to share that information with us. And if they don't tell us about their cross-contamination status, we are unable to assign them an icon. So, when a company or product is listed without an icon, that does not necessarily mean, for example, that the products are (or are not) made in a shared facility; it just means that the company wouldn't tell us either way. Companies, unfortunately, are not required to share that information under current regulations; see Chapter 2 for more on the food labeling law.

Final Thoughts

This guide was created in response to a loose-leaf binder our company's founder used to carry. The binder was a collection of hundreds of gluten-free lists from hundreds of companies. It was a monster to carry and even worse to update. We're talking entire days spent calling companies and listening to bad hold music.

We've come a long way from loose-leaf binders and frantic calls to food companies right before dinner. And we hope that all this research we've done helps to make your life easier. We are the only guide that takes the time to give you these symbols, because we think they're relevant to good decision-making. Plus, you deserve the extra information. Please use it, and use it wisely.

LIMITATIONS OF THE GUIDE

While we hope that this guide makes gluten-free shopping easier, we do recognize that it has some limitations, which we would like to call out so that you can make informed shopping decisions.

Gluten-Free Lists

As mentioned in previous chapters, there is currently no FDA rule defining gluten-free and generally no consensus as to an exact definition. (Consider the controversies surrounding blue cheese and oats, just to name a few.) So when a company reports that its products are gluten-free, there is the possibility that their definition of gluten-free may differ from yours.

In addition, the information published in this guide for each food item has been obtained directly from that item's manufacturer, the entity that licensed the manufacturing, or an affiliate, unless otherwise noted. It's impossible for us to verify the accuracy of the information companies report to us.

Always Read Labels

It's important to keep in mind that product formulations and ingredient sourcing can and do change without notice, companies can make mistakes on their gluten-free list, and people compiling and categorizing large volumes of information (like the content for this guide) can make mistakes, as well. For these reasons, Triumph Dining cannot assume any liability for the correctness or accuracy of any information presented in this guide. You should read labels every time you make a purchase and regularly contact companies to confirm the gluten-free status of the products you consume.

Contact the Company with Questions

Please contact companies directly with any questions or for updates. Any information provided in this guide was obtained from the company (unless otherwise noted), and they will always be your best source of information on their products.

A Question of Semantics

Since there is still no FDA regulation defining the term "gluten-free" and no requirement that companies report the possibility of cross-contamination, as consumers, we're still very much on our own. A company may claim its products are "gluten-free" and free of "cross-contamination," but since there's no universally accepted definition of either term, you may still not be getting the whole story. Therefore, a product's appearance in this guide does not mean that the product is entirely free of gluten (besides, that would likely be an impossible standard, as the most sophisticated commercially-available tests for gluten do not measure to 0 ppm). However, you may find our symbols useful in deciding whether a product is suitable for you. Please see page 21 for more details.

This guide is largely a compilation of the information provided by over 1,000 companies when consumers reach out to them to ask about the gluten-free status of their products.

Common Sense is Your Best Guide

A guide like this should never be a replacement for your own knowledge, common sense and diligence. This guide is intended as a starting point only, and not a final determination that a listed product is gluten-free, suitable for the gluten-free diet, or safe for you personally to consume. It is not a substitute for reading labels and contacting companies. Rather, this guide is designed to help you hone in on the products most likely to be suitable for the gluten-free diet, so that you can focus your label-reading and company-contacting efforts on the most promising products, without wasting dozens and dozens of hours chasing dead ends. Always exercise caution when using any lists, even this one or ones directly from a brand. People make mistakes, so if something doesn't feel right, it probably isn't.

Some Final Notes

The information published in this guide is intended for use in the United States and with products manufactured with the intent to be sold in the United States only. Products sold or intended to be sold outside the United States may have completely different ingredients than their U.S. counterparts, and may not be gluten-free.

This guide is for limited educational purposes only and is not medical advice. If you have questions about the gluten-free diet, what ingredients are appropriate to consume, whether or not particular items are appropriate for your consumption, etc., please consult with your physician.

For the foregoing reasons, Triumph Dining cannot assume any liability for any losses or damages resulting from your use of this product listing. It's up to you to determine whether a product is appropriate based on your individual dietary needs. For more information about a particular company's testing practices, standards and thresholds, please contact that company directly.

Use of this guide indicates your acknowledgement of and agreement to these terms.

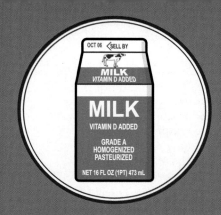

DAIRY & EGGS

Butter

Bashas'
Butter - Salted
Butter - Unsalted

Borden
Borden Butter (All)

Cabot
Cabot Products (All)

Crystal Farms
60/40 Butter Blend
Salted Butter
Unsalted Butter

Darigold
Darigold (All)

Falfurrias
Butter (All)

Food Club (Marsh)
Butter AA Quarters
Butter AA Unsalted Quarters

Fresh & Easy ()
Butter

Great Value (Wal-Mart)
Salted Butter Quarters
Unsalted Butter Quarters

Haggen
Butter AA Carton Quarters

Horizon Organic (i)
Horizon Organic (All BUT Ice Cream Sandwiches)

Hotel Bar ()
Butter (All)

Hy-Vee
Sweet Cream Butter Quarters
Sweet Cream Butter Solid

Sweet Cream Whipped Butter
Unsalted Sweet Butter Quarters

Keller's Creamery
Butters (All)

Kroger (i)
Butter

Land O'Lakes ()
Butter

Meijer
Butter AA Quarters

Mid-America Farms ()
Butter (All)

Oberweis Dairy
Salted Butter
Unsalted Butter

Organic Valley (i)
Butter - Cultured, Unsalted
Butter - European Cultured
Butter - Pasture Cultured
Butter - Salted
Butter - Whipped, Salted

Plugrá
European Style Butter

Prairie Farms
Butter

Price Chopper
Salted Organic Butter
Unsalted Organic Butter

Publix ()
Butter - Salted
Butter - Unsalted
Butter - Whipped, Salted
Butter - Whipped, Unsalted
Sweet Cream Butter

Straus Family Creamery
Butter (All)

Vermont Butter & Cheese Creamery
Vermont Butter & Cheese Creamery
(All)

Winn-Dixie ()
Salted Butter
Unsalted Butter
Whipped Butter

BUTTERMILK

Axelrod
Buttermilk

Darigold
Darigold (All)

Friendship Dairies
Friendship Dairies (All)

Hood
Buttermilk

Marsh
2% Buttermilk

Organic Valley ⓘ
Buttermilk

Penn Maid
Buttermilk

Prairie Farms
Buttermilk

Saco
Saco (All)

CHEESE & CHEESE SPREADS

4C
100% Imported Cheese (All)

Alouette
Al Elegante Roasted Garlic/Pesto
Al Elegante Roasted Sweet Pepper/Olive
Tapenade
Al Elegante Sundried Tomato & Garlic
Baby Brie - Herb
Baby Brie - Plain
Berries & Cream Spreadable Cheese
Blue Cheese Crumbles
Brie Wedge, Plain
Brie Wedge, Smoked

Creamy Onion & Shallots Spreadable
Cheese
Crème de Brie - Herb
Crème de Brie - Original
Créme Fraîche
Feta Crumbles
Feta Garlic & Herb Crumbles
Feta Mediterranean Crumbles
Garlic & Herbs Spreadable Cheese
Goat Cheese Crumbles
Goat Cheese Provencal Crumbles
Gorgonzola Cheese Crumbles
Light Cucumber Dill Spreadable Cheese
Light Garlic & Herbs Spreadable Cheese
Peppercorn Parmesan Spreadable
Cheese
Petite Brie, Plain
Savory Vegetable Spreadable Cheese
Spinach Artichoke Spreadable Cheese
Sundried Tomato Spreadable Cheese
Sweet & Spicy Pepper Medley
Spreadable Cheese

Athenos
Blue Cheese Crumbled Natural
Chunk Mild
Chunk with Basil & Tomato
Chunk with Black Peppercorn
Chunk with Garlic & Herb
Crumbled Mild
Crumbled with Black Peppercorn
Crumbled with Roasted Bell Peppers &
Garlic
Feta Crumbled Reduced Fat
Feta Crumbled Reduced Fat with
Tomato & Basil
Feta Crumbled Traditional
Feta Crumbled with Basil & Tomato
Feta Crumbled with Basil & Tomato
Natural
Feta Crumbled with Garlic & Herb
Feta Crumbled with Lemon/Garlic &
Oregano
Feta Traditional Chunk Packed In Brine
Natural
Gorgonzola Crumbled Natural
Traditional Feta Crumbled Natural

Bashas'

Cheddar & Monterey Jack Cheese Finely Shredded
Cheddar Cheese Finely Shredded
Cheddar Extra Sharp Bar Chunk
Cheddar Medium Bar Chunk
Cheddar Mild Bar Chunk
Cheddar Mild Chunk
Cheddar Sharp
Cheddar Sharp Bar Chunk
Cheddar Shredded (Zipper)
Cheddar Shredded Sharp (Zipper)
Cheddar Sliced Shingle Chunk
Cheese - Cheddar - Medium
Cheese - Cheddar - Sharp
Cheese - Mild Cheddar
Cheese - Monterey Jack
Cheese - String
Cheezy Does It - Processed Spread Loaf
Colby & Monterey Jack Cheese Finely Shredded
Colby & Monterey Jack Cheese Shredded
Colby Chunk
Colby Jack Bar
Colby Jack Chunk
Colby Jack Sliced Shingle
Deluxe American Cheese Slices
Finely Shredded Colby Jack
Finely Shredded Italian Blend
Finely Shredded Mexican Blend
Finely Shredded Mild Cheddar
Finely Shredded Mozzarella
Finely Shredded Nacho/Taco
Finely Shredded Sharp Cheddar
Grated Parmesan & Romano Cheese
Grated Parmesan Cheese
Hot Pepper Jack Chunk
Medium Cheddar Chunk
Mexican Style Cheese - 2% Milk - Reduced Fat
Mexican Style Cheese - Shredded
Mild Cheddar Cheese - 2% Milk, Reduced Fat
Monterey Jack Bar
Monterey Jack Chunk
Mozzarella Bar
Mozzarella Cheese - 2% Milk - Reduced Fat
Mozzarella Chunk
Mozzarella Shredded
Mozzarella Shredded (Zipper)
Muenster Chunk
Muenster Slice Shingle
Pasteurized Processed Cheese Product, American (Individually Wrapped Slices)
Pasteurized Processed Cheese Product, Nonfat, American (Individually Wrapped Slices)
Pasteurized Processed Cheese Product, Reduced Fat, Sharp (Individually Wrapped Slices)
Pepperjack Chunk
Pepperjack Slices Shingle
Pizza Finely Shredded 4 Cheese (Zipper)
Pizza Style Cheese - Shredded
Processed American Cheese - Sliced
Provolone Sliced Shingle
Ricotta Cheese Low Fat
Shredded Cheddar
String Cheese
Swiss Cheese - Shredded
Swiss Chunk

BelGioioso Cheese

Cheeses (All)

Bett's ⚇

Bett's (All)

Biazzo

Biazzo (All)

Boar's Head

Cheeses (All)

Bongards

Cheese (All)

Borden

Borden Cheese Products (All BUT Borden Applewood Bacon Cheddar Flavor Single Sensations)

Cabot

Cabot Products (All)

Cache Valley

Cheese (All)

Central Market Classics (Price Chopper)

Brick Baby Swiss
New York Cheddar
New York Extra Sharp Cheddar
Vermont Cheddar
Vermont Extra Sharp Cheddar

Chavrie ☺

Chavrie Log
Chavrie Log, Herb
Chavrie with Basil/Roasted Garlic
Chavrie, Original

Cracker Barrel ✎

Cheese Sticks - Extra Sharp Cheddar 2% Milk Reduced Fat
Cheese Sticks - Natural Extra Sharp Cheddar White
Cheese Sticks - Natural Sharp Cheddar
Cracker Cuts - Extra Sharp Cheddar Cheese Cuts
Cracker Cuts - Extra Sharp Cheddar Reduced Fat Cheese Cuts with 2% Milk
Cracker Cuts - Natural Baby Swiss
Emmentaler Swiss
Extra Sharp
Extra Sharp Cheddar
Extra Sharp Cheddar 2% Milk Reduced Fat Shredded
Extra Sharp Cheddar Shredded
Extra Sharp-White Cheddar
Fontina
Havarti
Natural Cheddar Vermont Sharp-White
Natural Extra Sharp Cheddar
Natural Extra Sharp Cheddar 2% Milk Reduced Fat
Natural Extra Sharp White Cheddar Reduced Fat
Natural Sharp Cheddar
Natural Sharp Cheddar 2 Stacks Slices
Natural Sharp Cheddar 2% Milk Reduced Fat
Natural Sharp Cheddar Slices
Natural Sharp White Cheddar Reduced Fat

Natural Vermont's Sharp White Cheddar 2% Milk Reduced Fat
Sharp Cheddar Shredded
Sharp-White Cheddar
White Colby

Crystal Farms

2% Individually Wrapped Slices
Aerosol Cheese (All)
American Deluxe Sliced
American Individually Wrapped Slices
Blue Cheese
Cheese Spread Loaf
Cold Packs
Fat Free Individually Wrapped Slices
Gorgonzola
Jar Cheese (All)
Natural Cheeses - Chunks (All)
Natural Cheeses - Shreds (All)
Parmesan Shaker
Pepper Jack Individually Wrapped Slices
Ricotta (All)
Romano Shaker
Sharp Individually Wrapped Slices
Shredded Parmesan
Shredded Romano
Stick Cheeses
String Cheese
Swiss Individually Wrapped Slices

Dofino ☺

Cheeses (All)

Finlandia Cheese

Finlandia (All)

Food Club (Marsh)

Cheddar New York Sharp Bar (Colored)
Cheese Food - 2% Individually Wrapped Slices
Cheese Product with Calcium - Individually Wrapped Slices
Colby Chunk
Colby Jack Bar
Colby Jack Chunk
Colby Jack Longhorn Half Moon
Colby Jack Slices Shingle
Colby Longhorn Halfmoon
Extra Sharp Cheddar - Chunk
Finely Shredded Colby Jack

Finely Shredded Italian Blend (6 Cheese)

Finely Shredded Mexican Blend (4 Cheese)

Finely Shredded Mild Cheddar

Finely Shredded Mozzarella

Finely Shredded Nacho/Taco

Finely Shredded Pizza 4 Cheese Blend

Finely Shredded Sharp Cheddar

Low Moisture Part Skim Mozzarella Bar

Low Moisture Part Skim Mozzarella Shredded

Low Moisture Part Skim Mozzarella Shredded (Zipper)

Medium Cheddar - Chunk

Mild Cheddar - Bar

Mild Cheddar - Chunk

Mild Cheddar - Shredded 2%

Monterey Jack Bar

Mozzarella Shingle Slice

Muenster Slice Shingle

Parmesan Finely Shredded

Pepperjack Chunk

Pepperjack Slices Shingle

Processed Cheese - Fat Free Individually Wrapped Slices

Provolone Slices Shingle

Sharp Cheddar - Bar

Sharp Cheddar - Chunk

Sharp Cheddar - Shredded

Sharp Cheese Food - 2% Individually Wrapped Slices

Shredded Cheddar

Swiss Cheese Food - 2% Individually Wrapped Slices

Swiss Chunk

Swiss Finely Shredded

Swiss Slice Shingle

Fresh & Easy ()
Cheeses

Friendship Dairies
Friendship Dairies (All)

Giant Eagle
2% Cheese Food - Individually Wrapped Slices

Blue Crumbled Cheese

Cheese Food - Individually Wrapped Slices

Chunk Colby Jack Cheese

Chunk Extra-Sharp Cheddar Cheese

Chunk Low-Moisture Part-Skim Mozzarella

Chunk Mild Cheddar Cheese

Chunk Monterey Jack

Chunk NY Extra - Sharp Cheddar Cheese

Chunk NY Sharp Cheddar Cheese

Chunk NY White Cheddar

Chunk Pepper Jack

Chunk Pepper Jack Cheese

Chunk Sharp Cheddar Cheese

Chunk Swiss Cheese

Colby - High Moisture

Deluxe Sliced American

Easy Melt

Fancy Shred Colby Jack

Fancy Shred Mild Cheddar

Fancy Shred Parmesan

Fancy Shred RBST Free 2% Mexican

Fancy Shred Sharp Cheddar

Fancy Shred Swiss

Fancy Shred Taco Cheese

Fat Free Cheese Food - Individually Wrapped Slices

Feta Crumbled Cheese

Gorgonzola Crumbled Cheese

Lite String Cheese

Mozzarella Ball

Pepper Jack Cheese Spread - Individually Wrapped Slices

Reduced Fat Blue Crumbled Cheese

Reduced Fat Feta Crumbled Cheese

Sharp 2% Cheese Food - Individually Wrapped Slices

Sharp Fat Free Cheese Food - Individually Wrapped Slices

Shredded 4 Cheese Italian

Shredded 4 Cheese Mexican

Shredded Mexican Blend

Shredded Mild Cheddar

Shredded Mozzarella

Shredded RBST Free 2% Mild Cheddar

Shredded RBST Free 2% Mozzarella

Shredded Sharp Cheddar

Shredded Whole Milk Mozzarella
Sliced Colby Jack Cheese
Sliced Muenster
Sliced Pepper Jack Cheese
Sliced Provolone Cheese
Sliced Sharp Cheddar
Sliced Swiss Cheese
String Cheese

Great Value (Wal-Mart)

100% Parmesan Grated Cheese
2% Milk American Deluxe Reduced Fat Pasteurized Process Cheese with Added Calcium
2% Milk Reduced Fat Mild Cheddar Cheese Chunk
2% Milk Reduced Fat Sharp Cheddar Cheese Chunk
American Pasteurized Prepared Cheese Product Singles
American Reduced Fat Pasteurized Process Cheese Food Singles
Cheese Wow American Cheese
Cheese Wow Cheddar Cheese
Cheese Wow Pepper Jack Cheese
Colby And Monterey Jack Cheese Chunk
Colby And Monterey Jack Cheese Cubes
Deluxe American Pasteurized Process Cheese Singles
Deluxe White American Pasteurized Process Cheese Singles
Extra Sharp Cheddar Cheese Chunk
Fancy Shredded Colby & Monterey Jack Cheese
Fancy Shredded Fiesta Blend Cheese
Fancy Shredded Italian Blend Cheese
Fancy Shredded Low-Moisture Part-Skim Mozzarella Cheese
Fancy Shredded Mild Cheddar Cheese
Fancy Shredded Mozzarella Cheese
Fancy Shredded Parmesan Blend
Fancy Shredded Parmesan Cheese
Fancy Shredded Pizza Blend Cheese
Fancy Shredded Sharp Cheddar Cheese
Fancy Shredded Swiss Cheese
Fancy Shredded Taco Blend Cheese

Fat Free Pasteurized Process Cheese Product Singles
Feather Shredded Colby & Monterey Jack Cheese
Feather Shredded Mild Cheddar Cheese
Feather Shredded Mozzarella Cheese
Longhorn Style Colby Cheese Chunk
Longhorn Style Mild Cheddar Cheese Chunk
Medium Cheddar Cheese Chunk
Medium Cheddar Chunk
Melt 'n Dip Pasteurized Processed Cheese Spread
Mild Cheddar Cheese Chunk
Mild Cheddar Cheese Cubes
Monterey Jack Cheese Chunk
Mozzarella Cheese Chunk
Muenster Cheese Chunk
Natural Colby Cheese Chunk
Pepper Jack Cheese Chunk
Pepper Jack Cheese Cubes
Sharp Cheddar Cheese Chunk
Sharp Cheddar Chunk
Shredded Mild Cheddar Cheese
Shredded Mozzarella Cheese
Shredded White Sharp Cheddar Cheese
Sliced Mild Cheddar Cheese
Sliced Mozzarella Cheese
Sliced Pepper Jack Cheese
Sliced Provolone Cheese
Sliced Swiss Cheese
Swiss Cheese Chunk
White American Pasteurized Prepared Cheese Product Singles
White Mild Cheddar Cheese Chunk
White Sharp Cheddar Cheese Chunk

Haggen

4 Cheese Mexican Blend
Cheddar Extra Sharp Chunk
Cheddar Medium Chunk
Cheddar Mild Chunk
Cheddar Sharp Chunk
Cheddar Sharp Loaf
Cheese Product Individually Wrapped Slices
Colby Jack - Shredded
Colby Jack Bar

Colby Jack Chunk
Colby Jack Loaf
Colby Longhorn Halfmoon
Finely Mexican Blend - Shredded
Finely Shredded Colby Jack
Finely Shredded Italian Pizza
  Mozzarella/Cheddar
Finely Shredded Parmesan
Hot Pepper Jack Chunk
Medium Cheddar Bar
Medium Cheddar Loaf
Medium Cheddar Sliced
Monterey Jack Chunk
Mozzarella - Shredded
Mozzarella Chunk - Low Moisture, Part
  Skim
Mozzarella Loaf
Parmesan Grated
Pepperjack Cheese Bar
Processed Cheese Fat Free - Individually
  Wrapped Slices
Ricotta Cheese - Low Fat
Ricotta Cheese - Part Skim
Shredded Cheddar
String Cheese
Swiss Cheese Bar
Swiss Chunk

Heini's
Cheese (All)

Heluva Good
Shredded Cheese (All)
Solid Block Style Cheese (All)
String Cheese

Horizon Organic ⓘ
Horizon Organic (All BUT Ice Cream
  Sandwiches)

Hy-Vee
American Singles
American Singles 2% Milk
Colby 1/2 Moon Longhorn Cheese
Colby Cheese
Colby Hunk Cheese
Colby Jack 1/2 Moon Longhorn Cheese
Colby Jack Cheese
Colby Jack Cheese Cubes
Colby Jack Hunk Cheese
Colby Jack Slices

Colby Longhorn Cheese
Colby Slice Singles
Extra Sharp Cheddar Cheese
Fancy Shredded 6 Italian Cheese
Fancy Shredded Cheddar Jack Cheese
Fancy Shredded Colby Jack Cheese
Fancy Shredded Mild Cheddar 2%
  Cheese
Fancy Shredded Mild Cheddar Cheese
Fancy Shredded Mozzarella 2% Milk
Fancy Shredded Mozzarella Cheese
Fat Free Singles
Fat Free Swiss Cheese Slices
Finely Shredded Colby Jack Cheese
Finely Shredded Mild Cheddar Cheese
Grated Parmesan Cheese
Grated Parmesan Romano Cheese
Hot Pepper Cheese
Lil' Hunk Colby Jack Cheese
Lil' Hunk Mild Cheddar Cheese
Medium Cheddar Cheese
Medium Cheddar Longhorn Cheese
Mild Cheddar Cheese
Mild Cheddar Cheese Cubes
Mild Cheddar Hunk Cheese
Mild Cheddar Slices
Monterey Jack Cheese
Monterey Jack Hunk Cheese
Mozzarella Cheese
Mozzarella Hunk Cheese
Muenster Cheese
Muenster Cheese Slices
Pepper Jack Cheese
Pepper Jack Cheese Cubes
Pepper Jack Hunk Cheese
Pepper Jack Singles
Pepper Jack Slices
Provolone Cheese
Provolone Cheese Slices
Sharp Cheddar Cheese
Sharp Cheddar Hunk Cheese
Sharp Cheddar Longhorn Cheese
Shredded Colby Jack Cheese
Shredded Mexican Blend Cheese
Shredded Mild Cheddar Cheese
Shredded Mozzarella Cheese
Shredded Parmesan Cheese
Shredded Pizza Cheese

Shredded Sharp Cheddar Cheese
Shredded Taco Cheese
Sliced Low-Moisture Part-Skim
  Mozzarella
Swiss Cheese
Swiss Singles
Swiss Slices

Jarlsberg 🏅
Jarlsberg (All)

Kerrygold
Cheeses (All BUT Kerrygold Dubliner
  with Irish Stout)

Kraft Cracker Cuts ↝
Natural Baby Swiss 18 Ct

Kraft Deli Deluxe ↝
American 2% Milk Slices
American Slices
American White Slices
Sharp Cheddar 2% Milk Slices
Sharp Cheddar Slices
Swiss Slices

Kraft Deli Fresh ↝
Colby Jack Slices
Mild Cheddar Slices
Mozzarella Slices Low Moisture
Natural Swiss Slices
Pepper Jack Spicy Slices
Provolone Slices
Sharp Cheddar Slices
Swiss 2% Milk Reduced Fat Slices
Swiss Slices

Kraft Easy Cheese ↝
American
Cheddar
Sharp Cheddar

Kraft ↝
Parmesan & Romano Medium 100%
  Grated Cheese
Parmesan 100% Grated Cheese
Parmesan Original Grated Cheese
Parmesan Reduced Fat Grated Cheese
Parmesan Shredded Cheese
Parmesan, Romano & Asiago Shredded
  Cheese
Romano 100% Grated Cheese

Kraft Natural Cheese ↝
Cheddar & Monterey Jack Marbled

Cheddar Bacon
Cheddar Extra Sharp
Cheddar Medium
Cheddar Mild
Cheddar Sharp
Colby
Colby & Monterey Jack
Colby & Monterey Jack Marbled
Colby Longhorn Style
Extra Sharp Cheddar
Extra Sharp Cheddar Cheese Sticks
Medium Cheddar
Mild Cheddar
Mild Cheddar Cheese Sticks
Mild Cheddar Longhorn Style 2% Milk
Mild Cheddar Natural Shredded
Monterey Jack
Mozzarella Low-Moisture Part-Skim
Organic Cheddar
Pepper Jack
Roasted Garlic Cheddar
Sharp Cheddar
Sharp Cheddar 2% Milk Reduced Fat
  Cheese Sticks
Smoky Swiss & Cheddar

Kraft Natural Cheese Sticks ↝
Extra Sharp Cheddar
Mild Cheddar
Sharp Cheddar 2% Milk Reduced Fat

Kraft Natural Crumbles ↝
Blue Cheese
Feta Cheese
Italian Style
Mediterranean Style
Mexican Style 2% Milk Reduced Fat
Mozzarella
Reduced Fat-Colby & Monterey Jack
Sharp Cheddar
Three Cheese-Monterey Jack/Colby &
  Cheddar

Kraft Natural Shredded Cheese ↝
Cheddar & Monterey Jack Cheese
  Shreds
Cheddar Mild Cheese Shreds
Cheddar Sharp Cheese Shreds
Colby & Monterey Jack Cheese Shreds

Colby & Monterey Jack Finely Shredded Cheese Shreds
Finely Shredded Sharp Cheddar
Italian Style Five Cheese Cheese Shreds
Mexican Cheddar Jack
Mexican Cheddar Jack with Jalapeno Peppers
Mexican Four Cheese Cheese Shreds
Mexican Taco
Mild Cheddar Finely Shredded Cheese Shreds
Monterey Jack Cheese Shreds
Mozzarella & Parmesan Finely Shredded
Mozzarella Low Moisture Cheese Shreds
Mozzarella Low-Moisture Finely Shredded Cheese Shreds
Mozzarella Low-Moisture Part-Skim Cheese Shreds
Organic Cheddar Cheese Shreds
Organic Mozzarella Cheese Shreds
Pizza Four Cheese Cheese Shreds
Pizza Mozzarella & Cheddar Cheese Shreds
Sharp Cheddar Finely Shredded Cheese Shreds
Swiss Cheese Shreds

Kraft Singles
Aged Swiss
American 2% Milk 2/3 Oz Slices
American Fat Free 2/3 Oz Slices
American Slices
American White
Pepperjack 2% Milk 2/3 Oz Slices
Select American Slices
Sharp Cheddar
Sharp Cheddar 2% Milk 2/3 Oz Slices
Sharp Cheddar Fat Free 2/3 Oz Slices
Swiss 2% Milk 2/3 Oz Slices
Swiss Fat Free 2/3 Oz Slices
White American 2% Milk 2/3 Oz Slices
White American Fat Free 2/3 Oz Slices
White American Slices

Kraft String-Ums
Mozzarella String Cheese

Kroger
Bar Cheeses
Cubed Cheeses

Shredded Cheeses
Sliced Cheeses

Land O'Lakes
Natural Cheeses
Process Cheese

Laughing Cow, The
Laughing Cow (All)

Lifeway
Lifeway (All)

Light n' Lively
Fat Free Cottage Cheese
Free Fat Free Cottage Cheese
Lowfat Cottage Cheese
Lowfat Snack Size Cottage Cheese

Litehouse
Bleu Cheese Crumbles
Heart of Bleu Cheese
Monarch Mountain Gorgonzola Crumbles

Lucini Italia
Lucini Italia (All BUT Russian Tomato Vodka Sauce and Minestrone Soup)

Maggio
Mozzarella (Solid Block)
Ricotta Cheese

Marsh
Cheddar Extra Sharp Bar (Colored)
Cheddar Medium Bar (Colored)
Cheddar Sharp Bar (Colored)
Colby Jack Cheese Cube
Low Moisture Part Skim Mozzarella Bar
Monterey Jack Bar
Pepper Jack Cheese Cube

Meijer
2% Individual American
2% Individual Sharp
American Cheese - Slices
American Cheese Spray (Aerosol)
Cheddar - Extra Sharp Bar
Cheddar - Fancy Shredded
Cheddar - Medium Bar
Cheddar - Midget Horn
Cheddar - Mild Bar
Cheddar - Mild Chunk
Cheddar - Sharp Bar
Cheddar - Sharp Chunk
Cheddar - Sharp Fancy Shredded

Cheddar - Sharp Shredded
Cheddar - Shredded (Zipper Pouch)
Cheddar - Shredded Sharp (Pouch)
Cheddar - Sliced Half Moon
Cheddar Jack Shredded (Pouch)
Cheddar/Monterey Jack Bar
Cheese Cheddar (Aerosol)
Cheese Sharp Cheddar (Aerosol)
Cheese Swiss (Individually Wrapped)
Cheezy Does It - Jalapeno
Cheezy Does It - Spread Loaf
Colby Bar
Colby Chunk
Colby Fancy Shredded
Colby Jack Bar
Colby Jack Fancy Shredded
Colby Jack Sliced Shingle
Colby Longhorn Full Moon
Colby Longhorn Half Moon (Sliced)
Colby Longhorn Sliced
Colby Midget Horn
Fancy Italian Blend Shredded
Fancy Mexican Blend Shredded
Fancy Shredded Colby Jack
Fancy Shredded Mild Cheddar
Fancy Shredded Mozzarella
Fancy Shredded Nacho/Taco
Fat Free Sharp Individual Slices
Hot Pepper Jack Chunk
Individually Wrapped Sliced Pepper
Low Moisture Part Skim Mozzarella Bar
Low Moisture Part Skim Mozzarella
 Shredded
Low Moisture Part Skim Mozzarella
 Square
Low Moisture Part Skim String Cheese
Marble Cheddar (C&W Cheddar)
Mexican Blend - Shredded
Mexican Shredded
Monterey Jack Chunk
Mozzarella Shingle Slice
Mozzarella Shredded
Muenster Slice Shingle
Parmesan and Romano Cheese (Grated)
Parmesan Cheese (Grated)
Parmesan Cheese 1/3 Less Fat
Pepper Jack Bar
Pepperjack Sliced Stack Pack

Pizza Shredded Mozzarella/Cheddar
Provolone Stacked Slice
Ricotta Cheese - Part Skim
Ricotta Cheese - Whole Milk
String Cheese
Swiss Chunk
Swiss Slice Shingle
Swiss Sliced Sandwich/Cut

Mid-America Farms ()
Cheese (All)

Midwest Country Fare (Hy-Vee)
American Sandwich Slices
Shredded Cheddar Cheese
Shredded Mozzarella Cheese

Oberweis Dairy
Colby Cheese
Colby Jack Cheese
Mild Cheddar
Pepper Cheddar
Sharp Cheddar

Old Chatham Sheepherding Company
Camembert

Organic Valley ⓘ
Baby Swiss
Cheddar - Mild
Cheddar - Mild, Shredded
Cheddar - Raw Mild
Cheddar - Raw Sharp
Cheddar - Reduced Fat and Sodium
Cheddar - Sharp
Cheddar - Vermont Extra Sharp
Cheddar - Vermont Medium
Cheddar - Vermont Sharp
Colby
Feta
Mexican Blend - Shredded
Monterey Jack
Monterey Jack - Reduced Fat
Mozzarella
Mozzarella - Shredded, Low Moisture,
 Part Skim
Muenster
Pepper Jack
Provolone
Ricotta
Stringles - Cheddar

Stringles - Colby-Jack
Stringles - Mozzarella
Wisconsin Raw Milk Jack-Style

Pastene
Grated Parmesan Cheese
Grated Romano Cheese

Penn Maid
String Cheese

Pilgrims Choice
Cheese Products (All)

Polly-O Cheese ⌒
Cheese Pizza Mozzarella Provolone
   Romano Parmesan Shredded
Fat Free Cheese Ricotta
Lite Cheese Ricotta
Mozzarella Fat Free
Mozzarella Parmesan Finely Shredded
Mozzarella Part Skim
Mozzarella Shredded Fat Free
Mozzarella Shredded Lite
Mozzarella Shredded Part Skim
Mozzarella Shredded Whole Milk
   Cheese
Original Ricotta Cheese
Parmesan Grated
Part Skim Cheese Ricotta

Price Chopper
2% White Singles
2% Yellow Singles
Brick Mild Cheddar
Brick Monterey Jack
Brick Sharp Cheddar
Chunk Mild Cheddar
Chunk Muenster
Chunk New York Extra - Sharp Cheddar
Chunk Pepper Jack
Chunk Swiss
Chunk Vermont Sharp Cheddar
Colby Cheese
Deluxe White American Slices
Deluxe Yellow American Slices
Fancy Shredded Swiss
Fat Free White Singles
Fat Free Yellow Singles
Lite String Cheese
Mild Cheddar Stick
Monterey Jack

Monterey Jack/Jalapeno
Mozzarella Slices
Muenster Slices
Muenster Stick
Provolone Slices
Shredded 2% Reduced Fat Mild
   Cheddar
Shredded 2% Reduced Fat Mozzarella
Shredded 6-Cheese Blend
Shredded Fat Free Mozzarella
Shredded Mexican Blend
Shredded Mild Cheddar
Shredded Monterey Jack
Shredded Mozzarella
Shredded Mozzarella Part Skim
Shredded Pizza Blend
Shredded Sharp Cheddar
String Cheese
Swiss Slices
Swiss Stick
Vermont Sharp Cheddar
Wisonsin Sharp Cheddar

Publix ()
Asiago Wedge
Blue Crumbled
Cheddar - Extra Sharp (All Forms:
   Block, Chunk & Shreds)
Cheddar - Medium (All Forms: Block,
   Chunk & Shreds)
Cheddar - Mild (All Forms: Block,
   Chunk & Shreds)
Cheddar - Sharp (All Forms: Block,
   Chunk & Shreds)
Cheese Spread - Processed Cheese
Colby (All Forms: Block, Chunk &
   Shreds)
Colby Jack (All Forms: Block, Chunk &
   Shreds)
Creative Classic Queso Blanco
Creative Classic Queso de Freir
Crumbled Feta
Crumbled Goat
Crumbled Reduced Fat Feta
Deluxe American Cheese Slices
   (Processed Cheese)
Feta Chunk
Garden Jack Stick

Garlic and Herb Cheese Spread
Gorgonzola Crumbled
Horseradish Jack Stick
Imitation Mozzarella Cheese - Shredded (Processed Cheese)
Italian 6-Cheese Blend - Shredded
Mexican 4-Cheese Blend - Shredded
Monterey Jack & Cheddar - Shredded
Monterey Jack (All Forms: Block, Chunk & Shreds)
Monterey Jack with Jalapeño Peppers (All Forms: Block, Chunk & Shreds)
Mozzarella (All Forms: Block, Chunk & Shreds)
Muenster (All Forms: Block, Chunk & Shreds)
Parmesan Wedge
Parmesan, Grated
Provolone (All Forms: Block, Chunk & Shreds)
Reduced Fat Feta Chunk
Reduced Fat Pepper Jack
Ricotta
Salsa Jack Stick
Shredded Parmesan
Singles - Pasteurized Process American Cheese Food
Singles - Pasteurized Process American Cheese Food - Thick Slice
Singles - Pasteurized Process Swiss Cheese Food
Swiss (All Forms: Block, Chunk & Shreds)

Redwood Hill Farm
Redwood Hill Farm (All)

Sargento
Natural Cheese (All BUT Blue Cheese)

Soignon
Cheese (All)

Thumann's ✓
Cheese (All BUT Deep Fry Hot Dogs)

V & V Supremo
Cheese Products (All)
Requeson (All)

Valio
Cheese Products

Valu Time (Marsh)
Cheese Product - Individually Wrapped Slices

Velveeta ⌇
2% Milk
Mexican Mild
Pepper Jack
Regular
Slices
Slices Extra Thick 10 Ct.

Vermont Butter & Cheese Creamery
Vermont Butter & Cheese Creamery (All)

Winn-Dixie ()
American Pasteurized Process Cheese Product
Blue Cheese
Cheddar Jack
Cheddar, Extra Sharp
Cheddar, Medium
Cheddar, Mild
Cheddar, NY Extra Sharp
Cheddar, NY Sharp
Cheddar, Sharp
Colby
Colby Jack
Deluxe American Pasteurized Process Cheese Food
Feta
Gorgonzola
Grated Parmesan
Grated Parmesan and Romano
Italian Blend, Shredded
Mexican Blend
Monterey Jack
Monterey Jack with Jalapeno Peppers
Mozzarella
Muenster
Pasteurized Process Swiss Cheese Product
Pimiento Cheese - Chunky
Pimiento Cheese - Regular
Pimiento Cheese - with Jalapenos
Provolone
Reduced Fat American Pasteurized Process Cheese Product
Ricotta (All)

String Cheese
Swiss
White Cheddar

CHEESE, ALTERNATIVES

Lisanatti

MUNCHEEZE Snack Sticks American Style
MUNCHEEZE Snack Sticks Mozzarella Style
RiceCheeze Cheddar Style Chunks
RiceCheeze Mozzarella Style Chunks
RiceCheeze Pepper Jack Style Chunks
SENORA LUPE Chipotle Style Chunks
SENORA LUPE Jalapeno-Mild Style Chunks
SENORA LUPE Manchego Style Chunks
SENORA LUPE Quesadilla Style Chunks
SoySation 3 Cheese Blend Shreds
SoySation Cheddar Jalapeno Style Shreds
SoySation Cheddar Style Shreds
SoySation Cheddar Style Chunks
SoySation Cheddar Style Slices
SoySation Mozzarella Style Shreds
SoySation Mozzarella Style Chunks
SoySation Parmesan Style Shreds
SoySation Pepper Jack Style Chunks
SoySation Pepper Jack Style Slices
SoySation Swiss Style Slices
THE ORIGINAL Almond Cheddar Style Chunks
THE ORIGINAL Almond Garlic & Herb Style Chunks
THE ORIGINAL Almond Jalapeno Jack Style Chunks
THE ORIGINAL Almond Mozzarella Style Chunks

Rice
Rice (All)

Rice Vegan
Rice Vegan (All)

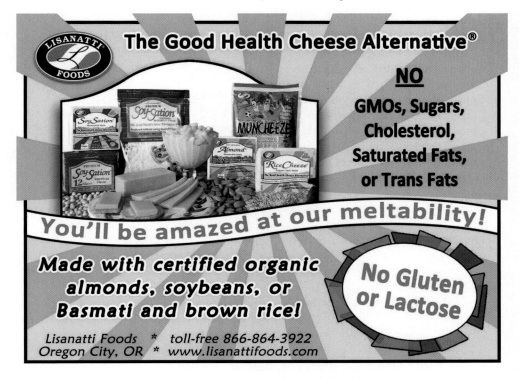

Soy Kaas
Soy Kaas (All BUT Soy Kaas Vegan)

Sunergia ()
Sunergia (All)

Valu Time (Marsh)
Imitation Cheddar Shredded
Imitation Mozzarella Shredded

Vegan
Vegan (All)

Vegan Gourmet ⓘ 🍴 ✓
Cheddar
Monterey Jack
Mozzarella Cheese Alternative
Nacho

Veggie
Veggie (All)

Veggy
Veggy (All)

COTTAGE CHEESE

Alta Dena ()
Cottage Cheese (All)

Axelrod
Cottage Cheese

Breakstone's ᔕ
Cottage Doubles Apples & Cinnamon
Lowfat
Cottage Doubles Blueberry Lowfat
Cottage Doubles Peach Lowfat
Cottage Doubles Pineapple Lowfat
Cottage Doubles Raspberry Lowfat
Cottage Doubles Strawberry Lowfat
Large Curd Lowfat 2% Milkfat Cottage
Cheese
Large Curd Smooth & Creamy 4%
Milkfat Min Cottage Cheese
Liveactive Lowfat with Mixed Berries 4
Oz Cottage Cheese
Liveactive Lowfat with Pineapple 4 Oz
Cottage Cheese
Small Curd 2% Milkfat Low Fat Snack
Size 4 Ct Cottage Cheese
Small Curd 4% Milkfat Min Cottage
Cheese
Small Curd 4% Milkfat Min Snack Size 4
Ct Cottage Cheese

Small Curd Fat Free Cottage Cheese
Small Curd Fat Free Snack Size 4 Ct
Cottage Cheese
Small Curd Low Fat with Pineapple 4 Oz
Cottage Cheese
Small Curd Lowfat 2% Milkfat Cottage
Cheese
Small Curd Smooth & Creamy 4%
Milkfat Min Cottage Cheese

Cabot
Cabot Products (All)

Darigold
Darigold (All)

Farmers' All Natural Creamery
Cottage Cheese

Food Club (Marsh)
Cottage Cheese - 1% Lowfat
Cottage Cheese - Large Curd
Cottage Cheese - Small Curd

Fresh & Easy ()
Cottage Cheese - Pineapple
Cottage Cheese - Regular

Friendship Dairies
Friendship Dairies (All)

Great Value (Wal-Mart)
1% Lowfat Small Curd Cottage Cheese
2% Lowfat Small Curd Cottage Cheese
2% Small Curd Cottage Cheese
4% Large Curd Cottage Cheese
4% Small Curd Cottage Cheese
Fat Free Small Curd Cottage Cheese

Haggen
Cottage Cheese 4% Large Curd
Cottage Cheese Lowfat 2%
Cottage Cheese Nonfat
Cottage Cheese Small Curd

Hood
Cottage Cheese (All)

Horizon Organic ⓘ
Horizon Organic (All BUT Ice Cream
Sandwiches)

Hy-Vee
1% Low Fat Small Curd Cottage Cheese
4% Large Curd Cottage Cheese
4% Small Curd Cottage Cheese

Knudsen 🦢
  Cottage Cheese On The Go Free Nonfat
  Cottage Cheese On The Go Lowfat with Pineapple
  Cottage Cheese On The Go Single Serve Lowfat
  Cottage Doubles Apples & Cinnamon Lowfat
  Cottage Doubles Blueberry Lowfat
  Cottage Doubles Peach Lowfat
  Cottage Doubles Pineapple Lowfat
  Cottage Doubles Raspberry Lowfat
  Cottage Doubles Strawberry Lowfat
  Free Nonfat Cottage Cheese
  Lowfat & Pineapple Cottage Cheese
  Small Curd 4% Milkfat Min Cottage Cheese
  Small Curd Cottage Cheese
  Small Curd Lowfat 2% Milkfat Cottage Cheese
  Small Curd Lowfat Cottage Cheese

Lactaid
  Lowfat Cottage Cheese

Midwest Country Fare (Hy-Vee)
  1% Small Curd Cottage Cheese
  4% Small Curd Cottage Cheese

Nancy's 🍸
  Nancy's (All)

Oberweis Dairy
  1% Cottage Cheese
  4% Cottage Cheese

Penn Maid
  Cottage Cheese

Prairie Farms
  Dry Curd Cottage Cheese
  Fat Free Cottage Cheese
  Large Curd Cottage Cheese
  Lowfat Cottage Cheese
  Small Curd Cottage Cheese

Publix ◯
  Fat Free (All Styles and Flavors)
  Large Curd, 4% Milkfat (All Styles & Flavors)
  Low Fat (All Styles & Flavors)
  Low Fat with Pineapple
  Small Curd, 4% Milkfat (All Styles & Flavors)

Winn-Dixie ◯
  Fat Free Cottage Cheese
  Lowfat Cottage Cheese
  Small & Large Curd Cottage Cheese - 4% milkfat

CREAM

Axelrod
  Cream
Darigold
  Darigold (All)
Food Club (Marsh)
  UPP Heavy Cream
  UPP Whipping Cream
Fresh & Easy ◯
  Whipping Cream
Giant Eagle
  Coffee Cream 18%
  Heavy Cream 36%
  Light Whipping Cream 30%
Great Value (Wal-Mart)
  Heavy Whipping Cream
  Light Cream
Hood
  Cream (All)
Horizon Organic ⓘ
  Horizon Organic (All BUT Ice Cream Sandwiches)
Kroger ⓘ
  Whipping Cream
Meijer
  Ultra Pasteurized Heavy Whipping Cream
Oberweis Dairy
  Heavy Whipping Cream
Organic Valley ⓘ
  Heavy Whipping Cream
Penn Maid
  Cream
Prairie Farms
  Whipping Cream
Publix ◯
  Heavy Whipping Cream
  Whipping Cream

Vermont Butter & Cheese Creamery
- Vermont Butter & Cheese Creamery (All)

Winn-Dixie ()
- Heavy Whipping Cream
- Whipping Cream

CREAM CHEESE

Bashas'
- Cream Cheese - Garden Vegetable
- Cream Cheese - Light Soft
- Cream Cheese - Neufchatel 1/3 Less Bar
- Cream Cheese - Soft Tub
- Cream Cheese - Soft Tub - Onion/Chive
- Cream Cheese - Soft Tub - Strawberry
- Cream Cheese Bar
- Whipped Cream Cheese

Breakstone's ～
- Temp Tee Whipped
- Temp Tee Whipped Cream Cheese

Crystal Farms
- Cream Cheese (All)

Fresh & Easy ()
- Cream Cheese - Regular
- Cream Cheese - Whipped

Great Value (Wal-Mart)
- Chive & Onion Cream Cheese Spread
- Cream Cheese Brick
- Cream Cheese Spread
- Fat Free Cream Cheese Brick
- Light Cream Cheese
- Neufchatel Cheese
- Strawberry Cream Cheese Spread
- Whipped Cream Cheese Spread

Horizon Organic (i)
- Horizon Organic (All BUT Ice Cream Sandwiches)

Hy-Vee
- 1/3 Less Than Fat Cream Cheese
- Blueberry Cream Cheese
- Fat Free Cream Cheese
- Fat Free Soft Cream Cheese
- Garden Vegetable Cream Cheese
- Honey Nut Cream Cheese
- Onion/Chive Cream Cheese
- Soft Cream Cheese
- Soft Light Cream Cheese
- Strawberry Cream Cheese
- Whipped Cream Cheese Spread

Kroger (i)
- Cream Cheeses

Nancy's ♨
- Nancy's (All)

Organic Valley (i)
- Cream Cheese
- Neufchatel

Philadelphia Cream Cheese ～
- Blueberry
- Cheesecake Cream Cheese Spread
- Chive & Onion Cream Cheese Spread
- Chive & Onion Light
- Cream Swirls Peaches 'n Cream
- Fat Free
- Garden Vegetable
- Honey Nut
- Light
- Light Garden Vegetable
- Neufchatel 1/3 Less Fat
- Original
- Pineapple
- Raspberry Cream Cheese Spread
- Regular
- Regular Cream Cheese Spread Original
- Regular Whipped
- Roasted Garlic Light
- Salmon
- Strawberry
- Strawberry Fat Free
- Strawberry Light
- Whipped
- Whipped Cinnamon 'n Brown Sugar
- Whipped Garlic 'n Herb
- Whipped Mixed Berry
- Whipped Ranch
- Whipped with Chives

Price Chopper
- Soft Cream Cheese

Publix ()
- Fat Free (All Styles)
- Light, Soft (All Styles, All Flavors)
- Neufchatel (All Styles, All Flavors)
- Regular - Soft (All Styles, All Flavors)
- Regular (All Styles, All Flavors)

Vegan Gourmet (i) ⛄ ✓
  Cream Cheese Alternative
Winn-Dixie ()
  Lite Cream Cheese
  Regular Cream Cheese
  Soft Cream Cheese

Egg Substitutes

All Whites
  All Whites (All)
Better'n Eggs
  Better'n Eggs (All)
Ener-G ⛄ ✓
  Egg Replacer
Fresh & Easy ()
  Egg Whites
Hy-Vee
  Egg Substitute - Refrigerated
Meijer
  Egg Substitute (Refrigerated)
Price Chopper
  Egg Whites
Publix ()
  Egg Stirs

Eggnog & Other Nogs

Darigold
  Darigold (All)
Hood
  Cinnamon Eggnog
  Gingerbread Eggnog
  Golden Eggnog
  Light Eggnog
  Pumpkin Eggnog
  Sugar Cookie EggNog
  Vanilla Eggnog
Kroger (i)
  Eggnog - Liquid
  Eggnog - Powdered
Oberweis Dairy
  Egg Nog
Organic Valley (i)
  Eggnog

Prairie Farms
  Eggnog
  Holiday (Boiled) Custard
  Holiday Nog
Publix ()
  Low Fat Egg Nog
  Original Egg Nog

Half & Half

Axelrod
  Half & Half
Darigold
  Darigold (All)
Fresh & Easy ()
  Half & Half
Giant Eagle
  Fat Free Half & Half
  Half & Half 10.5%
Great Value (Wal-Mart)
  Half & Half
Haggen
  UPP Half & Half Quart
Hood
  Simply Smart Fat Free Half & Half
Hy-Vee
  Fat Free Half & Half
  Half & Half
Meijer
  Ultra Pasteurized Heavy Half & Half
Oberweis Dairy
  Half and Half
Organic Valley (i)
  Half and Half
Penn Maid
  Half & Half
Prairie Farms
  Half & Half
Publix ()
  Half & Half
Winn-Dixie ()
  Fat Free Half & Half
  Half & Half

Hummus

Athenos 🌿
Artichoke & Garlic Hummus
Black Olive Hummus
Cucumber Dill Hummus
Greek Style Hummus
Original Hummus
Pesto Hummus
Roasted Eggplant Hummus
Roasted Garlic Hummus
Roasted Red Pepper Hummus
Scallion Hummus
Spicy Three Pepper Hummus

Fantastic World Foods
Original Hummus

Marzetti
Black Bean Hummus
Garden Hummus
Original Hummus
Roasted Garlic Hummus
Roasted Red Pepper Hummus

Sabra ◇
Sabra (All)

Tribe Hummus
Hummus (All)

Margarine & Spreads

Benecol
Benecol Spreads (All)

Brummel & Brown
Margarine (All)
Spreads (All)

Country Crock
Spread and Spreadable Butter Products (All)

Crystal Farms
Margarine and Spreads (All)

Earth Balance
Earth Balance (All)

Food Club (Marsh)
No'Ifs'Ands'Or'Butter'
Spread Quarters 65%

Great Value (Wal-Mart)
48% Vegetable Oil Soft Spread
Margarine Quarters

Haggen
Margarine - Soft Tub
Spread - 48% Crock
Spread - 70% Quarters

Hy-Vee
100% Corn Oil Margarine
Best Thing Since Butter
Rich & Creamy Soft Margarine
Soft Margarine
Soft Spread
Soft Spread Crock

I Can't Believe It's Not Butter!
Margarine and Spread Products (All)

Kroger ⓘ
Margarine
Vegetable Spreads

Meijer
Margarine Corn Oil Quarters
Margarine Soft Sleeve
Margarine Soft Tub
Spread 48% Crock
Spread 70% Quarters
Spread No Ifs Ands Or Butter

Olivio
Olivio (All)

Promise
Margarine and Spread Products (All)

Publix ◇
Corn Oil Margarine Quarters
Homestyle Spread - 48% Vegetable Oil
Homestyle Squeeze Spread - 60% Vegetable Oil
It Tastes Just Like Butter Spread - 70% Vegetable Oil
Original Spread Quarters - 70% Vegetable Oil

Milk, Chocolate & Flavored

Alta Dena ◇
Milk (All)

Axelrod
Chocolate Milk
Strawberry Milk

Darigold
Darigold (All)

Great Value (Wal-Mart)
1% Lowfat Chocolate Milk
1/2% Lowfat Chocolate Milk
2% Chocolate Milk

Hood
Calorie Countdown Dairy Beverages
(All Flavors & Fat Levels)
Chocolate Milk - Full Fat (All Sizes)
Chocolate Milk - Low Fat (All Sizes)
Simply Smart Fat Free Chocolate Milk

Horizon Organic ⓘ
Horizon Organic (All BUT Ice Cream
Sandwiches)

Hy-Vee
1% Chocolate Low Fat Milk

Marsh
Low Fat Chocolate Milk

Meijer
1% Chocolate Milk Lowfat
1% Chocolate Milk LowFat No Sugar
Added
1% Chocolate Milk Single Serve
Chocolate Milk
Strawberry Milk

Nesquik ⓘ
Ready-to-Drink Milk (All Flavors)

Oberweis Dairy
No Sugar Added Fat Free Vanilla Milk
No Sugar Added Lowfat Chocolate Milk
No Sugar Added Strawberry Milk
Reduced Fat Strawberry Milk
Reduced Fat Vanilla Milk

Organic Valley ⓘ
8 oz. Single Serves - Chocolate
8 oz. Single Serves - Strawberry
8 oz. Single Serves - Vanilla
Chocolate 2%

Over the Moon ◊
Milk (All)

Penn Maid
Chocolate Milk
Strawberry Milk

Prairie Farms
Candy Cane Milk
Chocolate Cherry Milk
Chocolate Milk

Chocolate Mint Milk
Cookies & Cream Milk
Fat Free Chocolate Milk
Irish Crème Milk
Lowfat Chocolate Milk
Pumpkin Spice Milk
Reduced Fat Chocolate Milk
Strawberry Milk
Vanilla Milk

Publix ◊
Chocolate Milk
Low Fat Chocolate Milk

Rosenberger's Dairies
Milk (All)

Straus Family Creamery
Milk (All)

Stremicks Heritage Foods
Organic Milk (All)

MILK, LACTOSE-FREE

Lactaid
Milk (All)

Meijer
Lactose Free Milk 2% with Calcium
Lactose Free Milk Fat Free with Calcium

Organic Valley ⓘ
Lactose Free Milk

SOUR CREAM

Alta Dena ◊
Sour Cream (All)

Axelrod
Sour Cream (Nonfat, Light, Regular)

Breakstone's ᴄ
All Natural Sour Cream
Free Fat Free Sour Cream
Grade A Pasteurized Homogenized Sour
Cream
Reduced Fat Sour Cream

Cabot
Cabot Products (All)

Cascade Fresh
Cascade Fresh (All)

Darigold
  Darigold (All)
Farmers' All Natural Creamery
  Sour Cream
Food Club (Marsh)
  Sour Cream
  Sour Cream Light
  Sour Cream Non Fat
Fresh & Easy ()
  Sour Cream
Friendship Dairies
  Friendship Dairies (All)
Great Value (Wal-Mart)
  Fat Free Sour Cream
  Light Sour Cream
  Sour Cream
Haggen
  Sour Cream
  Sour Cream - Light
  Sour Cream - Nonfat
Hood
  Sour Cream (All)
Hy-Vee
  Light Sour Cream
  Sour Cream
Knudsen ∽
  Fat Free Sour Cream
  Hampshire 100% Natural Sour Cream
  Hampshire Sour Cream
  Light Sour Cream
Kroger ⓘ
  Sour Cream
Nancy's ⅄
  Nancy's (All)
Oberweis Dairy
  Lite Sour Cream
  Sour Cream
Organic Valley ⓘ
  Lowfat Sour Cream
  Regular Sour Cream
Penn Maid
  Sour Cream - Light
  Sour Cream - Nonfat
  Sour Cream - Regular
Prairie Farms
  Fat Free Sour Cream

  Light Sour Cream
  Regular Sour Cream
Publix ()
  Fat Free Sour Cream (All Styles)
  Light Sour Cream (All Styles)
  Regular Sour Cream (All Styles)
V & V Supremo
  Sour Cream Products (All)
Vegan Gourmet ⓘ ⅄ ✓
  Sour Cream Alternative
Winn-Dixie ()
  Fat Free Sour Cream
  Light Sour Cream
  Regular Sour Cream

Soymilk & Milk Alternatives

Almond Breeze ⅄
  Almond Breeze (All)
Eden Foods ⓘ ✓
  EdenBlend - Organic
  Unsweetened Edensoy, Organic
Fresh & Easy ()
  Soy Milks
Great Value (Wal-Mart)
  Chocolate Soymilk
  Original Soymilk
  Vanilla Soymilk
HealthMarket (Hy-Vee)
  Organic Chocolate Soy Milk
  Organic Original Soy Milk
  Organic Unsweetened Soymilk -
    Refrigerated
  Organic Vanilla Soy Milk
Hy-Vee
  Chocolate Soy Milk
  Enriched Original Rice Milk
  Enriched Vanilla Rice Milk
  Original Soy Milk
  Refrigerated Organic Vanilla Soy Milk
  Refrigerated Original Soy Milk
  Vanilla Soy Milk
Kroger ⓘ
  Rice Drink - Plain
  Rice Drink - Vanilla
  Soy Drink - Plain

Soy Drink - Vanilla

Living Harvest ⓘ ✓
Tempt Hempmilk

Meijer
Organic Soymilk
Ricemilk Organic
Ricemilk Vanilla
Soymilk Chocolate
Soymilk Vanilla

MimicCreme
MimicCreme (All)

Organic Valley ⓘ
Chocolate Soymilk
Original Soymilk
Unsweetened Soymilk
Vanilla Soymilk

Pacific Natural Foods ⓘ
Hazelnut - Chocolate
Hazelnut - Original
Hemp - Chocolate
Hemp - Original
Hemp - Vanilla
Low Fat Rice - Plain
Low Fat Rice - Vanilla
Organic Almond Chocolate
Organic Low-Fat Almond - Original
Organic Low-Fat Almond - Vanilla
Organic Soy - Unsweetened
Organic Unsweetened Almond Original
Organic Unsweetened Almond Vanilla
Select Soy - Low Fat Plain
Select Soy - Low Fat Vanilla
Ultra Soy - Plain
Ultra Soy - Vanilla
Unsweetened Hemp - Original
Unsweetened Hemp - Vanilla

Publix ()
GreenWise Market Soy Milk - Chocolate
GreenWise Market Soy Milk - Plain
GreenWise Market Soy Milk - Vanilla

Rice Dream ✓
Carob
Enriched Original
Enriched Vanilla
Heartwise Original
Heartwise Vanilla
Horchata

Original
Supreme Chocolate Chai
Supreme Vanilla Hazelnut
Vanilla

Silk
Silk Soymilk (All)

Soy Dream ✓
Chocolate Enriched
Classic Original
Classic Vanilla
Original Enriched
Original Enriched, Refrigerated
Vanilla Enriched
Vanilla Enriched, Refrigerated

Winn-Dixie ()
Chocolate Soy Milk
Plain Soy Milk
Unsweetened Soy Milk
Vanilla Soy Milk

WHIPPED TOPPINGS

Axelrod
Aerosol Topping

Bashas'
UPP Whipped Heavy Cream
UPP Whipped Light Cream

Cabot
Cabot Products (All)

Cool Whip ⌇
Regular Extra Creamy Whipped
Topping
Regular Lite Whipped Topping
Regular Whipped Topping

Crowley Foods
Aerosol Topping

Crystal Farms
Aerosol Whip Cream

Food Club (Marsh)
UPP Whipped Cream Aerosol

Great Value (Wal-Mart)
Aerosol Extra Creamy Sweetened
Whipped Cream
Aerosol Sweetened Whipped Light
Cream

Haggen
Dairy UPP Whipped Cream
UPP Heavy Whipping Cream

Hood
Instant Whipped Cream
Sugar Free Light Whipped Cream

Meijer
Ultra Pasteurized Non Dairy (Aerosol)
Ultra Pasteurized Whip Cream
(Aerosol)

Penn Maid
Aerosol Topping

Publix ()
Whipped Heavy Cream (Aerosol Can)
Whipped Light Cream (Aerosol Can)
Whipped Topping - Fat Free (Aerosol
Can)

YOGURT

Alta Dena ()
Yogurt (All)

Axelrod
Yogurt

Bashas'
Yogurt - Blended Peach
Yogurt - Blended Strawberry
Yogurt - Blended Strawberry Banana
Yogurt - Fruit on the Bottom - Black
Cherry
Yogurt - Fruit on the Bottom -
Blueberry
Yogurt - Fruit on the Bottom - Peach
Yogurt - Fruit on the Bottom -
Strawberry
Yogurt - Fruit on the Bottom -
Strawberry Banana
Yogurt - Lowfat Plain
Yogurt - Lowfat Vanilla
Yogurt - Nonfat Light Strawberry
Yogurt - Probiotic Peach
Yogurt - Probiotic Strawberry

Brown Cow
Brown Cow Products (All)

Cabot
Cabot Products (All)

Cascade Fresh
Cascade Fresh (All)

Chobani
Chobani (All)

Cultural Revolution
Yogurt (All)

Dannon
Plain Activia (24 oz. container)
Plain Lowfat
Plain Natural
Plain Nonfat

Darigold
Darigold (All)

FAGE Total Yogurt
FAGE Total Yogurt (All)

Food Club (Marsh)
Yogurt Blended Blueberry
Yogurt Blended Cherry
Yogurt Blended Peach
Yogurt Blended Pineapple Orange
Banana
Yogurt Blended Raspberry
Yogurt Blended Strawberry
Yogurt Blended Strawberry Banana
Yogurt Blended Strawberry Rhubarb
Yogurt Drinkable Mixed Berry
Yogurt Drinkable Strawberry
Yogurt Lite Banana Cream
Yogurt Lite Blackberry
Yogurt Lite Blueberry
Yogurt Lite Cherry
Yogurt Lite Cherry Vanilla
Yogurt Lite Key Lime
Yogurt Lite Lemon Chiffon
Yogurt Lite Peach
Yogurt Lite Raspberry
Yogurt Lite Strawberry
Yogurt Lite Strawberry Banana
Yogurt Lite Strawberry Kiwi
Yogurt Lite Vanilla
Yogurt Lowfat Blended Strawberry
Yogurt Lowfat Blended Vanilla
Yogurt Nonfat Plain

Fresh & Easy ()
Lowfat Yogurt - Blueberry
Lowfat Yogurt - Peach
Lowfat Yogurt - Pina Colada

Lowfat Yogurt - Strawberry
Lowfat Yogurt - Vanilla
Nonfat Yogurt - Black Cherry
Nonfat Yogurt - Peach
Nonfat Yogurt - Raspberry
Nonfat Yogurt - Strawberry
Nonfat Yogurt - Vanilla
Plain Greek Yogurt

Friendship Dairies
Friendship Dairies (All)

Giant Eagle
Blended Lowfat Blackberry Yogurt
Blended Lowfat Blueberry Yogurt
Blended Lowfat Mixed Berry Yogurt
Blended Lowfat Peach Yogurt
Blended Lowfat Raspberry Yogurt
Blended Lowfat Red Cherry Yogurt
Blended Lowfat Strawberry Yogurt
Blended Lowfat Strawberry/Banana Yogurt
Blended Lowfat Vanilla Yogurt
Fat Free Fruit On The Bottom Black Cherry Yogurt
Fat Free Fruit On The Bottom Blueberry Yogurt
Fat Free Fruit On The Bottom Mixed Berry Yogurt
Fat Free Fruit On The Bottom Peach Yogurt
Fat Free Fruit On The Bottom Raspberry Yogurt
Fat Free Fruit On The Bottom Strawberry Yogurt
Light Banana Crème Yogurt
Light Blackberry Yogurt
Light Blueberry Yogurt
Light Key Lime Yogurt
Light Lemon Chiffon Yogurt
Light Mixed Berry Yogurt
Light Orange Crème Yogurt
Light Peach Yogurt
Light Raspberry Lemonade Yogurt
Light Raspberry Yogurt
Light Strawberry Yogurt
Light Strawberry/Banana Yogurt
Light Vanilla Yogurt
Lowfat Plain Yogurt

Nonfat Plain Yogurt

Great Value (Wal-Mart)
Benefit Blueberry Probiotic Light Nonfat Yogurt
Benefit Peach Probiotic Light Nonfat Yogurt
Benefit Raspberry Probiotic Light Nonfat Yogurt
Benefit Strawberry Probiotic Light Nonfat Yogurt
Benefit Vanilla Probiotic Light Nonfat Yogurt
Blended Banana Yogurt
Blended Black Cherry Lowfat Yogurt
Blended Blueberry Lowfat Yogurt
Blended Cherry Vanilla Lowfat Yogurt
Blended Key Lime Lowfat Yogurt
Blended Mango Lowfat Yogurt
Blended Mixed Berry Lowfat Yogurt
Blended Peach Lowfat Yogurt
Blended Pina Colada Lowfat Yogurt
Blended Raspberry Lowfat Yogurt
Blended Strawberry Banana Lowfat Yogurt
Blended Strawberry Lowfat Yogurt
Blended Vanilla Lowfat Yogurt
Fat Free Plain Nonfat Yogurt
Light Banana Cream Nonfat Yogurt
Light Banana Cream Pie Nonfat Yogurt
Light Black Cherry Nonfat Yogurt
Light Blueberry Nonfat Yogurt
Light Lemon Chiffon Nonfat Yogurt
Light Mixed Berry Nonfat Yogurt
Light Peach Nonfat Yogurt
Light Raspberry Nonfat Yogurt
Light Strawberry Banana Nonfat Yogurt
Light Strawberry Nonfat Yogurt
Light Vanilla Nonfat Yogurt

Haggen
Lite Blueberry Yogurt
Lite Cherry Yogurt
Lite Mixed Berry Yogurt
Lite Peach Yogurt
Lite Raspberry Yogurt
Lite Strawberry Yogurt
Lite Vanilla Yogurt
Lowfat Blueberry Yogurt

Lowfat Cherry Yogurt
Lowfat Key Lime Yogurt
Lowfat Mixed Berry Yogurt
Lowfat Orange Crème Yogurt
Lowfat Peach Yogurt
Lowfat Raspberry Yogurt
Lowfat Strawberry Yogurt
Lowfat Vanilla Yogurt

Horizon Organic ⓘ
Horizon Organic (All BUT Ice Cream Sandwiches)

Hy-Vee
Banana Cream Nonfat Yogurt
Black Cherry Low Fat Yogurt
Blueberry Low Fat Yogurt
Blueberry Nonfat Yogurt
Cherry Nonfat Yogurt
Cherry-Vanilla Low Fat Yogurt
Fat Free Plain Yogurt
Key Lime Pie Fat Free Yogurt
Lemon Chiffon Nonfat Yogurt
Lemon Low Fat Yogurt
Mixed Berry Low Fat Yogurt
Nonfat Vanilla Yogurt
Peach Nonfat Yogurt
Peach Yogurt
Plain Low Fat Yogurt
Raspberry Low Fat Yogurt
Raspberry Nonfat Yogurt
Strawberry Banana Low Fat Yogurt
Strawberry Banana Nonfat Yogurt
Strawberry Low Fat Yogurt
Strawberry Nonfat Yogurt
Yogurt To Go - Strawberry
Yogurt To Go - Strawberry & Blueberry
Yogurt To Go - Strawberry/Banana & Cherry

La Yogurt
La Yogurt (All)

Meijer
Blended Boysenberry
Blended Strawberry
Blended Tropical Fruit
Fruit on the Bottom Blueberry
Fruit on the Bottom Peach
Fruit on the Bottom Raspberry
Fruit on the Bottom Strawberry

Lite Banana Crème
Lite Black Cherry
Lite Blueberry
Lite Cherry-Vanilla
Lite Coconut Cream
Lite Lemon Chiffon
Lite Mint Chocolate
Lite Peach
Lite Raspberry
Lite Strawberry
Lite Strawberry-Banana
Lite Vanilla
Lowfat Blended Cherry
Lowfat Blended Mixed Berry
Lowfat Blended Peach
Lowfat Blended Pina Colada
Lowfat Vanilla
Strawberry-Banana
Tube-Yo-Lar Strawberry/Blueberry
Tube-Yo-Lar Tropical Punch/Raspberry
Tube-Yo-Lar Watermelon/Strawberry/Banana

Mountain High Yoghurt
Yoghurt Products (All)

Nancy's ⚕
Nancy's (All)

Nature's Basket (Giant Eagle)
Organic Lowfat Blueberry
Organic Lowfat Peach
Organic Lowfat Raspberry
Organic Lowfat Strawberry
Organic Lowfat Vanilla

Oberweis Dairy
100-Calorie Yogurt (All Flavors)
Plain Nonfat Yogurt
Yogurt (All Flavors)

Old Chatham Sheepherding Company ⚕
Yogurts

Organic Valley ⓘ
Berry Yogurt
Plain Yogurt
Vanilla Yogurt

Penn Maid
Yogurt

Prairie Farms
Fat Free Yogurt (All Flavors)

Lowfat Yogurt (All Flavors)

Publix ()

Apple Pie Light - Fat Free Yogurt

Banana Crème Pie Light - Fat Free Yogurt

Banana Fruit On The Bottom Yogurt

Black Cherry Creamy Blend Yogurt

Black Cherry Fruit On The Bottom Yogurt

Black Cherry with Chocolate - Limited Edition

Blackberry Fruit On The Bottom Yogurt

Blueberry - No Sugar Added Yogurt

Blueberry Creamy Blend Yogurt

Blueberry Fruit on the Bottom Yogurt

Blueberry Light - Fat Free Yogurt

Cappuccino Light - Fat Free Yogurt

Caramel Crème Light - Fat Free Yogurt

Cherry Fruit On The Bottom Yogurt

Cherry Light - Fat Free Yogurt

Cherry Vanilla Light - Fat Free Yogurt

Coconut Crème Pie Light - Fat Free Yogurt

Cranberry Raspberry - No Sugar Added Yogurt

Creamy Blends Black Cherry & Mixed Berry - Multi Pack

Creamy Blends Blueberry & Strawberry Banana - Multi Pack

Creamy Blends Peach and Strawberry - Multi Pack

Egg Nog - Limited Edition Yogurt

Fat Free Light "Active" Peach Yogurt

Fat Free Light "Active" Strawberry Yogurt

Fat Free Light "Active" Vanilla Yogurt

Guava Fruit On The Bottom Yogurt

Honey Almond Light - Fat Free Yogurt

Key Lime Pie Light - Fat Free Yogurt

Kids Blue Raspberry & Cotton Candy - Multi Pack

Kids Grape Bubblegum & Watermelon - Multi Pack

Kids Strawberry & Blueberry - Multi Pack

Kids Strawberry Banana & Cherry - Multi Pack

Lemon Chiffon Light - Fat Free Yogurt

Mandarin Orange Light - Fat Free Yogurt

Mango Fruit On The Bottom Yogurt

Mixed Berry Fruit On The Bottom Yogurt

Peach - No Sugar Added Yogurt

Peach Creamy Blend Yogurt

Peach Fruit On The Bottom Yogurt

Peach Light - Fat Free Yogurt

Piña Colada Light - Fat Free Yogurt

Pineapple Fruit On The Bottom Yogurt

Pumpkin Pie - Limited Edition Yogurt

Raspberry Fruit On The Bottom Yogurt

Raspberry Light - Fat Free Yogurt

Strawberry - No Sugar Added Yogurt

Strawberry Creamy Blend Yogurt

Strawberry Fruit On The Bottom Yogurt

Strawberry Light - Fat Free Yogurt

Strawberry with Chocolate - Limited Edition

Strawberry/Banana Fruit On The Bottom Yogurt

Strawberry/Banana Light - Fat Free Yogurt

Tropical Blend Fruit On The Bottom Yogurt

Vanilla - No Sugar Added Yogurt

Vanilla Creamy Blend Yogurt

Vanilla Light - Fat Free Yogurt

Redwood Hill Farm

Redwood Hill Farm (All)

Silk

Silk Live! Soy Yogurt (All)

Skyr.is ⓘ

Blueberry

Plain

Vanilla

Stonyfield Farm ✓

Stonyfield Farm (All BUT YoBaby Plus Fruit & Cereal, Frozen Yogurt, and Ice Cream)

Straus Family Creamery

Plain Yogurts (All)

Wallaby Yogurt Company

Yogurt (All)

WholeSoy & Co. ⓘ ✓
Soy Yogurt (All)

Winn-Dixie ⟨⟩
Banana Cream Pie Fat Free Yogurt
Black Cherry Fat Free Yogurt
Blueberry Fat Free Yogurt
Blueberry Lowfat Yogurt
Key Lime Pie Fat Free Yogurt
Mixed Berry Fat Free Yogurt
No Sugar Added Strawberry Yogurt
Peach Fat Free Yogurt
Peach Lowfat Yogurt
Pina Colada Fat Free Yogurt
Pineapple Cherry Lowfat Yogurt
Pineapple Lowfat Yogurt
Plain Lowfat Yogurt
Raspberry Fat Free Yogurt
Raspberry Lowfat Yogurt
Strawberry Fat Free Yogurt
Strawberry Lowfat Yogurt
Vanilla Fat Free Yogurt
Vanilla Lowfat Yogurt

Yoplait ✓
99% Fat Free Creamy Harvest Peach Large Size Yogurt
99% Fat Free Creamy Strawberry Banana Large Size Yogurt
99% Fat Free Creamy Strawberry Large Size Yogurt
All Natural Fat Free Plain Yogurt
Delights Parfait Chocolate Raspberry
Delights Parfait Crème Caramel
Delights Parfait Lemon Torte
Delights Parfait Triple Berry Crème
Fiber One Key Lime Pie Yogurt
Fiber One Peach Yogurt
Fiber One Strawberry Yogurt
Fiber One Vanilla Yogurt
Fridge Pack Light Key Lime Pie and Vanilla Yogurt
Fridge Pack Light Strawberry and Light Blueberry Patch Yogurt
Fridge Pack Light Strawberry and Light Harvest Peach Yogurt
Fridge Pack Original Strawberry and Original Harvest Peach Yogurt
Fridge Pack Original Strawberry and Original Mixed Berry Yogurt
Fridge Pack Original Strawberry and Strawberry Banana Yogurt
Fridge Pack Original Strawberry Yogurt
Go-Gurt Banana Split/Strawberry Milkshake Yogurt
Go-Gurt Berry Blue Blast/Chill Out Cherry Yogurt
Go-Gurt Cool Cotton Candy/Burstin' Melon Berry Yogurt
Go-Gurt iCarly Special Edition Rad Raspberry/Paradise Punch Yogurt
Go-Gurt Sponge Bob Special Edition Strawberry Riptide/Bikini Bottom Berry Yogurt
Go-Gurt Strawberry Banana Burst/ Watermelon Meltdown Yogurt
Go-Gurt Strawberry Kiwi Kick/Chill Out Cherry Yogurt
Go-Gurt Strawberry Splash/Berry Blue Blast Yogurt
Go-Gurt Strawberry Splash/Cool Cotton Candy Yogurt
Greek Yogurt - Blueberry
Greek Yogurt - Honey Vanilla
Greek Yogurt - Plain
Greek Yogurt - Strawberry
Kids Banana and Vanilla Yogurt
Kids Strawberry and Strawberry Vanilla Yogurt
Kids Strawberry Banana and Peach Yogurt
Light Apple Turnover Yogurt
Light Apricot Mango Yogurt
Light Banana Cream Pie Yogurt
Light Blackberry Yogurt
Light Blueberry Patch Yogurt
Light Boston Cream Pie Yogurt
Light Fat Free Creamy Strawberry Large Size Yogurt
Light Fat Free Creamy Vanilla Large Size Yogurt
Light Harvest Peach Yogurt
Light Key Lime Pie Yogurt
Light Lemon Cream Pie Yogurt
Light Orange Crème Yogurt

Light Pineapple Upside Down Cake Yogurt
Light Raspberry Cheesecake Yogurt
Light Red Raspberry Yogurt
Light Strawberries 'N Bananas Yogurt
Light Strawberry Orange Sunrise Yogurt
Light Strawberry Shortcake Yogurt
Light Strawberry Yogurt
Light Thick & Creamy French Vanilla Yogurt
Light Thick & Creamy Key Lime Pie Yogurt
Light Thick & Creamy Lemon Meringue Yogurt
Light Thick & Creamy Mixed Berry Yogurt
Light Thick & Creamy Orange Crème Yogurt
Light Thick & Creamy Strawberry Yogurt
Light Very Cherry Yogurt
Light Very Vanilla Yogurt
Light White Chocolate Strawberry Yogurt
Light Yogurt Warehouse Multipack (Boston Cream Pie, Key Lime Pie)
Light Yogurt Warehouse Multipack (Strawberry, Harvest Peach)
Light Yogurt Warehouse Multipack (Strawberry, Harvest Peach, Blueberry)
Light Yogurt Warehouse Multipack (Strawberry, Peach, Vanilla)
Original Banana Crème Yogurt
Original Blackberry Harvest Yogurt
Original Boysenberry Yogurt
Original Cherry Orchard Yogurt
Original Coffee Yogurt
Original French Vanilla Yogurt
Original Harvest Peach Yogurt
Original Key Lime Pie Yogurt
Original Lemon Burst Yogurt
Original Mango Yogurt
Original Mixed Berry Yogurt
Original Mountain Blueberry Yogurt
Original Orange Crème Yogurt
Original Pear Yogurt
Original Pina Colada Yogurt

Original Pineapple Yogurt
Original Red Raspberry Yogurt
Original Strawberry Banana Yogurt
Original Strawberry Cheesecake Yogurt
Original Strawberry Kiwi Yogurt
Original Strawberry Yogurt
Original Yogurt Warehouse Multipack (Strawberry)
Original Yogurt Warehouse Multipack (Strawberry, Peach)
Original Yogurt Warehouse Multipack (Strawberry, Peach, Blueberry)
Original Yogurt Warehouse Multipack (Strawberry, Peach, Vanilla)
Ro-Gurt Special Edition Shaggy's Like Cool Punch & Rawberry Yogurt
Simply…Go-Gurt Strawberry Yogurt
Splitz Rainbow Sherbet Yogurt
Splitz Strawberry Banana Split Yogurt
Splitz Strawberry Sundae Yogurt
Thick & Creamy Blackberry Harvest Yogurt
Thick & Creamy Key Lime Pie Yogurt
Thick & Creamy Peaches 'N Cream Yogurt
Thick & Creamy Royal Raspberry Yogurt
Thick & Creamy Strawberry Banana Yogurt
Thick & Creamy Strawberry Yogurt
Thick & Creamy Vanilla Yogurt
Trix Strawberry Banana Bash/Raspberry Rainbow Yogurt
Trix Strawberry Kiwi/Cotton Candy Yogurt
Trix Strawberry Punch/Watermelon Burst Yogurt
Trix Triple Cherry/Wildberry Blue Yogurt
Trix Very Berry Watermelon/Berry Bolt Yogurt
Whips Chocolate Raspberry Yogurt
Whips Chocolate Yogurt
Whips Key Lime Pie Yogurt
Whips Lemon Burst Yogurt
Whips Orange Crème Yogurt
Whips Peaches 'N Cream Yogurt
Whips Raspberry Yogurt

Whips Strawberry Mist Yogurt
Whips Vanilla Crème Yogurt
Yoplus Blackberry Pomegranate Yogurt
Yoplus Blueberry Acai Yogurt
Yoplus Cherry Yogurt
Yoplus Peach Yogurt
Yoplus Strawberry Yogurt
Yoplus Vanilla Yogurt

MISCELLANEOUS

Lifeway ♉
Lifeway (All)

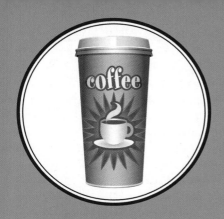

BEVERAGES

BEER

Bard's Tale Beer ✓
Bard's Gold

Green's
Discovery Amber Ale
Endeavour Dubble Ale
Quest Tripel Ale

Lakefront Brewery ⓘ ✓
New Grist

Redbridge ⓘ ✓
Redbridge Beer

Sprecher Brewing Co.
Mbege
Shakparo

St. Peter's Brewery
Sorghum Beer

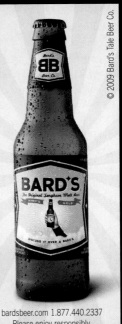

Carbonated Drinks

7Up
7Up (All)
A&W
A&W (All)
Adirondack Beverages
Adirondack Beverages (All)
Barq's
Barq's Root Beer
Caffeine Free Barq's Root Beer
Diet Barq's Red Crème Soda
Diet Barq's Root Beer
Big Shot
Big Shot (All)
Boylan Bottling Co.
Boylan Bottling Co. (All)
Canada Dry
Canada Dry (All)
Cascadia
Cascadia (All)
Chek (Winn-Dixie) ()
Black Cherry Soda
Caffeine Free Cola
Cherry Cola
Club Soda
Cola
Cream Soda
Diet Kountry Mist Soda
Diet Lemon-Lime Soda
Diet Orange Soda
Diet Root Beer
Diet Strawberry Soda
Diet Vanilla Coke
Dr. Chek
Ginger Ale
Grape Soda
Green Apple Soda
Kountry Mist Soda
Lemon-Lime Soda
Orange Pineapple Soda
Orange Soda
Peach Soda
Premium Draft Style Root Beer
Punch
Red Alert Soda
Red Cream Soda

Root Beer
Seltzer Water
Strawberry Soda
Vanilla Cola
China Cola
China Cola
ClearFruit
ClearFruit (All)
Coca-Cola Company, The
Caffeine Free Coca-Cola Classic
Caffeine Free Diet Coke
Cherry Coke
Cherry Coke Zero
Coca-Cola Classic
Coca-Cola Zero
Diet Cherry Coke
Diet Coke
Diet Coke Plus
Diet Coke Sweetened with Splenda
Diet Coke with Lime
Vanilla Coke
Vanilla Coke Zero
Crush
Crush (All)
Deja Blue
Deja Blue
Diet Rite
Diet Rite (All)
Double-Cola
Ski
Dr. Pepper
Dr. Pepper (All)
Efferve
Efferve (All)
Fanta
Fanta Grape
Fanta Orange
Fanta Orange Zero
Faygo
Faygo (All)
Fresca
Fresca
Ginger People, The
Ginger Beer
Lemon Ginger Beer

Great Value (Wal-Mart)
Limeade

GuS Grown-Up Soda
GuS Grown-Up Soda (All flavors)

Hansen's
Soda (All) ♀

Hires
Hires (All)

Hy-Vee
Cherry Cola
Club Soda
Cola
Diet Cola
Diet Dr. Hy-Vee
Diet Orange
Diet Tonic
Dr. Hy-Vee
Fruit Punch
Gingerale
Grape
Heee Haw
Lemon Lime
Orange
Root Beer
Seltzer Water
Sour
Strawberry
Tonic Water

IBC
IBC (All)

Izze ⓘ
Izze Beverages (All)

Kristian Regale
Sparkling Apple Juice
Sparkling Apple Lite Juice
Sparkling Black Currant Juice
Sparkling Lingonberry Juice
Sparkling Orange Juice
Sparkling Peach Juice
Sparkling Pear Juice
Sparkling Pear Lite Juice
Sparkling Pomegranate Juice

Kroger ⓘ
Big K Soft Drinks

LaCROIX
LaCROIX (All)

Martinelli's ⓘ
Martinelli's (All)

Meijer
Diet Caffeine-Free Encore Red
Diet Cherry Encore
Diet Encore Blue
Diet Encore Red
Encore Blue
Encore Cherry Red
Encore Red
Red Pop

Mountain Dew
Carbonated Beverages (All)

Mug
Mug Root Beer (All)

Ohana
Ohana

Orangina
Orangina (All)

Pennsylvania Dutch Birch Beer
Pennsylvania Dutch Birch Beer - Diet
Pennsylvania Dutch Birch Beer -
Regular

Pepsi
Pepsi-Cola Products (All)

Perrier ♀
Sparkling Mineral Water (All)

Prestige (Winn-Dixie) ◌
Clearly Prestige Country Strawberry
Sparkling Water Beverage
Clearly Prestige Key Lime Sparkling
Water Beverage
Clearly Prestige Mandarin Orange
Sparkling Water Beverage
Clearly Prestige Mellow Peach Sparkling
Water Beverage
Clearly Prestige White Grape Sparkling
Water Beverage
Clearly Prestige Wild Cherry Sparkling
Water Beverage

Price Chopper
Black Cherry
Citrus Dew
Club Soda
Cola
Cream Soda

Diet Cola
Diet Ginger Ale
Diet Lemon/Lime
Diet Orange
Diet Raspberry Ginger Ale
Diet Root Beer
Dr. Sparkle
Ginger Ale
Grape
Lemon/Lime
Lemon/Lime Seltzer
Orange Seltzer
Orange Soda
Plain Seltzer
Raspberry Gingerale
Root Beer

Publix ()
Black Cherry Soda
Cherry Cola
Citrus Hit Soda
Club Soda
Cola
Cream Soda
Diet Cola
Diet Ginger Ale
Diet Tonic Water
Ginger Ale
Grape Soda
Lemon Lime Seltzer
Lemon Lime Soda
Orange Soda
Raspberry Seltzer
Root Beer
Tonic Water

RC Cola
RC Cola (All)

Reed's
Ginger Brews

Ritz (Beverage)
Ritz Soda (All)

Schweppes
Schweppes (All)

Shasta
Shasta (All Flavors)

Sierra Mist
Carbonated Beverages (All)

Slice
Carbonated Beverages

Sonoma Sparkler
Sonoma Sparkler (All)

Sprecher Brewing Co.
Sodas

Sprite
Sprite
Sprite Zero

Squirt
Squirt (All)

St. Nick's
St. Nicks (All)

Stewart's
Stewart's (All)

Sundrop
Sundrop (All)

Sunkist
Sunkist (All)

Vernors
Vernors (All)

Virgil's
Cream Sodas
Root Beer

Waist Watcher
Waist Watcher Beverages (All)

Welch's (Dr. Pepper/Snapple Group)
Soda Products (All)

Zevia
Natural Diet Soda (All Flavors)

CHOCOLATE DRINKS

Yoo-hoo
Yoo-hoo

CIDER (ALCOHOLIC)

Ace Cider
Ace Cider (All)

J.K. Scrumpy's Orchard Gate Gold
Ciders (All)

Magners Irish Cider
Magners Irish Cider (All)

Original Sin Hard Cider
Original Sin Hard Apple Cider

Original Sin Hard Pear Cider

Samuel Smith's Organic Cider
Samuel Smith's Organic Cider

Strongbow
Strongbow

Woodchuck Draft Cider ♀ ✓
Woodchuck 802 Dark & Dry Draft
Cider
Woodchuck Amber Draft Cider
Woodchuck Granny Smith Draft Cider
Woodchuck Pear Draft Cider
Woodchuck Raspberry Cider

Woodpecker Cider ♀ ✓
Woodpecker Cider

Wyder's Cider ♀ ✓
Wyder's Hard Cider (All Varieties)

COFFEE DRINKS & MIXES

Ambassador Organics
Ambassador Organics (All)

Audubon Coffee ♀
Coffee (All)

Bashas'
Coffee - Ground - Classic Roast
Coffee - Ground - Decaf Classic Roast
Coffee - Ground - Decaf Original Roast
Coffee - Ground - French Roast
Coffee - Ground - Original Roast
Coffee - Ground - Special Roast
Coffee - Instant - Classic Roast
Colombian Coffee
Decaffeinated Coffee

Black Mountain Gold Coffee ♀
Coffee (All)

Caffe D'vita ()
Caffe D'vita Products (All)

CDM
Coffee & Chicory
Decaf Coffee & Chicory
Medium Roast Coffee & Chicory

Chock Full O' Nuts
Coffee Products (All)

Don Francisco's Coffee
Coffee (All)

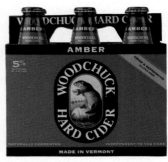
Eight O'Clock Coffee
Coffee (All)

Equal Exchange
Coffee (All) ♀

Flavia
Coffees (All)

Folgers
Coffees (All)

Food Club (Marsh)
Coffee - Can Classic Roast (Red)
Coffee - Can Decaf (Green) Ezo
Coffee - French Roast Ezo
Coffee - Instant (Red)
Coffee - Instant Decaf (Green)
Coffee - Lite, 50/50 Blend (Light Blue)
Ezo

French Market Coffee
Coffee & Chicory City Roast
Coffee & Chicory Creole Roast
Coffee & Chicory Decaf
Pure Chicory
Pure Dark Roast Restaurant Blend
Pure French Roast

Restaurant Blend
Union Coffee & Chicory City Roast

Fresh & Easy ()
Coffee (Assorted Varieties)

General Foods International ～
Café Francais
Café Vienna
Café Vienna Sugar Free
Cappuccino Coolers French Vanilla
Cappuccino Coolers Hazelnut
Chai Latte
Crème Caramel
Dark Mayan Chocolate Latte
French Vanilla Cafe
French Vanilla Café Sugar Free
French Vanilla Café Sugar Free Decaf
Hazelnut Belgian Cafe
Hazelnut Café
Hot Cappuccino Café Mocha
Hot Cappuccino French Vanilla
Italian Cappuccino
Mocha Latte
On The Go Cafe Mocha Sugar Free
On The Go Hazelnut Cappuccino Sugar
 Free
On The Go Vanilla Latte Sugar Free
Orange Spice Latte
Peppermint Mocha Latte
Pumpkin Spice Latte
Raspberry Truffle Latte
Suisse Mocha
Suisse Mocha Café
Suisse Mocha Café Sugar Free
Suisse Mocha Café Sugar Free Decaf
Swiss White Chocolate
Vanilla Bean Latte
Vanilla Bean Latte Decaf
Vanilla Caramel Latte
Vanilla Nut Café
Viennese Chocolate Café

Giant Eagle
Coffee Singles
Colombian Coffee
Decaf Coffee Singles
Decaf Colombian Coffee
Decaf Instant Original Blend Coffee
Decaf Original Blend Coffee

French Roast Coffee
French Vanilla Coffee
Hazelnut Coffee
Instant Original Blend Coffee
Lite Coffee
Original Blend Coffee

Great Value (Wal-Mart)
100% Arabica Instant Coffee
100% Arabica Premium Ground Coffee
100% Colombian Naturally
 Decaffeinated Premium Ground
 Coffee
100% Colombian Premium Ground
 Coffee
French Roast 100% Arabica Coffee
Naturally Decaffeinated Instant Coffee

Green Mountain Coffee
Coffees (All)

Haggen
Coffee - 100% Colombian
Coffee - Decaf
Coffee - French Roast
Coffee - Premium Blend

Harmony Bay
Harmony Bay (All)

Hy-Vee
100% Colombian Coffee
Breakfast Blend Coffee
Coffee
Decaffeinated Coffee
Decaffeinated Instant Coffee
French Roast Coffee
Instant Coffee

Illy
Coffee (All)

JFG Coffee & Tea
Bonus Blend
Bonus Blend Decaf
Decaf Instant Coffee
Gourmet/Restaurant Blend
Instant Coffee
JFG Decaf
JFG Lite
Rich French Roast
Special

Kroger ⓘ
Coffee - Instant

Coffee - Unflavored Ground
Coffee - Whole

Maxwell House ⌒
Cafe Collection Cappuccino
Cafe Collection Decaffeinated Pods
Cafe Collection French Roast Pods
Cafe Collection Hazelnut Pods
Cafe Collection House Blend Pods
Decaffeinated Instant Coffee Singles Bags
House Blend
Instant Original
Master Blend Ground
Original Decaffeinated Filter Packs
Original Decaffeinated Ground
Original Filter Packs
Original Singles

Meijer
Coffee - Decaf
Coffee - French Roast
Coffee - French Roast Ground
Coffee - Ground Colombian
Coffee - Ground Lite 50%
Coffee - Ground Lite 50% Decaf
Coffee - Regular

Millstone ()
Ground Coffee (All BUT Flavored Coffee Products)
Roast Coffee (All BUT Flavored Coffee Products)

Mountain Blend ⓘ
Instant Coffee

Nescafé ⓘ
Classic Instant Coffee
Taster's Choice Instant Coffee (Flavored & Non-Flavored)

Newman's Own Organics () ⓘ
Coffees (All)

Organic Coffee Company, The ♀
Coffee (All)

Pacific Natural Foods ⓘ
Organic Simply Coffee - Latte
Organic Simply Coffee - Mocha
Organic Simply Coffee - Vanilla Latte

POM Wonderful ♀
POM Wonderful (All)

Publix ()
Coffee (All Varieties)

Rogers Family Coffee Company, The ♀
Coffees (All)

San Francisco Bay Coffee Company ♀
Coffee (All)

Sanka ⌒
Naturally Decaffeinated

Seattle's Best Coffee
Coffee (All)

Stewarts
Coffee

Van Houtte
Pure Roasted Coffee - Ground (All)
Pure Roasted Coffee - Whole Bean (All)

Yuban ⌒
100% Arabica Hazelnut Single Serve 16 Ct Pods
100% Colombian Decaffeinated Single Serve 16 Ct
100% Colombian Single Serve 18 Ct Pods
Dark Roast Coffee 100% Columbian
Instant Coffee 100% Columbian
Organic Rich Medium Roast Coffee 100% Columbian
Original Coffee 100% Columbian

CREAMERS & FLAVORINGS

Bashas'
Creamer Powdered French Vanilla
Creamer Powdered Hazelnut
Creamer Powdered Non-Dairy

Coffee-Mate ⓘ
Coffee-Mate Liquid (Flavored & Non-Flavored)
Coffee-Mate Powder (Flavored & Non-Flavored)

Cremora
Cremora

Flavia
Specialty Swirls (All)

Food Club (Marsh)
Creamer Powder - Fat Free

Creamer Powdered
Fat Free French Vanilla Non Dairy
    Creamer
Fat Free Hazelnut Non Dairy Creamer
French Vanilla Non Dairy Creamer
Hazelnut Non Dairy Coffee Creamer
UPP Creamer Non Dairy

Fresh & Easy ()
Soy Creamer

Giant Eagle
Non Dairy Creamer

Great Value (Wal-Mart)
Coffee Creamer
French Vanilla Coffee Creamer

Haggen
Powdered Creamer

Hood
Country Creamer
Fat Free Country Creamer

Hy-Vee
Fat Free French Vanilla Coffee Creamer
    - Refrigerated
Fat Free Hazelnut Coffee Creamer -
    Refrigerated
Hazelnut Coffee Creamer - Refrigerated

International Delight
International Delight (All)

Luzianne
Liquid Flavoring - Peach Mango
Liquid Flavoring - Raspberry

Meijer
Creamer French Vanilla
Creamer Hazelnut
Organic Creamer
Ultra Pasteurized Nondairy Creamer

MimicCreme
MimicCreme (All)

Publix ()
Coffee Creamer
Fat Free Non-Dairy Creamer
Non-Dairy Creamer (Powder)
Non-Dairy French Vanilla Flavored
    Creamer (Powder)
Non-Dairy Lite Creamer (Powder)

Silk
Silk Creamer (All)

Torani
Torani (All BUT Classic Caramel, Sugar
    Free Classic Caramel, Sugar Free
    French Vanilla, Toasted Marshmallow,
and Bacon)

Valu Time (Marsh)
Creamer Powdered

Winn-Dixie ()
Fat Free Non-Diary Coffee Creamer
Original Non-dairy Coffee Creamer

DIET & NUTRITIONAL DRINKS

Boost
Boost (All BUT Chocolate Malt)

Elations
Elations (All)

Ensure
Ensure (All)
Ensure High Calcium (All)
Ensure High Protein (All)
Ensure Plus (All)
Ensure Plus HN - Vanilla

Fibersouce HN
Fibersource HN

FUZE
Fuze (All Flavors)

Gatorade ()
Nutrition Shakes (All Flavors)

Glucerna
Glucerna - Vanilla
Glucerna Shakes (All Flavors)
Weight Loss Shake (All Flavors)

Hy-Vee
Chocolate Nutritional Supplement
Chocolate Nutritional Supplement Plus
Vanilla Nutritional Supplement
Vanilla Nutritional Supplement Plus

Kroger (i)
Active Lifestyle Drink Sticks

Meijer
Chocolate Diabetic Nutritional Drink
Diet Quick Chocolate Extra Thin
Diet Quick Strawberry Extra Thin
Diet Quick Vanilla Extra Thin

Gluco-Burst - Chocolate Diabetic
Nutritional Drink
Gluco-Burst - Strawberry Diabetic
Nutritional Drink
Gluco-Burst - Vanilla Diabetic
Nutritional Drink
Strawberry Diabetic Nutritional Drink
Vanilla Diabetic Nutritional Drink

POM Wonderful ⚱
POM Wonderful (All)

Right Size
Right Size (All)

Tahiti Trader ⓘ
Tahiti Trader (All)

ENERGY DRINKS

4C
Totally Light Drink Mix Energy Rush
(All Flavors)

5-hour Energy ⚱
5-Hour Energy

AMP Energy Drink
AMP Energy Drinks (ALL)

FUZE
Fuze (All Flavors)

Gatorade ⚘
Energy Drink (All Flavors)

GURU Energy Drink ⓘ
GURU Energy Drink

No Fear
No Fear (All)

NOS
Energy Drinks

Red Bull
Red Bull Cola
Red Bull Energy Drink
Red Bull Sugarfree

Rip It
Rip It

Sambazon
Sambazon (All)

SoBe
SoBe (All)

FLAVORED OR ENHANCED WATER

Adirondack Beverages
Adirondack Beverages (All)

Crystal Bay
Crystal Bay (All)

Dasani
Dasani Essence
Dasani Lemon
Dasani Plus Cleanse + Restore
Dasani Plus Refresh + Revive

Fresh & Easy ⚘
Flavored Water - Coconut
Flavored Water - Cucumber
Flavored Water - Peppermint
Flavored Water - Strawberry
Vitamin Water - Acai Blue Pome
Vitamin Water - Black Cherry
Vitamin Water - Dragonfruit
Vitamin Water - Lemonade

Hy-Vee
Black Cherry Water Cooler
Black Cherry Water Refreshers
Key Lime Water Cooler
Kiwi Strawberry Water Cooler
Mixed Berry Water Cooler
Peach Melba Water Cooler
Peach Water Cooler
Raspberry Water Cooler
Strawberry Water Cooler
White Grape Water Cooler

Kellogg's ⚘
Special K Protein Water Mixes

Kroger ⓘ
Crystal Clear Flavored Waters

Meijer
Calcium Spring Water
Natural Calcium Spring Water

Price Chopper
Grape Spring Water
Lemon Spring Water
Raspberry Spring Water

Propel ⚘
Propel

Smartwater
Smartwater (All)

SoBe
SoBe (All)

VIO
Vibrancy Drinks (All)

Vitaminwater
Vitaminwater (All)
Vitaminwater Zero (All)

HOT COCOA & CHOCOLATE MIXES

Bashas'
Chocolate Flavor Drink Mix
Hot Cocoa - No Sugar
Hot Cocoa Mix
Hot Cocoa Mix Mini Marshmallows
Hot Cocoa Mix with Marshmallows

Best Friends Cocoa
Hot Cocoa (All)

Caffe D'vita ()
Caffe D'vita Products (All)

Food Club (Marsh)
Chocolate Flavor Drink Mix
Hot Cocoa
Hot Cocoa (Can)
Hot Cocoa with Marshmallows

Great Value (Wal-Mart)
Milk Chocolate Hot Cocoa Mix
Milk Chocolate Hot Cocoa Mix w/
Marshmallows

Green Mountain Coffee
Hot Cocoas (All)

Hy-Vee
Instant Chocolate Flavored Drink Mix
Instant Hot Cocoa Mix
No Sugar Added Instant Hot Cocoa Mix

Juanitas
Juanitas (All BUT Mole, Caldo de Pollo,
Chile Colorado, Chicken Veracruz,
Chile Verde, and Albondigas Soup)

Kroger ⓘ
Instant Cocoa

Land O'Lakes ()
Cocoa Classics Hot Cocoa Mixes (All)

Meijer
Chocolate Flavor Drink Mix
Cocoa Hot Instant Marshmallow

Hot Cocoa Mix
Hot Cocoa Mix No Sugar Added
Hot Cocoa Mix Sugar Free
Hot Cocoa Mix with Marshmallows
Organic Hot Cocoa Regular

Midwest Country Fare (Hy-Vee)
Hot Cocoa Mix
Instant Chocolate Flavored Drink Mix

Saco
Saco (All)

Sally's ☻
Sally's (All)

INSTANT BREAKFAST DRINKS

Kroger ⓘ
In An Instant Drink Powders

JUICE DRINK MIXES

4C
Instant Drink Mixes Sweetened with
Sugar (All)
Totally Light Drink Mixes Sweetened
with Splenda (All)

Alpine
Cider Drink Mixes (All)

Bashas'
Drink - Cranberry Raspberry
Drink Mix - Cherry
Drink Mix - Grape
Drink Mix - Lemonade
Drink Mix - Orange
Drink Mix - Punch
Drink Mix - Strawberry
Lemonade Sugar Free Drink Mix
Pink Lemonade Sugar Free Drink Mix
Raspberry Ice Sugar Free Drink Mix

Continental Mills ()
Alpine Spiced Cider - Original
Alpine Spiced Cider - Sugar Free

Country Time ✑
Lemonade Drink Mix
Lemonade Flavor Drink Mix
Lemonade Iced Tea Classic Drink Mix
Lemonade Iced Tea Raspberry Drink
Mix

Lemonade Lite Drink Mix
On The Go Lemonade 10 Packets Drink Mix
Pink Lemonade Drink Mix
Pink Lemonade Flavor Drink Mix
Pink Lemonade Lite Drink Mix
Raspberry Lemonade Drink Mix
Strawberry Lemonade Drink Mix

Crystal Light
Fusion Fruit Punch Fruit Drinks
Immunity Natural Cherry Pomegranate Drink Mix
Metabolism+ Peach Mango Green Tea Packets Drink Mix
On The Go Energy Wild Strawberry
On The Go Fruit Punch Sugar Free
On The Go Hunger Satisfaction Natural Strawberry Banana Drink Mix
On The Go Iced Tea Sugar Free Packets
On The Go Immunity Cherry Pomegranate
On The Go Lemonade Sugar Free Packets
On The Go Peach Tea Sugar Free Packets
On the Go Pink Lemonade
On The Go Raspberry Ice Sugar Free Packets
On The Go Raspberry Lemonade Sugar Free
On the Go Skin Essentials Pomegranate Lemonade
On The Go Sunrise Classic Orange
Pink Lemonade Sugar Free
Raspberry Ice Sugar Free Fruit Drinks
Raspberry Lemonade Sugar Free
Strawberry-Kiwi Sugar Free Fruit Drinks
Strawberry-Orange-Banana Sugar Free Lemonade
Sugar Free Lemonade
Sugar Free Lemonade Value Pack

Food Club (Marsh)
Drink Mix - Cherry
Drink Mix - Fruit Punch Sugar Free
Drink Mix - Grape
Drink Mix - Lemonade Canister

Drink Mix - Lemonade Sugar Free
Drink Mix - Orange
Drink Mix - Pink Lemonade Sugar Free
Drink Mix - Punch
Drink Mix - Raspberry Ice Sugar Free
Drink Stix - Iced Tea Sugar Free
Drink Stix - Lemonade Sugar Free
Drink Stix - Raspberry Ice Sugar Free

Hy-Vee
Splash Cherry Drink Mix
Splash Grape Drink Mix
Splash Lemonade Drink Mix
Splash Orange Drink Mix
Splash Tropical Fruit Punch Drink Mix

Kool-Aid
Black Cherry Unsweetened Soft Drink Mix
Cherry Sugar Free Soft Drink Mix
Cherry Sugar-Sweetened Soft Drink Mix
Cherry Unsweetened Soft Drink Mix
Fun Fizz Gigglin' Grape Drink Drops
Fun Fizz Laughin' Lemonade Drink Drops
Fun Fizz Partyin' Punch Drink Drops
Grape Sugar Free Soft Drink Mix
Grape Sugar-Sweetened Soft Drink Mix
Grape Unsweetened Soft Drink Mix
Invisible Changin' Cherry Sugar Sweetened Soft Drink Mix
Invisible Changin' Cherry Unsweetened Soft Drink Mix
Invisible Grape Illusion Sugar Sweetened Soft Drink Mix
Invisible Grape Illusion Unsweetened Soft Drink Mix
Lemonade Sugar-Sweetened Soft Drink Mix
Lemonade Unsweetened Soft Drink Mix
Lemon-Lime Unsweetened Soft Drink Mix
On The Go - Cherry Soft Drink Mix
On The Go - Tropical Punch Soft Drink Mix
On The Go - Tropical Punch Sugar Free Soft Drink Mix
Orange Sugar-Sweetened Soft Drink Mix

Orange Unsweetened Soft Drink Mix
Pink Lemonade Unsweetened Soft
  Drink Mix
Singles - Cherry Soft Drink Mix
Singles - Grape Soft Drink Mix
Singles - Orange Soft Drink Mix
Singles - Tropical Punch Soft Drink Mix
Soarin' Strawberry Lemonade
  Unsweetened Soft Drink Mix
Strawberry Sugar-Sweetened Soft Drink
  Mix
Strawberry Unsweetened Soft Drink
  Mix
Tropical Punch Soft Drink Mix
Tropical Punch Sugar Free Soft Drink
  Mix

Kool-Aid Mad Scientwists ∽
Raspberry Reaction Invisible
  Unsweetened Soft Drink Mix
Wild Watermelon Kiwi Invisible
  Unsweetened Soft Drink Mix

Kool-Aid Twists ∽
Berry Blue Unsweetened Soft Drink Mix
Blastin' Berry Cherry Unsweetened Soft
  Drink Mix
Ice Blue Raspberry Lemonade Sugar
  Sweetened Soft Drink Mix
Ice Blue Raspberry Lemonade
  Unsweetened Soft Drink Mix
Slammin' Strawberry Kiwi Unsweetened
  Soft Drink Mix
Watermelon Cherry Unsweetened Soft
  Drink Mix

Kroger ⓘ
Instant Spiced Cider

Marsh
Drink Mix Orange

Meijer
Crystal Quencher - Black Cherry
Crystal Quencher - Key Lime
Crystal Quencher - Kiwi Strawberry
Crystal Quencher - Peach
Crystal Quencher - Raspberry
Crystal Quencher - Tangerine Lime
Crystal Quencher - White Grape
Drink Mix - Breakfast Orange
Drink Mix - Cherry

Drink Mix - Grape
Drink Mix - Lemon Sugar Free
Drink Mix - Lemonade
Drink Mix - Lemonade Stix
Drink Mix - Orange
Drink Mix - Orange Free & Light
Drink Mix - Pink Lemonade
Drink Mix - Pink Lemonade Sugar Free
Drink Mix - Punch
Drink Mix - Raspberry Stix
Drink Mix - Raspberry Sugar Free
Drink Mix - Strawberry
Grape Juice Concentrate
Orange Juice (Shelf Stable)
Strawberry Flavor Drink Mix
White Grape Juice Cocktail Concentrate

Old Orchard
Old Orchard (All)

Tang ∽
Grape Drink Mix
Jamaica Hisibcus Makes 1 Quart Drink
  Mix
On The Go Orange 0.69 Oz Packets
  Drink Mix
Orange Drink Mix
Orange Kiwi Drink Mix
Orange Pineapple Drink Mix
Orange Strawberry Drink Mix
Orange Sugar Free Drink Mix
Orange with Fruit Pulp Makes 1 Quart
  Drink Mix
Strawberry with Fruit Pulp Makes 1
  Quart Drink Mix
Strawberry with Fruit Pulp Makes 6
  Quarts Drink Mix
Tangerine Strawberry Drink Mix
Tropical Passionfruit Drink Mix
Wild Berry Drink Mix

True Lemon
True Lemon (All)

JUICES & FRUIT DRINKS

American Beverage Corporation ✇
Fruit Flavored Drinks
Apple & Eve ✇
100% Juices (All)

Juice Beverages (All)

AriZona
Juice Products (All)

Axelrod
Orange Juice

Bashas'
Apple Juice
Apple Juice from Concentrate
Cranberry Apple Juice Cocktail
Cranberry Grape Juice Cocktail
Cranberry Juice Cocktail Lite
Cranberry Raspberry Juice Cocktail Lite
Fruit Mixed X-treme Cherry
Fruit Punch Sugar Free Drink Mix
Juice - Grape
Juice - Grape White
Prune Juice from Concentrate
Tomato Clam Juice Cocktail (bi-lingual)
Tomato Juice
Vegetable Juice Cocktail

Bionaturae
Nectars (All) ⓘ

Bolthouse Farms ⓘ
Bolthouse Farms Juices (All BUT Pear Merlot Fruit Juice)

Bom Dia ⓘ
Bom Dia Juices (All BUT Pear Merlot Fruit Juice)

Campbell's ⓘ
Healthy Request Tomato Juice
Low Sodium Tomato Juice
Organic Tomato Juice
Tomato Juice

Capri Sun ᔕ
Coastal Cooler/Strawberry Banana Blend
Coolers Variety Pack
Grape
Mountain Cooler Mixed Fruit
Orange
Pacific Cooler Mixed Fruit Blend
Red Berry/Strawberry Raspberry Blend
Splash Cooler Mixed Fruit Blend
Strawberry
Sunrise Berry Strawberry Tangerine Morning
Sunrise Orange Wake Up

Sunrise Tropical Morning
Surfer Cooler Mixed Fruit Blend
Tropical Punch Blend
Variety Pack
Wild Cherry Blend

Central Market Classics (Price Chopper)
Premium Apple Juice

Ceres
Juices (All)

Chek (Winn-Dixie) ◌
Lemonade

Clamato
Clamato (All BUT Red Eye)

Country Time (Dr. Pepper/Snapple Group)
Country Time (All)

Country Time ᔕ
Lemonade - Large Ready To Drink Pouches 6 Ct

Dei Fratelli
Dei Fratelli (All BUT Tomato Soup)

Dole ◌
100% Juice Products (All)

Earth Wise
Earth Wise (All)

Eden Foods ⓘ ✓
Apple Juice - Organic
Cherry Juice Concentrate - Organic
Concord Grape Juice, Organic

Florida's Natural
Premium Orange Juice
Ruby Red Grapefruit Juice

Food Club (Marsh)
Cranberry Apple (Rectangular Bottle)
Cranberry Grape (Rectangular Bottle)
Cranberry Grape Lite (Rectangular Bottle)
Cranberry Raspberry (Rectangular Bottle)
Cranberry Raspberry Lite
Juice - Apple, Not From Concentrate
Juice - Cranberry Blend 100% (Rectangle Bottle)
Juice - Cranberry Cocktail (Rectangle Bottle)

Juice - Cranberry Lite (Rectangle Bottle)
Juice - Cranberry White Strawberry
Juice - Grape (Rectangle Bottle)
Juice - Grape White (Rectangle Bottle)
Juice - Grapefruit (Rectangle Bottle)
Juice - Pineapple Can
Juice - Pomegranate Blend 100%
Juice - Pomegranate Blueberry Blend 100%
Juice - Prune, Not From Concentrate
Juice - Refrigerated Orange Premium
Juice - Refrigerated Orange Premium Groves Best
Juice - Refrigerated Orange Premium with Calcium
Juice - Refrigerated Orange Reconstituted Original
Juice - Refrigerated Orange Reconstituted Pulp Added
Juice - Ruby Red Grapefruit (Rectangular Bottle)
Juice - Ruby Red Tangerine (Rectangle Bottle)
Tomato Juice
Vegetable Juice
Vegetable Juice Cocktail

Fresh & Easy ()

100% Juice - Apple
100% Juice - Grape
100% Juice - Grapefruit
100% Juice - Pineapple
100% Juice - Prune
Antioxidant Juice - Blue Raspberry
Antioxidant Juice - Mango Acai
Antioxidant Juice - Pome Cranberry
Blended Juice - Breakfast Blend
Blended Juice - Cranberry
Blended Juice - Fruit Punch
Blended Juice - Lemonade
Blended Juice - Limeade
Blended Juice - Pome Blue
Fusio Juice - Acai Mixed Berry
Fusio Juice - Peach Mango
Fusio Juice - Strawberry Banana
Pure Juice - Black Cherry
Pure Juice - Blueberry
Pure Juice - Cranberry

Pure Juice - Pomegranate
Vegetable Juice - Low Sodium
Vegetable Juice - Regular
Vegetable Juice - Spicy
Vegetable Juice - Tomato

Ginger People, The

Ginger 'Gizer
Ginger Soother

Great Value (Wal-Mart)

100% Apple Juice
100% Cranberry Juice
100% Florida Grapefruit Juice
100% Grape Juice
100% Grape Peach Juice
100% Juice Apple Juice Punch Blend
100% Juice Fruit Punch
100% Juice Unsweetened Apple Juice
100% Orange Country Style Juice
100% Orange Juice
100% Orange Juice From Concentrate
100% Pure Orange Juice
100% Pure Orange Juice with Calcium
100% Tomato Juice
100% Vegetable Juice
100% White Grape Juice
Acai Mixed Berry 100% Vegetable & Fruit Juice
Apple Juice
Country Style Orange Juice
Cranberry Apple
Cranberry Apple Juice Cocktail
Cranberry Juice Cocktail
Fruit Punch
Grape Cranberry
Grape Cranberry Juice Cocktail
Grape Drink
Grape Punch
Guava Nectar w/Calcium
Kiwi Strawberry Punch
Lemon Berry Punch
Lemon Juice
Lemonade
Light Apple Juice Cocktail
Light Apple Juice Cocktail w/Splenda
Light Pomegranate Blueberry Vegetable & Fruit Juice

Light Strawberry Banana Vegetable & Fruit Juice
Orange Juice
Orange Juice w/Calcium
Orange Punch
Pineapple Juice
Pineapple Orange Juice
Pink Grapefruit Juice
Pink Lemonade
Pomegranate Blueberry 100% Vegetable & Fruit Juice
Prune Juice
Strawberry Banana 100% Vegetable & Fruit Juice
Strawberry Banana Nectar
Strawberry Banana Nectar w/Calcium
Tomato Juice
Unsweetened Pink Grapefruit Juice
Unsweetened White Grapefruit Juice
Vegetable Juice
Vegetable Juice with Vitamins A&C

Haggen

100% Cranberry Blend
100% White Grape Juice
Apple Cider from Concentrate
Apple Juice from Concentrate
Cranberry Juice Cocktail
Cranberry Raspberry Drink
Drink - Cranberry Apple
Drink - Cranberry Grape
Drink - Cranberry Lite
Drink - Cranberry Raspberry Lite
Grapefruit Juice
Orange Juice - Premium (Refrigerated)
Orange Juice - Premium with Calcium + Vit C (Refrigerated)
Orange Juice - Reconstituted (Refrigerated)
Orange Juice Reconstituted w/Calcium (Refrigerated)
Pineapple Juice
Prune Juice
Ruby Red Grapefruit Juice
Tangerine / Ruby Red Grapefruit Juice
Vegetable Juice Cocktail

Honest Ade

Honest Ade (All)

Honest Kids

Honest Kids (All)

Honest Mate

Honest Mate (All)

Honest Tea

Honest Tea (All)

Hood

Juice (All)

Hy-Vee

100% Apple Juice From Concentrate
100% Blueberry Pomegranate Juice
100% Cherry Pomegranate Juice
100% Cranberry Juice Blend
100% Cranberry/Apple Juice Blend
100% Cranberry/Raspberry Juice Blend
100% Grapefruit Juice From Concentrate with Added Calcium
100% Unsweetened Prune Juice From Concentrate
100% White Grape Juice From Concentrate
Apple Just Juice
Berry Just Juice
Calcium Fortified Apple Juice From Concentrate
Cherry Just Juice
Concord Grape Juice
Cranberry Apple Juice Cocktail From Concentrate
Cranberry Grape Juice Cocktail From Concentrate
Cranberry Grape Juice Lite
Cranberry Juice Cocktail From Concentrate
Cranberry Raspberry Juice Cocktail From Concentrate
Cranberry Raspberry Juice Lite
Cranberry Strawberry Juice Cocktail From Concentrate
Fruit Punch Coolers
Fruit Punch Just Juice
Grape Just Juice
Lemonade From Concentrate
Light Apple Cherry Juice Cocktail From Concentrate
Light Apple Juice Cocktail From Concentrate

Light Apple Kiwi Strawberry Juice Cocktail From Concentrate
Light Apple Raspberry Juice Cocktail From Concentrate
Light Grape Juice Cocktail From Concentrate
Lite Cranberry Juice
No Concentrate Country Style Orange Juice
No Concentrate Orange Juice
No Concentrate Orange Juice with Calcium
Not From Concentrate Ruby Red Grapefruit Juice
Orange Tangerine Just Juice
Ruby Red Grapefruit Juice Cocktail From Concentrate
Splash Apple Cranberry
Splash Cherry
Splash Fruit Punch
Splash Grape
Splash Lemonade
Splash Light Blue Fruit Punch
Splash Light Fruit Punch
Splash Light Grape Punch
Splash Light Orange Punch
Splash Orange
Splash Orange Pineapple
Splash Raspberry
Splash Strawberry
Splash Strawberry Kiwi Punch
Splash Tropical Punch
Tomato Juice From Concentrate
Tropical Punch Coolers
Vegetable Juice From Concentrate

Italian Volcano �
Italian Volcano (All)

Juicy Juice ⓘ
Juicy Juice (All Flavors)
Juicy Juice Harvest Surprise (All Flavors)

Kool-Aid Bursts ᗡ
Berry Blue Flavored Soft Drink
Berry Blue Soft Drink
Cherry Flavored Soft Drink
Cherry Soft Drink
Grape Flavored Soft Drink

Grape Soft Drink
Lime Soft Drink
Tropical Punch Soft Drink

Kool-Aid Jammers ᗡ
Blue Raspberry Juice Drink Pouches
Cherry Juice Drink Pouches
Grape Juice Drink Pouches
Green Apple Juice Drink Pouches
Kiwi Strawberry Juice Drink Pouches
Orange Juice Drink Pouches
Tropical Punch Juice Drink Pouches

Kroger ⓘ
Fruit Juices
Vegetable Juice

Langer Juice Company
Juice (All)

Manischewitz
Grape Juice

Martinelli's ⓘ
Martinelli's (All)

Meijer
Acai and Grape Juice Blend (Shelf Stable)
Apple Juice - Concentrate (Shelf Stable)
Apple Juice - Natural (Shelf Stable)
Apple Juice - PET (Shelf Stable)
Apple Juice (Shelf Stable)
Cherry Juice (Shelf Stable)
Cranberry Apple Juice Cocktail (Shelf Stable)
Cranberry Flavored with 2 Fruit Juices (Shelf Stable)
Cranberry Grape Cocktail (Shelf Stable)
Cranberry Grape Flavored with 2 Juices (Shelf Stable)
Cranberry Grape Juice Drink
Cranberry Grape Juice Light (Shelf Stable)
Cranberry Juice Cocktail (Shelf Stable)
Cranberry Juice Cocktail Light
Cranberry Raspberry 100% (Shelf Stable)
Cranberry Raspberry Cocktail (Shelf Stable)
Cranberry Strawberry Cocktail (Shelf Stable)

Cranberry/Raspbeery Juice with 3 Fruit Juices (Shelf Stable)

Drink - Berry Blend Splash (Shelf Stable)

Drink - Cranberry Raspberry (Shelf Stable)

Drink - Cranberry Strawberry (Shelf Stable)

Fruit Punch (Shelf Stable)

Fruit Punch Genuine (Shelf Stable)

Fruit Punch Light (Shelf Stable)

Grape Cranberry Juice Cocktail Light (Shelf Stable)

Grapefruit Juice (Shelf Stable)

Juice - Berry 100% (Shelf Stable)

Juice - Cherry 100% (Shelf Stable)

Juice - Cranapple Cocktail (Shelf Stable)

Juice - Cranberry White Cocktail (Shelf Stable)

Juice - Cranberry White Peach (Shelf Stable)

Juice - Grape (Shelf Stable)

Juice - Grape 100% Genuine (Shelf Stable)

Juice - Grape White (Shelf Stable)

Juice - Punch 100% Genuine (Shelf Stable)

Orange Juice (Refrigerated)

Orange Premium High Pulp Carafe (Refrigerated)

Orange Premium with Calcium (Refrigerated)

Orange Reconstituted (Refrigerated)

Orange Reconstituted + Pulp (Refrigerated)

Orange Reconstituted with Calcium (Refrigerated)

Organic Apple Juice (Shelf Stable)

Organic Concord Grape Juice (Shelf Stable)

Organic Cranberry Juice (Shelf Stable)

Organic Lemonade (Shelf Stable)

Pink Grapefruit Juice (Shelf Stable)

Pomegranate and Blueberry Blend (Shelf Stable)

Pomegranate and Cranberry Blend (Shelf Stable)

Prune Juice (Shelf Stable)

Raspberry Cranberry Juice Light (Shelf Stable)

Ruby Red Grapefruit Cocktail (Shelf Stable)

Ruby Red Grapefruit Cocktail Light 22% (Shelf Stable)

Ruby Red Grapefruit Juice (Shelf Stable)

Strawberry/Kiwi Splash (Shelf Stable)

Tangerine & Ruby Red (PGB)

Thirst Quencher - Fruit Punch

Thirst Quencher - Lemon Lime

Tropical Blend Splash (PGB)

White Cranberry Flavored Juice Blend (Shelf Stable)

White Cranberry Juice Cocktail (Shelf Stable)

White Cranberry Peach Cocktail (Shelf Stable)

White Cranberry Strawberry Juice Cocktail (Shelf Stable)

White Grape from Concentrate (Shelf Stable)

White Grape Peach Blend (Shelf Stable)

White Grape Raspberry Blend (Shelf Stable)

White Grapefruit Juice (Shelf Stable)

White Grapefruit Juice Cocktail

Midwest Country Fare (Hy-Vee)

100% Unsweetened Apple Cider from Concentrate

100% Unsweetened Apple Juice from Concentrate

Cranberry Apple Juice Cocktail

Cranberry Juice Cocktail

Cranberry Raspberry Juice

Minute Maid

Active Orange Juice

Kids + Apple

Kiwi-Strawberry Energy

Lemonade

Light Lemonade

Pomegranate Blueberry Juice

Pomegranate Lemonade

Mott's

100% Apple Juice

Naked Juice
 Naked Juice Products (All BUT Green
 Machine)

Nantucket Nectars
 Nantucket Nectars (All)

Nature Factor ✓
 Organic Coconut Water

Newman's Own ⓘ
 Gorilla Grape
 Grape Juice
 Lemonade
 Lightly Sweetened Lemonade
 Limeade
 Orange Mango Tango
 Organic Lemonade
 Pink Lemonade

Northland
 Juices (All)

Oberweis Dairy
 Fruit Punch
 Lemonade

Ocean Spray
 Beverages (All)

Odwalla
 Beverages (All BUT Super Protein
 Vanilla Al Mondo & Original
 Superfood)

Old Orchard
 Old Orchard (All)

Organic Valley ⓘ
 Orange Juice - Pulp-Added
 Orange Juice - Pulp-Free
 Orange Juice - with Calcium

Penn Maid
 Orange Juice

POM Wonderful ⚱
 POM Wonderful (All)

Prairie Farms
 Blue Raspberry Drink
 Fruit Punch Drink
 Grape Drink
 Lemon Drink
 Lemon Lime Drink
 Lemonade
 Orange Drink
 Orange Juice

 Pink Lemonade Drink

Price Chopper
 Cranberry Juice Blend
 Fruit Punch
 Organic Apple Juice
 Organic Grape Juice
 Pineapple Juice
 Tropical Punch

Publix ◌
 Apple Juice
 Cranberry Apple Juice Cocktail
 Cranberry Juice Cocktail
 Grape Juice
 Grape-Cranberry Juice Cocktail
 GreenWise Market 100% Organic Apple
 Juice
 GreenWise Market Organic Cranberry
 Juice
 GreenWise Market Organic Grape Juice
 GreenWise Market Organic Lemonade
 GreenWise Market Organic Tomato
 Juice
 Orange Juice from Concentrate
 Orange with Calcium Juice from
 Concentrate
 Premium Orange Juice - Calcium Plus
 Premium Orange Juice - Grove Pure
 Premium Orange Juice - Old Fashioned
 Premium Orange Juice - Original
 Premium Ruby Red Grapefruit
 Raspberry Cranberry Juice Cocktail
 Reduced Calorie Cranberry Juice
 Cocktail
 Ruby Red Grapefruit Juice
 Tomato Juice
 White Grape Juice

R.W. Knudsen
 R.W. Knudsen (All)

Raley's
 100% Apple Juice
 100% Cranberry Juice
 100% Cranberry-Concord Grape Juice
 100% Cranberry-Raspberry Juice
 100% Grape Juice
 100% Vegetable Juice
 100% White Grape Juice
 Acai Cherry Juice

Cranberry Apple Juice Cocktail
Cranberry Raspberry Juice Cocktail
Light Cranberry Juice Cocktail
Light Grape Juice
Light White Grape Juice
Pineapple Juice
Pomegranate Cranberry Juice
Prune Juice
Ruby Red Grapefruit Juice
Tomato Juice

Red Gold
Tomato Products (All)

Right Size
Right Size (All)

Sacramento
Tomato Products (All)

Sambazon
Sambazon (All)

Santa Cruz Organic
Organic Juices (All)

Simply Apple
Simply Apple

Simply Grapefruit
Simply Grapefruit

Simply Lemonade
Simply Lemonade
Simply Lemonade with Raspberry

Simply Limeade
Simply Limeade

Simply Orange
Orange Juice Country Stand Medium
Pulp with Calcium
Simply Orange with Mango
Simply Orange with Pineapple

Snapple
Snapple (All)

Ssips
Ssips (All)

Sunny D
Sunny D (All)

Sunsweet ♀
Sunsweet (All BUT Chocolate Covered
PlumSweets)

Tang ∿
Watermelon Wallop 10 Ct. Juice Drink

Tree Ripe
Tree Ripe (All)

Tree Top
Juices (All)

Tropicana
100% Juice Products (All)

V8 ⓘ
100% Vegetable Juice
Calcium Enriched Vegetable Juice
Essential Antioxidants Vegetable Juice
High Fiber Vegetable Juice
Low Sodium Vegetable Juice
Organic Vegetable Juice
Spicy Hot Vegetable Juice
Splash Berry Blend
Splash Diet Berry Blend
Splash Diet Tropical Blend
Splash Fruit Medley
Splash Mango Peach
Splash Strawberry Kiwi Blend
Splash Tropical Blend
V-Fusion Açai Mixed Berry
V-Fusion Cranberry Blackberry
V-Fusion Goji Raspberry
V-Fusion Light Acai Mixed Berry
V-Fusion Light Peach Mango
V-Fusion Light Pomegranate Blueberry
V-Fusion Light Strawberry Banana
V-Fusion Passionfruit Tangerine
V-Fusion Peach Mango
V-Fusion Pomegranate Blueberry
V-Fusion Strawberry Banana
V-Fusion Tropical Orange

Valu Time (Marsh)
Juice Apple
Juice Apple Cocktail
Tomato Juice

Vita Coco
100% Pure Coconut Water
Acai & Pomegranate Coconut Water
Passionfruit Coconut Water
Peach & Mango Coconut Water
Pineapple Coconut Water
Tangerine Coconut Water

Welch's
Welch's (All)

White House
White House (All)

Winn & Lovette (Winn-Dixie) ()
Black Cherry Juice
Cranberry Juice
Pomegranate Juice

Winn-Dixie ()
Apple Cider from Concentrate
Apple Juice from Concentrate
Cranberry Apple Juice Cocktail
Cranberry Juice Cocktail
Cranberry Raspberry Juice Cocktail
Grape Juice from Concentrate
Grapefruit Juice from Concentrate
Light Cranberry Grape Juice Cocktail
Light Cranberry Juice Cocktail
Light Grape Juice Cocktail
Orange Juice - Premium - Not from
  Concentrate
Orange Juice from Concentrate
Orange Juice from Concentrate with
  Calcium
Organic Apple Juice
Organic Grape Juice
Organic Lemonade
Organic Mango Acai Berry Juice Blend
Organic Orange Mango Juice Blend
Organic Tomato Juice
Pomegranate Blueberry Juice Blend
Pomegranate Cranberry Juice Blend
Pomegranate Juice Blend
Premium Apple Juice Not from
  Concentrate
Prune Juice from Concentrate
Prune Juice with Pulp from Concentrate
Ruby Red Grapefruit Juice
Ruby Red Grapefruit Juice Cocktail
Tomato Juice
Vegetable Juice Cocktail
White Grape Juice from Concentrate

Wyman's
Wyman's (All)

Zico
Zico (All)

MIXERS

American Beverage Corporation ♂
Non-Alcoholic Cocktail Mixes
Ready-to-Drink Cocktails

Baja Bob's
Baja Bob's Sugar-Free Cocktail Mixes
  (All)

Margaritaville
Margaritaville (All)

Mr. & Mrs. T
Mr. & Mrs. T (All BUT Premium
  Bloody Mary Mix)

Old Orchard
Old Orchard (All)

Rose's
Rose's (All)

Sacramento
Tomato Products (All)

Santa Barbara Olive Co.
Santa Barbara Olive Co. (All BUT Pasta
  Sauce and Salsa)

PROTEIN POWDER

Bob's Red Mill ♂ ✓
Hemp Protein Powder
Soy Protein Powder

Designer Whey ♂
Designer Whey (All)

Ensure
Ensure Powder - Vanilla

Fearn Natural Foods ⓘ
Soya Protein Isolate

Living Harvest ⓘ ✓
Living Harvest Protein Powder

Manitoba Harvest ♂ ✓
Manitoba Harvest Hemp Foods & Oils
  (All)

Sambazon
Sambazon (All)

Special K ()
Protein Water Mixes

SMOOTHIES & SHAKES

Betty Lou's
Chocolate Protein Shake
Orange Cream Protein Shake
Vanilla Protein Shake

Caffe D'vita ()
Caffe D'vita Products (All)

Cascade Fresh
Cascade Fresh (All)

Fresh & Easy ()
Smoothie - Powerhouse
Smoothie - Strawberry Banana
Smoothie - Strawberry Vitamin C
Booster
Smoothie - Vanilla Banana
Smoothie - Wellness Defence

Kellogg's ()
Special K Protein Shakes

Nesquik ⓘ
MilkShake

Old Orchard
Old Orchard (All)

Publix ()
Fat Free Light Mixed Berry Yogurt
Smoothie
Fat Free Light Strawberry Yogurt
Smoothie

Right Size
Right Size (All)

Special K ()
Protein Shakes

Stonyfield Farm ✓
Stonyfield Farm (All BUT YoBaby Plus
Fruit & Cereal, Frozen Yogurt, and Ice
Cream)

V8 ⓘ
Splash Smoothie - Strawberry Banana
Splash Smoothie - Tropical Colada

Yoplait ✓
Smoothie - Triple Berry

SPORTS DRINKS

Gatorade ()
Endurance Formula (All Flavors)
G2 (All Flavors)

Gatorade (All Flavors)

Hy-Vee
Berry Thunder Sports Drink
Fruit Punch Thunder Sports Drink
Glacial Ice Thunder Sports Drink
Lemon Lime Thunder Sports Drink
Orange Thunder Sports Drink

Meijer
Thirst Quencher Orange (Shelf Stable)

POM Wonderful 🏅
POM Wonderful (All)

POWERADE
POWERADE with ION4 (All Flavors)
POWERADE Zero with ION4 (All
Flavors)

TEA & TEA MIXES

4C
Instant Iced Tea Mixes Sweetened with
Sugar (All)
Light Instant Iced Tea Mixes Sweetened
with Splenda (All)
Totally Light Iced Tea Mixes Sweetened
with Splenda (All)

Ambassador Organics
Ambassador Organics (All)

Bashas'
Green Tea 100% Natural
Green Tea Decaffeinated
Iced Tea Mix
Instant Tea
Tea Bags
Tea Bags - Decaffeinated

Bentley's
Tea (All)

Bigelow Tea
Bigelow Teas (All BUT Blueberry
Harvest Herb Tea, Chamomile Mango
Herb Tea, & Cinnamon Spice Herb
Tea)

Boston Tea
Tea (All)

Bromley Tea Company, The
Bromley Products (All)

Caffe D'vita ( )
  Caffe D'vita Products (All)
Carrington
  Tea (All)
Celestial Seasonings
  Acai Mango Sweet Zinger Ice Tea
  Acai Mango Zinger
  African Orange Mango Red Tea
  Antioxidant Supplement Green Tea
  Antioxidant Supplement Plum White
    Tea
  Authentic Green Tea
  Bengal Spice
  Black Cherry Berry
  Blackberry Pomegranate Antioxidant
    Max Green Tea
  Blood Orange Star Fruit Antioxidant
    Max Green Tea
  Blueberry Breeze Green Tea
  Blueberry Cool Brew Iced Tea
  Caffeine Free Herbal Tea
  Candy Cane Lane
  Chamomile
  Cinnamon Apple Spice
  Country Peach Passion
  Cranberry Apple Zinger
  Decaf India Spice Chai
  Decaf Mandarin Orchard Green Tea
  Decaf Mint Green Tea
  Decaf Sleepytime Lemon Jasmine Green
    Tea
  Decaf Sweet Coconut Thai Chai
  Decaf White Tea
  Decaffeinated Green Tea
  Dragon Fruit Melon Antioxidant Max
    Green Tea
  Echinacea Complete Care Wellness Tea
  Gen Mai Cha Green Tea
  Goji Berry Pomegranate Green Tea
  Honey Lemon Ginseng Green Tea
  Honey Vanilla Chai
  Honey Vanilla Chamomile
  Imperial White Peach White Tea
  India Spice Chai
  Lemon Zinger
  Madagascar Vanilla Red Tea
  Mandarin Orange Spice

  Mint Magic
  Morning Thunder
  Moroccan Pomegranate Red Tea
  Nutcracker Sweet
  Peach Cool Brew Iced Tea
  Peppermint
  Perfectly Pear White Tea
  Raspberry Cool Brew Iced Tea
  Raspberry Gardens Green Tea
  Raspberry Sweet Zinger Ice Tea
  Raspberry Zinger
  Red Zinger
  Safari Spice Red Tea
  Senna Sunrise Wellness Tea
  Sleepytime
  Sleepytime Extra Wellness Tea
  Sleepytime Sinus Soother Wellness Tea
  Sleepytime Throat Tamer Wellness Tea
  Sleepytime Vanilla
  Sweet Apple Chamomile
  Tangerine Orange Sweet Zinger Ice Tea
  Tangerine Orange Zinger
  Tension Tamer
  Tropic of Strawberry
  Tropical Fruit Cool Brew Iced Tea
  True Blueberry
  Tummy Mint Wellness Tea
  Wild Berry Sweet Zinger Ice Tea
  Wild Berry Zinger
Choice Organic Teas
  Tea (All)
Crystal Light 〰
  Antioxidant Raspberry Green Tea Sugar
    Free Iced Tea
  Decaffeinated Lemon Iced Tea
  Lemon Iced Tea Sugar Free Iced Tea
  On The Go Antioxidant Honey Lemon
    Green Tea
  On The Go Antioxidant Raspberry
    Green Tea
  On the Go Skin Essentials White Peach
    Tea
  Peach Sugar Free Iced Tea
  Raspberry Sugar Free Iced Tea
  Sugar Free Iced Tea
Eden Foods ⓘ ✓
  Chamomile Herb Tea - Organic

Genmaicha Tea - Organic
Hoijicha Chai Roasted Green Tea, Organic
Kukicha Twig Tea - Organic
Lotus Root Tea
Mu 16 Herb Tea
Organic Matcha - Green Tea Powder
Organic Matcha - Green Tea Powder Kit
Sencha Ginger Green Tea, Organic
Sencha Green Tea, Organic
Sencha Mint Green Tea, Organic
Sencha Rose Green Tea, Organic

Equal Exchange
Tea (All)

Flavia
Teas (All)

Food Club (Marsh)
Tea Bags
Tea Bags Green
Tea Bags Green Decaf
Tea Instant

Fresh & Easy ()
Tea Bags (Assorted Varieties)

Great Value (Wal-Mart)
Decaffeinated Tea 100% Natural
Family Size Decaffeinated Tea 100% Natural
Family Size Tea 100% Natural
Green Tea with Ginseng And Honey

Green Mountain Coffee
Teas (All)

Hy-Vee
Chai Black Tea
Chamomile Herbal Tea
Cinnamon Apple Herbal Tea
Decaffeinated Green Tea
Decaffeinated Tea Bags
Dream Easy Herbal Tea
Earl Gray Black Tea
English Breakfast Black Tea
Family Size Tea Bags
Green Tea Bags
Instant Tea
Jasmine Green Tea
Orange & Spice Specialty Tea
Peppermint Herbal Tea
Pomegranate White Tea Bags

Rooibos Red Herbal Tea
Strawberry Herbal Tea Bags
Tea Bags

JFG Coffee & Tea
Family Tea Bags
Tea Bags

Kroger (i)
Tea - Bagged
Tea - Instant

Lipton
Black Tea
Decaf
Green Tea
Herbal
Pyramid
Regular (Orange Pekoe)

Luzianne
Decaf Tea Bags
Flavored Tea Bags - Lemon
Flavored Tea Bags - Peach
Flavored Tea Bags - Raspberry
Tea Bags

Meijer
Iced Tea Mix
Instant Tea
Tea Bags - Decaffeinated
Tea Bags - Green
Tea Bags - Green Decaffeinated

Midwest Country Fare (Hy-Vee)
Black Tea

Mighty Leaf Tea ()
Mighty Leaf Tea (All)

Nash Brothers
Organic Tea

Newman's Own Organics () (i)
Teas (All)

Numi
Numi (All)

Oregon Chai (i)
Oregon Chai (All BUT Vanilla Dry Mix)

Orient Emporium Tea Co.
Jasmine Sumana Tea

Original Ceylon Tea Company, The
Teas and Tea Bags (All)

Price Chopper
Black Tea Bags

Publix ()
Decaffeinated Tea Bags
Tagless Tea Bags
Tea Bags (All Varieties)

Republic of Tea, The
Republic of Tea, The (All BUT Coconut
Cocoa)

Rishi Tea
Tea (All)

St. Dalfour ⓘ
Organic Teas (All)

Stewarts
Tea

Taylors of Harrogate ♀
Tea (All)

Tazo
Teas (All BUT Green Ginger,
Honeybush, Lemon Ginger & Tea
Lemonade)

Teekanne
Herbal Wellness Teas (For Pomegranate
Delight, check ingredients because of
new formula release.)

Tetley
Tetley (All)

Traditional Medicinals Tea ⓘ
Teas (All BUT PMS Tea and St. John's
Good Mood Tea)

Twinings ♀
Herbal Infusions (All)
Teas (All)

Uncle Lee's Tea ♀
Teas (All)

Valu Time (Marsh)
Tea Bags Tagless

Winn-Dixie ()
Decaffeinated Tea Bags
Tea Bags

TEA DRINKS

AriZona
Teas (All)

Enviga
Berry Sparkling Green Tea
Sparkling Green Tea

FUZE
Fuze (All Flavors)

Gold Peak
Gold Peak Flavors

Good Earth Tea
Teas (All)

Great Value (Wal-Mart)
Diet Green Tea with Ginseng And
Honey
Ready To Drink Sweetened Tea
Sugar Free Sweet Iced Tea
Sweet Iced Tea

Honest Ade ♀
Honest Ade (All)

Honest Kids ♀
Honest Kids (All)

Honest Tea ♀
Honest Tea (All)

Hy-Vee
Diet Green Tea with Citrus
Green Tea with Citrus
Green Tea with Pomegranate
Honey Lemon Ginseng Green Tea
Thirst Splashers Raspberry Tea

Luzianne
Ready to Drink Diet Peach Tea
Ready to Drink Green with Mint Sweet
Tea
Ready to Drink Lemon Sweet Tea
Ready to Drink Raspberry Sweet Tea
Ready to Drink Sweet Tea

Minute Maid
Pomegranate Flavored Tea

Nestea (Coca-Cola Company, The)
Citrus Green Tea
Diet Citrus Green Tea
Diet Lemon
Lemon Sweet
Red Tea
Sweetened Lemon Tea

Newman's Own ⓘ
Lemon Aided Ice Tea

Numi
Numi (All)

Oberweis Dairy
Lemon Tea

Pacific Natural Foods ⓘ
    Organic Simply Mate - Citrus Lychee Yerba Mate
    Organic Simply Mate - Lemon Ginger Yerba Mate
    Organic Simply Mate - Peach Passion Yerba Mate
    Organic Simply Mate - Traditional Yerba Mate
    Organic Simply Tea - Kiwi Mango Green Tea
    Organic Simply Tea - Peach Green Tea
    Organic Simply Tea - Tangerine Green Tea
    Organic Simply Tea - Unsweetened Green Tea
    Organic Simply Tea - Wild Berry Green Tea

POM Wonderful ⚇
    POM Wonderful (All)

Prairie Farms
    Iced Tea

Snapple
    Snapple (All)

SoBe
    SoBe (All)

Ssips
    Ssips (All)

Swiss Premium ()
    Tea (All)

Winn-Dixie ()
    Organic Sweet Black Tea with Lemon
    Organic Sweet Green Tea
    Organic Sweet Red Tea with Mango and Mandarin Orange
    Organic Sweet White Tea with Raspberry
    Organic Unsweetened Green Tea
    Organic Unsweetened Red Tea with Pomegranate

Betty Crocker®

For those of you who said you'd give your right arm, we have some bittersweet news.

Gluten-Free Dessert Mixes from Betty Crocker.
The wait is over. Now you're free to share and enjoy the cakes, cookies and brownies you've been missing with Betty Crocker gluten free dessert mixes. Available in your neighborhood grocery store.

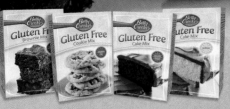

BAKE LIFE SWEETER™
www.bettycrocker.com/glutenfree

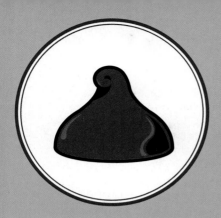

BAKING AISLE

BAKING CHIPS & BARS

Baker's 🌀
- Bittersweet Baking Chocolate
- German's Sweet Chocolate Bar
- Premium White Squares Baking Chocolate
- Real Dark Semi-Sweet Dipping Chocolate
- Real Milk Dipping Chocolate
- Semi-Sweet Baking Chocolate
- Semi-Sweet Chocolate Chunks
- Unsweetened Squares Baking Chocolate

Bashas'
- Chocolate Chips Real Semi-Sweet

Candiquik
- Candiquik (All)

Ener-G ☃ ✔
- Chocolate Chips

Enjoy Life Foods ☃ ✔
- Semi-Sweet Chocolate Chips

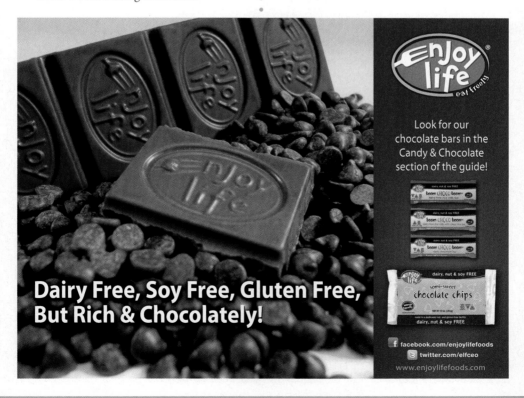

Dairy Free, Soy Free, Gluten Free, But Rich & Chocolately!

Look for our chocolate bars in the Candy & Chocolate section of the guide!

semi-sweet chocolate chips
dairy, nut & soy FREE

facebook.com/enjoylifefoods
twitter.com/elfceo
www.enjoylifefoods.com

Food Club (Marsh)
- Baking Chips - Milk Chocolate
- Baking Chips - Peanut Butter
- Baking Chips - Semisweet Chocolate
- Baking Chips - Vanilla

Great Value (Wal-Mart)
- Semi Sweet Chocolate Chips

Guittard
- Chocolate Products (All)

Haggen
- Semi Sweet Chocolate Baking Chips

Hershey's
- Semi-Sweet Baking Chocolate
- Semi-Sweet Chocolate Chips
- Unsweetened Baking Chocolate

Hy-Vee
- Butterscotch Baking Chips
- Milk Chocolate Baking Chips
- Mini Semi Sweet Chocolate Chips
- Peanut Butter Baking Chips
- Semi Sweet Chocolate Chips
- Vanilla Flavored White Baking Chips

Kroger ⓘ
- Butterscotch Morsels
- Chocolate Chunks
- Milk Chocolate Chips
- Peanut Butter Chips
- Semi Sweet Chips
- White and Chocolate Bark Coating

Log House
- Almond Bark

Manischewitz
- Chocolate Morsels

Meijer
- Butterscotch Baking Chips
- Chocolate Chips Semi-Sweet
- Milk Chocolate Chips
- Peanut Butter Chips
- White Baking Chips

Midwest Country Fare (Hy-Vee)
- Chocolate Flavored Chips

Nestlé Toll House ⓘ
- Milk Chocolate & Peanut Butter Swirled Morsels

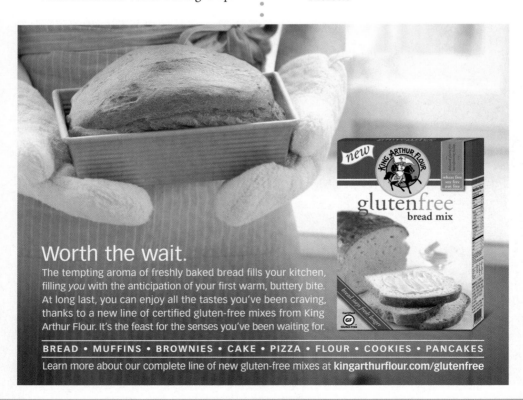

Milk Chocolate Morsels
Peanut Butter & Milk Chocolate Morsels
Premier White Morsels
Semi-Sweet Chocolate & Premier White
  Swirled Morsels
Semi-Sweet Chocolate Chunks
Semi-Sweet Chocolate Mini Morsels
Semi-Sweet Morsels

Plymouth Pantry
Almond Bark

Price Chopper
Milk Chocolate Chips

Publix ()
Butterscotch Morsels
Milk Chocolate Morsels
Semi-Sweet Chocolate Morsels

Saco
Saco (All)

Tropical Source ✓
Semi-Sweet Chocolate Chips ⅋

Valu Time (Marsh)
Baking Chips Chocolate Flavor

BAKING MIXES

Arrowhead Mills ✓
Bake with Me Gluten-Free Chocolate
  Cupcake Mix
Bake with Me Gluten-Free Vanilla
  Cupcake Mix
Gluten-Free All Purpose Baking Mix
Gluten-Free Brownie Mix
Gluten-Free Chocolate Chip Cookie
  Mix
Gluten-Free Pancake & Waffle Mix
Gluten-Free Vanilla Cake Mix

Authentic Foods ⅋
Authentic Foods (All)

Betty Crocker ✓
Gluten-Free Brownie Mix ⅋
Gluten-Free Chocolate Chip Cookie
  Mix ⅋
Gluten-Free Devil's Food Cake Mix ⅋
Gluten-Free Yellow Cake Mix ⅋

Bi Aglut
Bi Aglut (All)

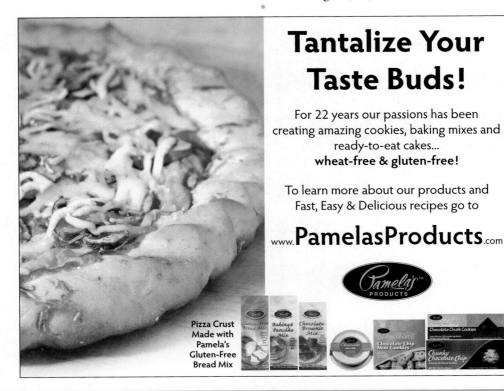

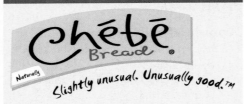

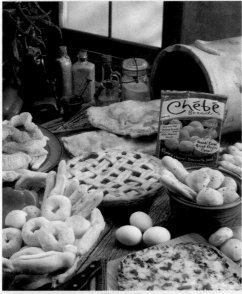

Bisquick
Bisquick Gluten Free

Bob's Red Mill
GF Biscuit Mix
GF Brownie Mix
GF Chocolate Cake Mix
GF Chocolate Chip Cookie Mix
GF Cinnamon Raisin Bread Mix
GF Cornbread Mix
GF Hearty Whole Grain Bread Mix
GF Homemade Wonderful Bread Mix
GF Pancake Mix
GF Pizza Crust Mix
GF Shortbread Cookie Mix
GF Vanilla Cake Mix

Breads From Anna
Apple Pancake & Muffin Mixes
Banana Bread Mix
Bread Mix
Bread Mix (All-Purpose Flour Blend)
Cranberry Pancake & Muffin Mix
Herb Bread Mix
Maple Pancake & Muffin Mix
Pie Crust Mix
Pumpkin Bread Mix

Chebe
Chebe All-Purpose Bread Mix
Chebe Cinnamon Roll Mix
Chebe Focaccia Bread Mix
Chebe Garlic Onion Breadstick Mix
Chebe Mix for Pizza Crust
Original Chebe Bread Mix

Cherrybrook Kitchen
Gluten-Free Dreams Chocolate Cake Mix
Gluten-Free Dreams Chocolate Chip Cookies Mix
Gluten-Free Dreams Chocolate Chip Pancake Mix
Gluten-Free Dreams Fudge Brownie Mix
Gluten-Free Dreams Pancake Mix
Gluten-Free Dreams Sugar Cookie Mix
Gluten-Free Dreams Yellow Cake Mix

Chi-Chi's
Fiesta Sweet Corn Cake Mix

Dowd & Rogers ✓
   Dowd & Rogers (All)

El Torito ⓘ
   Sweet Corn Cake Mix

Ener-G ♀ ✓
   Corn Mix
   Potato Mix
   Rice Mix

Gillian's Foods ♀
   Gillian's Foods (All)

Gluten-Free Pantry, The
   Brown Rice Pancake & Waffle Mix
   Chocolate Chip Cookie Mix
   Chocolate Truffle Brownie Mix
   Decadent Chocolate Cake Mix
   Favorite Sandwich Bread Mix
   French Bread & Pizza Mix
   Muffin & Scone Mix
   Old Fashioned Cake & Cookie Mix
   Perfect Pie Crust Mix
   Yankee Cornbread and Muffin Mix

Hodgson Mill ♀
   Apple Cinnamon Baking Mix ✓
   Gluten-Free Bread Mix ✓
   Gluten-Free Brownie Mix ✓
   Gluten-Free Chocolate Cake Mix ✓
   Gluten-Free Cookie Mix ✓
   Gluten-Free Pancake & Waffle Mix ✓
   Gluten-Free Pizza Crust Mix ✓
   Gluten-Free Yellow Cake Mix ✓
   Multi Purpose Baking Mix ✓

Hol-Grain
   Chocolate Brownie Mix
   Pancake & Waffle Mix

King Arthur ♀ ✓
   Gluten-free Bread Mix
   Gluten-free Brownie Mix
   Gluten-free Chocolate Cake Mix
   Gluten-free Cookie Mix
   Gluten-free Muffin Mix
   Gluten-free Pancake Mix
   Gluten-free Pizza Crust Mix

Kinnikinnick Foods ♀
   Kinnikinnick Foods (All)

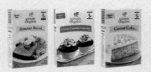
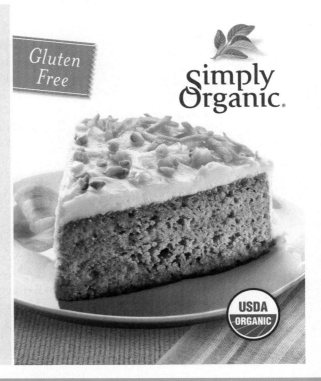

Larrowe's
Buckwheat Pancake Mix

Maple Grove Farms
Gluten-Free Pancake Mix

Namaste Foods ♀ ✓
Baking Mixes (All)
Biscuit Mix
Waffle/Pancake Mix

Orgran ✓
All Purpose Pastry Mix
Apple & Cinnamon Pancake Mix
Bread Mix - White
Bread Mix - Wholemeal
Buckwheat Pancake Mix
Cake Mix Range (All)
Chocolate Mousse Mix
Cornbread & Muffin Mix
Custard Mix
Pizza & Pastry Mix

Pamela's Products ✓
Baking & Pancake Mix
Chocolate Brownie Mix
Chocolate Cake Mix
Chocolate Chunk Cookies Baking Mix
Classic Vanilla Cake Mix
Cornbread & Muffin Mix
Gluten-Free Bread Mix
Single Serve Baking & Pancake Mix
Single Serve Brownie Mix

Schar ♀ ✓
Classic White Bread Mix

Simply Organic ♀ ✓
Organic Banana Bread Mix
Organic Carrot Cake Mix
Organic Chai Spice Scone Mix
Organic Cocoa Biscotti Mix
Organic Cocoa Brownie Mix
Organic Cocoa Cayenne Cupcake Mix
Organic Pancake & Waffle Mix

BAKING POWDER

Bob's Red Mill ♀ ✓
Baking Powder

Clabber Girl
Baking Powder

Davis Baking Powder
Baking Powder

Durkee
Baking Powder

Ener-G ♀ ✓
Baking Powder

Hain Pure Foods
Gluten-Free Featherweight Baking
Powder

Hearth Club
Baking Powder

Hy-Vee
Double Acting Baking Powder

Kroger ⓘ
Baking Powder

Rumford
Baking Powder

Spice Islands
also see Durkee

Tone's
also see Durkee

BAKING SODA

Arm & Hammer
Baking Soda

Bashas'
Baking Soda

Bob's Red Mill ♀ ✓
Baking Soda

Durkee
Baking Soda

Ener-G ♀ ✓
Baking Soda Substitute

Food Club (Marsh)
Baking Soda

Haggen
Baking Soda

Hy-Vee
Baking Soda

Kroger ⓘ
Baking Soda

Meijer
Baking Soda

Spice Islands
also see Durkee

Tone's
  also see Durkee

Bread Crumbs & Other Coatings

Ener-G
  Bread Crumbs
  Broken Melba Toast
Gillian's Foods
  Gillian's Foods (All)
Glutino
  Breadcrumbs
Hol-Grain
  Brown Rice Bread Crumbs
  Chicken Coating Mix
  Onion Ring Batter Mix
  Tempura Batter Mix
Katz Gluten Free
  Katz Gluten Free (All)
Kinnikinnick Foods
  Kinnikinnick Foods (All)
Luzianne
  Seafood Coating Mix
Orgran
  All Purpose Rice Crumbs
  Crumbs Corn Crispy
Schar
  Bread Crumbs
Shabtai Gourmet Gluten-Free Bakery
  Pread Crumbs - Gluten Free Bread
    Crumb Substitute
Southern Homestyle
  Corn Flake Crumbs
  Tortilla Crumbs
Sunbird
  Tempura Batter
Williams
  Bag-N-Bake Chicken

Cocoa Powder

Guittard
  Chocolate Products (All)
Hershey's
  Unsweetened Powdered Cocoa

Hy-Vee
  Baking Cocoa
Kroger
  Baking Cocoa
Saco
  Saco (All)

Coconut

Baker's
  Angel Flake Sweetened Coconut
Bashas'
  Coconut Flakes
Great Value (Wal-Mart)
  Sweetened Coconut Flakes
  Sweetened Flaked Coconut
Haggen
  Coconut Flakes
Hy-Vee
  Sweetened Flake Coconut
Kroger
  Coconut - Regular
  Coconut - Sweetened
Let's Do...Organic
  Organic Coconut Flakes
  Organic Reduced Fat Shredded Coconut
  Organic Shredded Coconut
Publix
  Coconut Flakes

Corn Syrup

Bashas'
  Syrup - Lite Corn
Brer Rabbit
  Syrup - Full
  Syrup - Light
Food Club (Marsh)
  Syrup - Lite Corn
Golding Farms
  Light Corn Syrup
Karo
  Karo Syrups (All)
Meijer
  Syrup - Lite Corn

CORNMEAL

Arrowhead Mills ✓
Blue Corn Meal
Yellow Corn Meal

Bob's Red Mill ⅄ ✓
GF Medium Cornmeal

Fresh & Easy ()
Yellow Cornmeal

Kinnikinnick Foods ⅄
Kinnikinnick Foods (All)

Publix ()
Plain Yellow Corn Meal

EXTRACTS AND FLAVORINGS

Amore
Amore (All)

Authentic Foods ⅄
Authentic Foods (All)

Bashas'
Lemon Juice

Butter Buds
Butter Buds (All)

C. F. Sauer Company, The ()
Pure Extracts (All)

Durkee
Liquid Extracts (All)
Liquid Flavorings (All)

Food Club (Marsh)
Juice - Lemon
Juice - Lemon Squeeze Bottle
Juice - Lime Squeeze Bottle

Great Value (Wal-Mart)
100% Lemon Juice

Haggen
Lemon Juice Squeeze Bottle
Vanilla Extract

Hy-Vee
Imitation Vanilla
Lemon Juice From Concentrate

Kroger ⓘ
Extracts
Flavorings

McCormick
Extracts (All)

Meijer
Imitation Vanilla
Lemon Juice (Shelf Stable)
Lemon Juice Squeeze Bottle (Shelf Stable)
Lime Juice (Shelf Stable)
Vanilla Extract

Midwest Country Fare (Hy-Vee)
Imitation Vanilla Flavoring

Molly McButter ⓘ ⅄
Molly McButter Products (All)

Nielsen-Massey ✓
Nielsen-Massey (All)

Price Chopper
Lemon Juice
Squeeze Lemon Juice

Publix ()
Almond Extract
Lemon Extract
Vanilla Extract

Raley's
Recons Lemon Juice

ReaLemon
ReaLemon (All)

Spice Islands
also see Durkee
Specialty - Vanilla Bean

Stubb's ⓘ ✓
Hickory Liquid Smoke
Mesquite Liquid Smoke

Tone's
also see Durkee

TryMe
TryMe Liquid Smoke

Valu Time (Marsh)
Vanilla - Imitation

Winn-Dixie ()
Reconstituted Lemon Juice

Woeber
Woeber (All)

Wright's Liquid Smoke
Liquid Smoke - Hickory
Liquid Smoke - Mesquite

Flax Meal

Bob's Red Mill ♈ ✓
Flaxseed Meal
Golden Flaxseed Meal
Organic Brown Flaxseed Meal
Organic Golden Flaxseed Meal
Hodgson Mill ♈
Milled Flax Seed ✓
Organic Golden Flax Seed ✓

Flours & Flour Mixes

Ancient Harvest
Quinoa Flour ♈
Arrowhead Mills ✓
Brown Rice Flour
Buckwheat Flour
Long Grain Brown Rice Flour
Millet Flour
Soy Flour
White Rice Flour
Authentic Foods ♈
Authentic Foods (All)
Bi Aglut
Bi Aglut (All)
Bisquick ♈ ✓
Bisquick Gluten Free
Bob's Red Mill ♈ ✓
Almond Meal/Flour
Black Bean Flour
Brown Rice Flour
Fava Bean Flour
Garbanzo Bean Flour
GF All Purpose Baking Flour
GF Corn Flour
GF Oat Flour
Green Pea Flour
Hazelnut Flour/Meal
Millet Flour
Millet Grits/Meal
Organic Amaranth Flour
Organic Brown Rice Flour
Organic Coconut Flour
Organic Quinoa Flour
Organic White Rice Flour
Potato Flour

Sorghum Flour
Sweet White Rice Flour
Tapioca Flour
Teff Flour
White Bean Flour
White Rice Flour
Dowd & Rogers ✓
Dowd & Rogers (All)
Ener-G ♈ ✓
Brown Rice Flour
Gluten Free Gourmet Blend
Potato Flour
Potato Starch Flour
Rice Bran
Sweet Rice Flour
Tapioca Flour
White Rice Flour
Fearn Natural Foods ⓘ
Brown Rice Baking Mix
Natural Soya Powder
Rice Baking Mix
Rice Flour
Fresh & Easy ()
Rice Flour
Gillian's Foods ♈
Gillian's Foods (All)
Gluten-Free Pantry, The
All-Purpose Baking Flour
Hodgson Mill ♈
Gluten-Free All Purpose Flour ✓
King Arthur ♈ ✓
Gluten-free Multi-Purpose Flour
Kinnikinnick Foods ♈
Kinnikinnick Foods (All)
Let's Do...Organic ✓
Organic Coconut Flour
Lundberg Family Farms ♈ ✓
Brown Rice Flour
Brown Rice Flour - Organic
Manitoba Harvest ♈ ✓
Manitoba Harvest Hemp Foods & Oils
(All)
Mochiko ♈
Mochiko Blue Star Sweet Rice Flour
Montina ♈
All-Purpose Flour Blend

Brown Rice Flour Blend
Pure Baking Flour Supplement

Namaste Foods 🍴
Flour Blend

Pocono
Buckwheat Flour

Tom Sawyer
All Purpose Gluten-Free Flour (All)

FOOD COLORING

Durkee
Food Coloring (All)

Hy-Vee
Assorted Food Coloring

Kroger ⓘ
Food Colors

Spice Islands
also see Durkee

Tone's
also see Durkee

FROSTING

Betty Crocker ✓
Butter Cream Rich & Creamy Frosting
Butter Cream Whipped Frosting
Cherry Rich & Creamy Frosting
Chocolate Rich & Creamy Frosting
Chocolate Whipped Frosting
Coconut Pecan Rich & Creamy Frosting
Cream Cheese Rich & Creamy Frosting
Cream Cheese Whipped Frosting
Creamy White Rich & Creamy Frosting
Dark Chocolate Rich & Creamy Frosting
Fluffy White Whipped Frosting
Lemon Rich & Creamy Frosting
Milk Chocolate Rich & Creamy Frosting
Milk Chocolate Whipped Frosting
Rainbow Chip Rich & Creamy Frosting
Strawberry Mist Whipped Frosting
Triple Chocolate Fudge Chip Rich &
   Creamy Frosting
Vanilla Rich & Creamy Frosting
Vanilla Whipped Frosting
Whipped Cream Whipped Frosting

Cake Mate
Gels (All)
Icings (All)

Duncan Hines
Caramel
Chocolate Butter Cream
Classic Chocolate
Classic Vanilla
Cream Cheese
Dark Chocolate Fudge
Fluffy White
Lemon Supreme
Milk Chocolate
Strawberry Cream
Vanilla Butter Cream
Whipped Chocolate
Whipped Cream Cheese
Whipped Vanilla

Fresh & Easy ⟨⟩
Chocolate Frosting (Glass Jar)

Grainless Baker, The 🍴
The Grainless Baker (All)

Namaste Foods 🍴
Frostings (All)

Pamela's Products ✓
Confetti Frosting Mix
Dark Chocolate Frosting Mix
Vanilla Frosting Mix

Pillsbury
Frosting (All BUT Coconut Pecan)

HONEY

Bashas'
Honey
Honey Squeeze Bear

BeeMaid
Honey (All)

Central Market Classics (Price Chopper)
Blueberry Honey
Buckwheat Honey
Organic Blossom Honey

Dutch Gold Honey
Dutch Gold Honey (All)

Food Club (Marsh)
- Honey - Inverted Squeeze Bottle
- Honey - Squeeze Bear

Fresh & Easy ()
- Orange Blossom Honey
- Organic Honey
- Regular Honey
- Whipped Honey
- Wild Raw Honey

Golding Farms ()
- Clover Honey

Great Value (Wal-Mart)
- Clover Honey

Haggen
- Honey
- Honey Inverted Squeeze Bottle
- Honey Squeeze Bear

Hy-Vee
- Honey

Madhava ⚇
- Honey (All)

Meijer
- Honey
- Honey Squeeze Bear
- Honey Squeeze Bottles

Mountain Ridge ()
- Pure Raw Honey

Naturally Healthy ()
- Pure Honey

Price Chopper
- Honey
- Honey Bears

Publix ()
- Clover Honey
- GreenWise Market Organic Honey
- Orange Blossom Honey
- Wildflower Honey

Really Raw Honey
- Honey (All)

St. Dalfour ⓘ
- Honey 7 oz (Both Varieties)

Valu Time (Marsh)
- Honey

Wholesome Sweeteners ⚇
- Organic Amber and Raw Honey

MARSHMALLOWS

Bashas'
- Marshmallow Crème
- Marshmallows Miniature
- Marshmallows Regular

Food Club (Marsh)
- Marshmallow Creme
- Marshmallows Mini
- Marshmallows Regular

Great Value (Wal-Mart)
- Marshmallow Creme
- Marshmallows
- Marshmallows Miniature
- Miniature Flavored Marshmallows
- Miniature Marshmallows

Haggen
- Marshmallow Crème
- Marshmallows - Mini
- Marshmallows - Regular

Hy-Vee
- Colored Miniature Marshmallows
- Marshmallows
- Miniature Marshmallows

Jet-Puffed ᔕ
- Chocomallows Marshmallows
- Funmallows Miniature Marshmallows
- Marshmallow Creme
- Marshmallows
- Miniature Choco Mallows Marshmallows
- Miniature Marshmallows
- Miniature Strawberry Mallows Marshmallows
- Starmallows Vanilla Marshmallows
- Strawberrymallows Marshmallows
- Swirl Mallows Caramel & Vanilla Marshmallows
- Toasted Coconut Marshmallows

Kroger ⓘ
- Colored Marshmallows
- Large Marshmallows
- Marshmallow Cream
- Miniature Marshmallows

Manischewitz
- Marshmallow Cups
- Marshmallows

Marshmallow Fluff
- Marshmallow Fluff

Meijer
- Marshmallows - Mini
- Marshmallows - Mini Flavored
- Marshmallows - Regular

Publix ◊
- Marshmallows

Solo
- Marshmallow Crème
- Toasted Marshmallow Crème

Valu Time (Marsh)
- Marshmallow Creme

Winn-Dixie ◊
- Marshmallows - Mini
- Marshmallows - Regular

MARZIPAN

Solo
- Almond Paste
- Marzipan

MILK, CONDENSED

Eagle Brand
- Sweetened Condensed Milk

Food Club (Marsh)
- Milk Sweetened Condensed

Great Value (Wal-Mart)
- Fat Free Sweetened Condensed Milk
- Sweetened Condensed Milk

Hy-Vee
- Sweetened Condensed Milk

Meijer
- Milk - Sweetened Condensed

Nestlé Carnation ⓘ
- Sweetened Condensed Milk

MILK, EVAPORATED

Bashas'
- Milk - Evaporated Tall

Food Club (Marsh)
- Milk Evaporated

Great Value (Wal-Mart)
- Evaporated Fat Free Milk
- Evaporated Milk
- Fat Free Evaporated Skimmed Milk

Hy-Vee
- Evaporated Milk
- Fat Free Evaporated Milk

Meijer
- Milk - Evaporated Lite Skimmed
- Milk - Evaporated Small
- Milk - Evaporated Tall

Nestlé Carnation ⓘ
- Evaporated Milk
- Fat Free Evaporated Milk
- Low Fat Evaporated Milk

PET Milk
- Evaporated Milk (All)

Valu Time (Marsh)
- Milk Evaporated Filled

MILK, INSTANT OR POWDERED

Bashas'
- Milk - Instant

Hy-Vee
- Instant Non Fat Dry Milk

Kroger ⓘ
- Milks - Powdered

Meijer
- Milk - Instant

Nestlé Carnation ⓘ
- Instant Nonfat Dry Milk

Organic Valley ⓘ
- Buttermilk Blend Powder
- Nonfat Dry Milk Powder

Publix ◊
- Instant Nonfat Dry Milk

Saco
- Saco (All)

Winn-Dixie ◊
- Instant Nonfat Dry Milk

MOLASSES

Brer Rabbit
- Molasses - Blackstrap

Molasses - Full
Molasses - Mild

Crosby's
Molasses

Golding Farms ()
Molasses

Grandma's Molasses
Original
Robust

Holly Sugar
Molasses (All)

Imperial Sugar
Molasses (All)

Plantation Molasses
Barbados Molasses
Blackstrap Molasses
Certified Organic Blackstrap
Holiday Blackstrap Molasses

Savannah Gold
Molasses (All)

Wholesome Sweeteners ♒
Organic Blackstrap Molasses

OIL & OIL SPRAYS

Alter Eco Fair Trade
Alter Eco Fair Trade (All)

Annie's Naturals ⓘ ✓
Basil Flavored Olive Oil
Dipping Oil Herb Flavored Olive Oil
Roasted Garlic Flavored Extra Virgin
Olive Oil
Roasted Pepper Flavored Olive Oil

B.R. Cohn ♒
Olive Oils (All)

Bashas'
Canola Oil
Cooking Spray - Baker's Release
Cooking Spray - Canola Butter Flavor
(Aerosol)
Cooking Spray - Canola Oil (Aerosol)
Cooking Spray - Olive Oil Extra Virgin
Corn Oil
Oil - Canola
Oil - Corn
Oil - Olive

Oil - Peanut
Oil - Vegetable
Oil Blended Canola/Vegetable
Olive Oil 100% Extra Virgin
Olive Oil 100% Mild in Taste
Vegetable Oil - Soybean

Bionaturae
Extra Virgin Olive Oil ♒

Blue Plate
Oil

Colavita
Oil (All)

Crisco
Crisco (All BUT Crisco Spray with
Flour)

Eden Foods ⓘ ✓
Hot Pepper Sesame Oil
Olive Oil - Extra Virgin - Spanish
Safflower Oil - Organic
Sesame Oil - Extra Virgin - Organic
Soybean Oil - Organic
Toasted Sesame Oil

Emeril's
Buttery Cooking Spray
Canola Oil Cooking Spray

Filippo Berio ♒
Olive Oil (All)

Food Club (Marsh)
Cooking Spray - Butter
Cooking Spray - Canola
Cooking Spray - Evoo
Oil Canola
Oil Corn
Oil Olive Extra Virgin
Oil Olive Mild
Oil Olive Pure
Oil Vegetable

Fragata
Fragata (All BUT Imitation Bacon Bits)

Grand Selections (Hy-Vee)
100% Pure & Natural Olive Oil
Extra Virgin Olive Oil
Olive Oil Lemon

Great Value (Wal-Mart)
100% Extra Virgin Olive Oil
Blended Canola Oil

Canola Oil
Canola Oil Blend
Corn Oil
Extra Virgin Olive Oil
Light Tasting Olive Oil
Olive Oil
Pure Canola Oil
Pure Corn Oil, Bilingual
Pure Vegetable Oil

Haggen
Canola Oil
Canola/Vegetable Oil Blend
Cooking Spray - Butter
Cooking Spray - Evoo
Corn Oil
Oil - Corn
Oil - Olive Extra Virgin
Oil - Olive Extra Virgin (Premier Label)
Oil - Olive Milder
Oil - Olive Pure
Vegetable Cooking Spray
Vegetable Oil

House Of Tsang ⓘ
Hot Chili Sesame Oil
Mongolian Fire Oil
Sesame Oil
Wok Oil

Hy-Vee
100% Pure Canola Oil
100% Pure Vegetable Oil
Natural Blend Oil

Kroger ⓘ
Canola Oil
Corn Oil
Olive Oil
Sunflower Oil
Vegetable Oil

Lee Kum Kee
Blended Sesame Oil (All Sizes)
Pure Sesame Oil (All Sizes)

Living Harvest ⓘ ✓
Living Harvest Hemp Oil

Lucini Italia ⟨⟩ ✓
Lucini Italia (All BUT Russian Tomato
  Vodka Sauce and Minestrone Soup)

MacNut Oil
MacNut Oil

Manischewitz
Cooking Sprays (All Varieties)
Vegetable Oil

Manitoba Harvest ⚥ ✓
Manitoba Harvest Hemp Foods & Oils
  (All)

Mario
Mario (All BUT Imitation Bacon Bits)

Mazola
Oils & Sprays (All)

Meijer
Cooking Spray - Butter
Cooking Spray - Extra Virgin Olive Oil
Cooking Spray - Vegetable Oil
Oil - Blended Canola/Vegetable
Oil - Canola
Oil - Corn
Oil - Olive
Oil - Olive 100% Pure - Classic
Oil - Olive Extra Virgin
Oil - Olive Extra Virgin - Italian Classic
Oil - Olive Infused Garlic & Basil Italian
Oil - Olive Infused Roasted Garlic
Oil - Olive Milder Tasting
Oil - Olive Spicy Red Pepper
Oil - Peanut
Oil - Sunflower
Oil - Vegetable
Olive - Italian Select Premium Extra
  Virgin

Midwest Country Fare (Hy-Vee)
100% Pure Vegetable Oil
Vegetable Oil

Nash Brothers
Premium Olive Oil

Newman's Own Organics ⟨⟩ ⓘ
Olive Oil

O Olive Oil ⚥
Oils (All)

Olivado
Olivado (All)

Olivio
Olivio (All)

PAM
Butter Flavor PAM
Olive Oil PAM

Freeze-Dried Dill
Freeze-Dried Garlic
Freeze-Dried Italian Herb Blend
Freeze-Dried Oregano
Freeze-Dried Parsley
Freeze-Dried Poultry Herb Blend
Freeze-Dried Red Onion
Freeze-Dried Salad Herb Blend
Freeze-Dried Spring Onion

Louisiana Fish Fry ()
Blackened Fish Seasoning
Cajun Seasoning
Chinese Red Pepper Seasoning
Crawfish Crab and Shrimp Boil
Fish Fry All Natural
Fish Fry New Orleans Style with Lemon
Fish Fry Seasoned
Spices (All)

Luzianne
Cajun Seasoning

Lydia's Organics 🖑
Lydia's Organics (All)

Manischewitz
Salt

McCormick
Single Ingredient Herbs (All)
Single Ingredient Spices (All)

Meijer
Black Pepper
Chili Powder
Cinnamon
Garlic Powder
Garlic Salt
Mild Taco
Minced Onion
Onion Salt
Oregano Leaves
Paprika
Parsley Flakes
Salt Iodized
Salt Plain
Seasoned Salt
Spaghetti Mix
Taco Seasoning

Midwest Country Fare (Hy-Vee)
Chili Powder
Chopped Onion

Garlic Powder
Garlic Salt
Ground Black Pepper
Ground Cinnamon
Italian Seasoning
Onion Powder
Parsley Flakes
Pure Ground Black Pepper
Seasoned Salt

Morton
Canning & Pickling Salt
Coarse Kosher Salt
Garlic Salt
Hot Salt
Iodized Table Salt
Lite Salt Mixture
Nature's Seasons Seasoning Blend
Plain Table Salt
Popcorn Salt
Salt & Pepper Shakers
Salt Substitute
Sausage & Meat Loaf Seasoning
Sea Salt (Fine and Coarse)
Seasoned Salt
Smoke Flavored Sugar Cure
Sugar Cure (Plain)
Tender Quick

Mrs. Dash ⓘ 🖑
Mrs. Dash (All)

Nash Brothers
Organic Spices

No Salt
No Salt Salt Substitute

Nueva Cocina ⓘ
Picadillo Seasoning
Taco Fresco Seasoning
Taco Seasoning with Chipotle

NU-Salt
NU-Salt (All)

Ortega
40% Less Sodium Taco Mix
Chipotle Mix
Guacamole Mix
Jalapeno & Onion Mix
Taco Seasoning
Taco Seasoning - Hot & Spicy

Oven Fry ✐

Fish Fry For Fish Seasoned Coating

Polaner

Ready To Use Wet Spices - Basil

Ready To Use Wet Spices - Garlic

Ready To Use Wet Spices - Jalapenos

Price Chopper

Iodized Salt

Regular Salt

Publix ()

Adobo Seasoning with Pepper

Adobo Seasoning Without Pepper

Black Pepper

Chili Powder

Cinnamon

Garlic Powder

Garlic Powder with Parsley

Garlic Salt

Ground Ginger

Ground Red Pepper

Italian Seasonings

Lemon & Pepper

Minced Onion

Onion Powder

Paprika

Parsley Flakes

Salt

Seasoned Salt

Taco Seasoning Mix

Whole Basil Leaves

Whole Bay Leaves

Whole Black Pepper

Whole Oregano

Sally's ⚕

Sally's (All)

Simply Asia

Beef & Broccoli Seasoning Mix

General Tso Steamers

Kung Pao Steamers

Spice Hunter ⓘ

Herbs (All BUT Grill Shakers Rib Seasoning)

Spice Blends (All BUT Grill Shakers Rib Seasoning)

Spices (All BUT Grill Shakers Rib Seasoning)

Spice Islands

also see Durkee

Grilling Gourmet & World Flavors (All)

Salt-Free (All)

Specialty - Beau Monde

Specialty - Chili Powder

Specialty - Crystallized Ginger

Specialty - Fines Herbs

Specialty - Garlic Pepper Seasoning

Specialty - Italian Herb Seasoning

Specialty - Old Hickory Smoked Salt

Specialty - Saffron

Specialty - Summer Savory

Spike ⓘ

5Herb Magic!

Garlic Magic!

Hot 'n Spicy Magic!

Onion Magic!

Original Magic!

Salt Free Magic!

Vegit Magic!

Stubb's ⓘ ✓

Bar-B-Q Rub

Chile-Lime Rub

Herbal Mustard Rub

Rosemary Ginger Rub

Sun Luck

Classic Stir Fry

Five Spice Powder

Hot & Spicy Stir Fry Sauce

Hot Mustard Powder

Sweet & Sour Mix

Teriyaki Marinade

Sunbird ⓘ

Asian Skillet Classics - Sweet & Sour Pork

Beef & Broccoli

Chinese Chicken Salad

Chop Suey

Chow Mein

Fried Rice

General Tso's Chicken

Honey Sesame Chicken

Hot & Spicy Fried Rice

Hot & Spicy Kung Pao
Hot & Spicy Szechwan
Lemon Chicken Stir Fry
Mongolian Beef
Oriental Vegetable Stir Fry
Phad Thai
Spare Rib
Spicy Orange Beef
Stir Fry
Sweet & Sour
Thai Chicken
Thai Fried Rice
Thai Red Curry
Thai Spicy Beef
Thai Stir Fry

Swanson (Williams Food) ⓘ
Swanson Chicken Salad

Taste of Thai, A
Taste of Thai, A (All)

Tone's
also see Durkee

Tradiciones ⓘ
Carne Adovada
Chimichurri
Green Mole
Guajillo Enchilada
Red Mole

TryMe
Tiger Seasoning

Wagners ⓘ
Hollandaise

Weber
Beer Can Chicken Seasoning
Burgundy Beef Rub
Burgundy Beef Seasoning
Chicago Steak Grinder
Chicago Steak Seasoning
Classic BBQ Rub
Classic BBQ Seasoning
Cracked Black Pepper and Herb Rub
Gourmet Burger Seasoning
Kick 'N Chicken Grinder
Kick 'N Chicken Seasoning
Mango Lime Seasoning
New Orleans Cajun Seasoning

Roasted Garlic & Herb Grinder
Roasted Garlic & Herb Seasoning
Seasoning Salt
Six Pepper Fusion Grinder
Smokey Mesquite Seasoning
Summer Citrus Rub
Sweet and Savory Salmon Rub
Tex Mex Fiesta Rub
Tex Mex Fiesta Seasoning
Twisted Citrus-Garlic Grinder
Veggie Grill Seasoning
Zesty Lemon Grinder
Zesty Lemon Seasoning

Wick Fowler's
Taco Seasoning

Williams ⓘ
Chili with Onions
Chipotle Chili
Chipotle Taco
Country Store Chili Soup
Country Store Tortilla Soup
Fancy Chili
Original Chili
Taco
Tex-Mex Chili
Tex-Mex Taco - Hot
White Chicken Chili

Woeber
Woeber (All)

SPRINKLES

Cake Mate
Sprinkles (All)

Kroger ⓘ
Rainbow Sprinkles
Sugar Sprinkles

Let's Do... ✔
Carnival Sprinkelz
Chocolatey Sprinkelz
Confetti Sprinkelz

Mr. Sprinkles ()
Mr. Sprinkles (All)

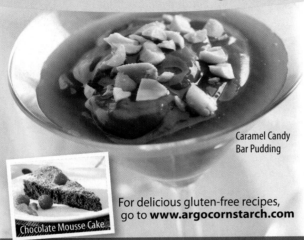
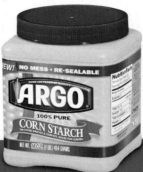
STARCHES

Argo
Corn Starch

Armour
Armour Cream Corn Starch

Authentic Foods
Authentic Foods (All)

Benson's
Corn Starch

Bob's Red Mill ✔
Arrowroot Starch
Corn Starch
Potato Starch

Canada
Corn Starch

Clabber Girl
Cornstarch

Durkee
Arrowroot

Eden Foods ⓘ ✔
Kuzu Root Starch

Hodgson Mill
Pure Corn Starch

Hy-Vee
Cornstarch

Kingsford
Corn Starch

Kinnikinnick Foods
Kinnikinnick Foods (All)

Kroger ⓘ
Corn Starch

Let's Do…Organic ✔
Organic Cornstarch
Organic Tapioca Starch

Meijer
Corn Starch

Rumford
Cornstarch

SUGAR & SUGAR SUBSTITUTES

Alter Eco Fair Trade
Alter Eco Fair Trade (All) ⓘ

Authentic Foods ⚇
Authentic Foods (All)

Bashas'
Sucrolose
Sugar
Sugar - Confectioners
Sugar - Granulated
Sugar - Light Brown
Sugar - Substitute

Billington's ⚇
Dark Brown Molasses Sugar
Demerara Sugar
Light Muscovado Sugar
Natural Sugar Crystals

C&H Sugar
Sugar (All)

Dixie Crystals
Sugar Products (All)

Domino
Sugars (All)

Eden Foods ⓘ ✓
Sweet Sorghum, Organic

Equal
Equal

Food Club (Marsh)
Aspartame Sweetner
Sugar
Sugar Confectioners
Sugar Light Brown
Sugar Substitute

Giant Eagle
Granulated Sugar
Sucralose Sugar Substitute

Great Value (Wal-Mart)
Altern No Calorie Sweetener
Calorie Free Sweetener
Confectioners Powdered Sugar
Extra Fine Granulated Sugar
Light Brown Sugar
Pure Cane Sugar

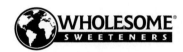

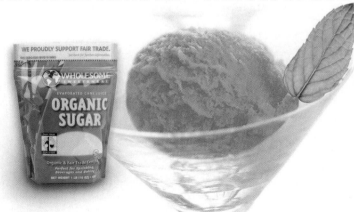

FAIR TRADE CERTIFIED™ ORGANIC SUGARS

Fair Trade Certified™ Organic & Natural Sugars, Syrups, Nectars & Honey.

Haggen
Confectioners Sugar
Dark Brown Sugar
Light Brown Sugar
Sugar

Holly Sugar
Sugar Products (All)

Hy-Vee
Confectioners Powdered Sugar
Dark Brown Sugar
Delecta Sugar Substitute
Light Brown Sugar
Pure Cane Sugar

Imperial Sugar
Sugar Products (All)

Kroger ⓘ
Dark Brown Sugar
Granulated Sugar
Light Brown Sugar
Powdered Sugar
Sugar Substitutes

Madhava ⚭
Agave (All)

Maple Grove Farms
Granulated Maple Sugar

Meijer
Sugar
Sugar - Confectioners
Sugar - Dark Brown
Sugar - Light Brown

Midwest Country Fare (Hy-Vee)
Granulated Sugar
Light Brown Sugar
Powdered Sugar

Nash Brothers
Organic Sugar

NatraTaste
NatraTaste (All)

Nielsen-Massey ✔
Nielsen-Massey (All)

Nutrasweet
NutraSweet

Publix ()
Dark Brown Sugar
Granulated Sugar
Light Brown Sugar

Powdered - 10X Sugar
Powdered - 4X Sugar

PureVia
PureVia (All)

Savannah Gold
Sugar Products (All)

Splenda
Splenda Sweetener Products (All)

Stevia Extract in the Raw ⚭
Stevia Extract in the Raw

Sugar in the Raw ⚭
Sugar In The Raw

Sweet Leaf
SweetLeaf (All)

Sweet'N Low
Sweet'N Low

Truvia
Truvia

Valu Time (Marsh)
Sugar

Wholesome Sweeteners ⚭
Dark Muscovado Sugar
Demerara Sugar, Sucanat (All Types)
Light Muscovado Sugar
Organic Agave Syrups
Organic Can Syrups, Inverts, and Blends
  (All Types)
Organic Powdered Sugar
Organic Sucanat (All Types)
Organic Sugar / Organic Evaporated
  Cane Juice (All Types)
Sugar / Evaporated Cane Juice

Winn-Dixie ()
Granulated Sugar
Light Brown Sugar
Powdered Sugar, 10X

WHOLE GRAINS

Alter Eco Fair Trade
Alter Eco Fair Trade (All) ⓘ

Ancient Harvest
Black Quinoa ⚭
Inca Red Quinoa ⚭
Quinoa Flakes ⓘ ✔
Traditional Quinoa ⚭

Arrowhead Mills ✓
- Amaranth
- Buckwheat Groats
- Flax Seeds
- Hulled Millet
- Organic Golden Flax Seeds
- Quinoa

Bob's Red Mill ☒ ✓
- Brown Flaxseeds
- GF Quick Rolled Oats
- GF Rolled Oats
- GF Steel Cut Oats
- Golden Flaxseed
- Hulled Hemp Seed
- Hulled Millet
- Organic Amaranth Grain
- Organic Brown Flaxseed
- Organic Buckwheat Groats
- Organic Golden Flaxseeds
- Organic Kasha
- Organic Quinoa Grain
- Whole Grain Teff

Cream Hill Estates ✓
- Gluten-Free Rolled Oats/Flakes
- Gluten-Free Whole Grain Oat Flour

Eden Foods ⓘ ✓
- Buckwheat - Organic
- Millet - Organic
- Quinoa - Organic
- Red Quinoa - Organic

Fresh & Easy ()
- Quinoa

Hodgson Mill ☒
- Whole Brown Flax Seed ✓

Pocono
- Cream of Buckwheat
- Groats
- Kasha

Tom Sawyer
- Gluten-Free Oats (All)

Wolff's Kasha
- Kasha
- Whole Buckwheat Groats

RED STAR ✦

Brown & White Gluten-Free Bread

This recipe has been developed by the Gluten-Free Experts!

Wet Ingredients:
3 large eggs, lightly beaten
1 teaspoon cider vinegar
3 tablespoons canola oil
1½ cups + 2 tablespoons water

Dry Ingredients:
2 ¼ cups white rice flour
1 cup brown rice flour
1½ teaspoons xanthan gum
3 tablespoons sugar
1½ teaspoons salt

1 tablespoon egg replacer, optional
½ cup dry milk
2¼ teaspoons RED STAR® Active Dry Yeast

Conventional Method: Yeast may be used cold. All other ingredients should be room temperature (70°–80°F). Combine liquid ingredients in a mixing bowl and whisk together. All dry ingredients, including the RED STAR® Active Dry Yeast packet (¼ oz.), should be thoroughly blended together. Mixing them in a bowl with a wire whisk or shaking them in a gallon size, self-locking bag is suggested. Gluten-free flours are very fine and need to be well blended. Using a mixer, add dry ingredients to the wet, beat about 10 minutes. Check appearance of dough. Pour batter into greased bread pan. Allow batter to rise approximately 1 hour. Bake at 375° F for 45 to 60 minutes; use a toothpick to test for doneness.

Bread Machine Method: Combine wet ingredients; pour carefully into baking pan. Measure dry ingredients, including yeast; mix well to blend. Add to baking pan. Carefully set pan in bread maker. Select NORMAL/WHITE cycle or GLUTEN FREE CYCLE (if machine has one); start machine. After mixing action begins, help any unmixed ingredients into the dough with a spatula, keeping to edges and top of batter to prevent interference with the paddle. Remove pan from the machine when bake cycle is complete. Invert pan and shake gently to remove bread. Cool on a rack before slicing.

For more gluten-free recipes, go to www.redstaryeast.com or call 800-445-4746.

CAROL'S COLLECTION

YEAST

Bakipan ☒
- Active Dry Yeast
- Bread Machine Yeast
- Fast Rising Instant Yeast

Bob's Red Mill ☒ ✓
- Active Dry Yeast
- Nutritional Yeast

Fleischmann's Yeast
- Yeast

Gayelord Hauser ⓘ
- Brewers Yeast

Hodgson Mill ☒
- Active Dry Yeast
- Fast Rise Yeast

Kroger ⓘ
- Yeast Packets

Red Star Yeast ☒
- Active Dry Yeast (ADY)
- Bread Machine Yeast
- Quick Rise Yeast

SAF ♻
  Bread Machine Yeast
  Gourmet Perfect Rise
  Traditional Active Dry Perfect Rise Yeast

MISCELLANEOUS

Bob's Red Mill ♻ ✓
  Guar Gum
  Organic Textured Soy Protein
  Rice Bran
  Soy Lecithin Granules
  Textured Vegetable Protein (TVP)
  Xanthan Gum
Dream Whip 〰
  Whipped Topping Mix
Ener-G ♻ ✓
  Xanthan Gum
Fearn Natural Foods ⓘ
  Lecithin Granules
  Liquid Lecithin
  Soya Granules
Let's Do…Organic ✓
  Organic Tapioca Granules
  Organic Tapioca Pearls
  Organic Waffle Bowls

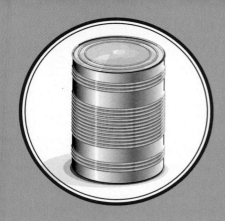

CANNED AND PACKAGED FOODS

Asian Specialty Items

Eden Foods ⓘ ✓
  Agar Agar Bars
  Agar Agar Flakes
  Arame
  Bonito Flakes
  Daikon Radish - Shredded and Dried
  Hiziki
  Kombu
  Lotus Root
  Maitake Mushrooms, Dried
  Mekabu
  Nori
  Pickled Daikon Radish
  Plum Balls
  Shiitake Muschrooms, Dried
  Shiro Miso - Organic
  Shiso Leaf Powder (Pickled Beefsteak
    Leaf)
  Sushi Nori
  Tekka (Miso Condiment)
  Toasted Nori Krinkles
  Ume Plum Concentrate (Bainiku Ekisu)
  Umeboshi Paste
  Umeboshi Plums
  Wakame
  Wakame, Instant Flakes
  Wasabi Powder
  Yansen (Dandelion Root Concentrate)

Sun Luck
  Bamboo Shoots - Sliced
  Bamboo Shoots - Strip
  Bean Sprouts (can)
  Phad Thai Rice Sticks, 3mm
  Sesame Seeds - Toasted
  Sesame Seeds - White
  Shiitake Mushrooms
  Stir Fry Vegetables
  Straw Mushrooms - Stiry Fry
  Straw Mushrooms - Whole/Peeled
  Waterchestnuts - Sliced
  Waterchestnuts - Whole

Beans, Baked

B&M Baked Beans
  B&M Baked Beans (All)
Bashas'
  Pork & Beans
Bush's Best
  Bush's Best Products (All BUT
    Chili Magic Chili Starter Line and
    Homestyle Chili Line)
Cattle Drive
  Cattle Drive Brown Sugar & Bacon
    Baked Beans
Eden Foods ⓘ ✓
  Baked Beans with Sorghum & Mustard
    - Organic
Food Club (Marsh)
  Canned Baked Beans
  Canned Baked Beans - Homestyle
  Canned Baked Beans - Maple Cured
  Canned Baked Beans - Vegetarian
  Canned Baked Beans with Onions
  Canned Pork And Beans
Fresh & Easy ()
  Organic Baked Beans
Great Value (Wal-Mart)
  Pork & Beans

Haggen
Pork and Beans

Hanover Foods ⓘ
Beans & Franks
Brown Sugar & Bacon Baked Beans
Homestyle Baked Beans
Pork & Beans
Vegetarian Baked Beans

HealthMarket (Hy-Vee)
Organic Baked Beans
Organic Maple & Onion Baked Beans

Heinz ⓘ
Vegetarian Beans

Hy-Vee
Home Style Baked Beans
Maple Cured Bacon Baked Beans
Onion Baked Beans
Original Baked Beans
Pork & Beans

Kid's Kitchen ⓘ
Beans & Wieners

Meijer
Pork and Beans

Midwest Country Fare (Hy-Vee)
Pork & Beans

Publix ⟨⟩
Baked Beans
Pork & Beans

Valu Time (Marsh)
Canned Pork And Beans

Wagon Master ⓘ ✓
Canned Items (All)

Winn-Dixie ⟨⟩
Baked Beans
Baked Beans with Bacon and Onion

Beans, Other

Allens ⓘ
Canned Products (All)

Bar Harbor ⓘ
Atlantic Soldier Beans with Pork
Atlantic Yellow Eye Beans with Pork
BH Vegetarian Soldier Beans
BH Vegetarian Yellow Eye Beans

Bashas'
Beans - Black
Beans - Blackeye Pea
Beans - Great Northern
Beans - Kidney
Beans - Lentil
Beans - Lima Baby
Beans - Lima Large
Beans - Mexican Style
Beans - Navy
Beans - Peas Green Split
Beans - Red, Small
Beans - White, Small
Butter Beans
Chili Beans
Dark Red Kidney Beans
Garbanzo Beans
Great Northern Beans
Pinto Beans

Casa Fiesta
Jalapeno Pinto Beans
Mexican Style Chili Beans
Pinto Beans

Eden Foods ⓘ ✓
Aduki Beans - Organic
Black Beans - Organic
Black Eyed Peas - Organic
Black Soybeans - Organic
Butter Beans (Baby Lima) - Organic
Cajun Rice & Small Red Beans - Organic
Cannellini (White Kidney) Beans - Organic
Caribbean Black Beans
Caribbean Rice & Black Beans - Organic
Curried Rice & Lentils - Organic
Garbanzo Beans (Chick Peas) - Organic
Great Northern Beans - Organic
Kidney Beans - Organic
Mexican Rice & Black Beans - Organic
Moroccan Rice & Garbanzo Beans - Organic
Navy Beans - Organic
Pinto Beans - Organic
Rice & Garbanzo Beans - Organic
Rice & Kidney Beans - Organic
Rice & Lentils - Organic
Rice & Pinto Beans - Organic

Small Red Beans - Organic

Fantastic World Foods
Instant Black Beans

Food Club (Marsh)
Canned Black Beans
Canned Butter Beans
Canned Chili Beans
Canned Dark Red Kidney Beans
Canned Garbanzo Beans
Canned Great Northern Beans
Canned Navy Beans
Canned Pinto Beans
Canned Red Beans

Fresh & Easy ()
Black Beans - No Salt Added
Black Beans - Organic
Black Beans - Regular
Butter Beans
Cannellini Beans
Chili Beans
Dark Red Kidney Beans - No Salt Added
Dark Red Kidney Beans - Regular
Garbanzo Beans - No Salt Added
Garbanzo Beans - Organic
Garbanzo Beans - Regular
Pinto Beans - Organic
Pinto Beans - Regular

Furmano's
Furmano's (All)

Great Value (Wal-Mart)
Baby Lima Beans
Black Beans
Chick Peas (Garbanzos), Bilingual
Great Northern Beans
Large Lima Beans
Lentils
Light Red Kidney Beans
Mayocoba Beans, Bilingual
Navy Beans
Pink Beans, Bilingual
Pinto Beans
Small Red Beans
Southern Ranch Beans

Haggen
Black Beans
Blackeye Beans
Dark Red Kidney Beans

Garbanzo Beans
Great Northern Beans
Hominy Gold Beans
Hominy White Beans
Kidney Beans
Lima Baby Beans
Pinto Beans

Hanover Foods ⓘ
3 Bean Salad
4 Bean Salad
Black Beans
Blackeye Peas
Butter Beans
Cannellini Beans
Chick Peas
Chili Beans
Great Northern Beans
Limagrands
Pink Beans
Pinto Beans
Red Beans
Redskin Kidney Beans (Light & Dark)
Seasoned Black Beans
Superfine Midget Green Butter Beans
Vegetarian Beans in Tomato Sauce

HealthMarket (Hy-Vee)
Organic Black Beans
Organic Dark Red Kidney Beans
Organic Pinto Beans

Hy-Vee
Baby Lima Beans
Black Beans
Black-Eyed Peas
Butter Beans
Chili Style Beans in Chili Gravy
Dark Red Kidney Beans
Garbanzo Beans (Chick Peas)
Great Northern Beans
Large Lima Beans
Lentils
Light Red Kidney Beans
Navy Beans
Pinto Beans
Red Beans
Red Kidney Beans

Joan of Arc
Black Beans

Butter Beans
Garbanzo Beans
Great Northern Beans
Light & Dark Red Kidney Beans
Pinto Beans
Red Beans

Kroger ⓘ
Unseasoned Beans - Canned

La Costena
La Costena (All BUT Jalapeno Hot Sauce)

Meijer
Beans - Lentil
Beans - Lima Large
Beans - Mexican Style
Beans - Navy
Beans - Peas Green Split
Beans - Pinto
Black Beans
Black Beans Organic
Blackeye Peas
Butter Beans
Garbanzo Beans
Garbanzo Beans - Organic
Great Northern Beans
Kidney Beans - Dark Red
Kidney Beans - Dark Red Organic
Kidney Beans - Light Red
Lima Beans
Pinto Beans
Pinto Beans - Organic
Red Beans

Midwest Country Fare (Hy-Vee)
Chili Style Beans

Ortega
Black Beans
Black Beans with Jalapenos

Pastene
Black Beans
Chick Peas
Lupini
Red Kidney Beans
White Kidney Beans

Publix ◌
Green Lima Beans
GreenWise Market Organic Black Beans

GreenWise Market Organic Garbanzo Beans
GreenWise Market Organic Kidney Beans, Dark Red
GreenWise Market Organic Pinto Beans
GreenWise Market Organic Soy Beans
Kidney Beans - Dark Red

Teasdale
Beans in Brine (All)
Organic Beans (All)

Valu Time (Marsh)
Canned Beans - Kidney Red
Canned Blackeye Peas

Winn-Dixie ◌
Garbanzo Beans
Green and White Lima Beans
Green Lima Beans
Kidney Beans - Dark Red
Kidney Beans - Light Red
Kidney Beans - Red
Mexican Style Chili Beans

BEANS, REFRIED

Amy's Kitchen ⓘ ✓
Refried Beans with Green Chiles
Refried Black Beans
Refried Black Beans - Light in Sodium
Traditional Refried Beans
Traditional Refried Beans - Light in Sodium
Vegetarian Refried Beans

Bashas'
Authentic Refried Beans
Refried Beans

Casa Fiesta
Refried Beans
Refried Beans with Green Chiles

Eden Foods ⓘ ✓
Refried Black Beans - Organic
Refried Black Soy & Black Beans - Organic
Refried Kidney Beans - Organic
Refried Pinto Beans - Organic
Spicy Refried Black Beans - Organic
Spicy Refried Pinto Beans - Organic

Fantastic World Foods
Instant Refried Beans
Food Club (Marsh)
Refried Beans
Refried Beans - Authenic
Refried Beans - Fat Free
Haggen
Refried Beans
Refried Beans - Fat Free
Refried Beans - Vegetarian
HealthMarket (Hy-Vee)
Organic Refried Beans
Hy-Vee
Black Refried Beans
Fat Free Refried Beans
Traditional Refried Beans
Vegetarian Refried Beans
La Costena
La Costena (All BUT Jalapeno Hot
Sauce)
Meijer
Refried Beans
Refried Beans - Fat Free
Refried Beans - Organic Black Bean
Refried Beans - Organic Black Bean/
Jalapeno
Refried Beans - Organic Roasted Chili/
Lime
Refried Beans - Organic Traditional
Refried Beans - Vegetarian
Ortega
Refried Beans - Fat Free
Refried Beans - Regular
Taco Bell ✎
Fat Free Refried Beans
Vegetarian Blend Refried Beans

BOUILLON

Bashas'
Soup Beef Bouillon Cube
Soup Beef Bouillon Instant
Better than Bouillon
All Natural Reduced Sodium Chicken
Base
Au Jus Base
Beef Base

Chicken Base
Chili Base
Clam Base
Fish Base
Ham Base
Kosher Line
Lobster Base
Organic Line
Turkey Base
Vegetarian Line
Edward & Sons ✓
Garden Veggie Bouillon Cubes
Low Sodium Veggie Bouillon Cubes
Not-Beef Bouillon Cubes
Not-Chick'n Bouillon Cubes
Food Club (Marsh)
Soup Bouillon Cube Beef
Soup Bouillon Instant Beef
Herb-Ox ⓘ
Beef
Chicken
Garlic Chicken
Vegetable
Hy-Vee
Beef Bouillon Cubes
Chicken Bouillon Cubes
Instant Beef Bouillon
Instant Chicken Bouillon
Lee Kum Kee
Chicken Bouillon Powder (All Sizes)
Kum Chun Chicken Bouillon Powder
(All Sizes)

BROTH & STOCK

Bar Harbor ⓘ
Clam Stock
Fish Stock
Lobster Stock
Seafood Stock
Bashas'
Broth - Beef
College Inn Broth ⓘ
Bold Stock Beef Sirloin
Garden Vegetable Variety
Organic Beef Broth Variety
White Wine & Herb Culinary Broth

Emeril's
Beef Stock
Chicken Stock
Vegetable Stock

Food Club (Marsh)
Beef Broth Ready to Serve Soup (Thin)
Chicken Broth - Fat Free, Low Sodium,
Thin
Soup Chicken Broth (Aseptic)

Great Value (Wal-Mart)
Beef Broth Ready To Serve
Chicken Broth Ready To Serve

Haggen
Chicken Broth (Aseptic)

Imagine
Organic Beef Flavored Broth
Organic Free Range Chicken Broth
Organic Low Sodium Beef Flavored
Broth
Organic Low Sodium Vegetable Broth
Organic No Chicken Broth
Organic Vegetable Broth

Kitchen Basics
Kitchen Basics (All)

Meijer
Broth - Chicken
Broth Chicken (First Line)

Nature's Basket (Giant Eagle)
Organic Broth - Chicken
Organic Broth - Low Sodium Chicken
Organic Broth - Vegetable

Pacific Natural Foods ⓘ
Natural Beef
Natural Free Range Chicken
Organic Beef
Organic Free Range Chicken
Organic Low Sodium Beef Broth
Organic Low Sodium Chicken
Organic Low Sodium Vegetable
Organic Mushroom
Organic Vegetable

Progresso ✓
Beef Flavored Broth
Chicken Broth
Reduced Sodium Chicken Broth

Shelton's
Chicken Broth Fat Free

Chicken Broth Regular
Organic Chicken Broth Fat Free
Organic Chicken Broth Regular

Swanson ⓘ
Beef Stock (Aseptic)
Chicken Broth (Aseptic & Canned)
Chicken Stock (Aseptic)
Natural Goodness Chicken Broth
(Aseptic & Canned)
Vegetable Broth (Canned)

CHILI & CHILI MIXES

Amy's Kitchen ⓘ ✓
Black Bean Chili
Medium Chili
Medium Chili - Light in Sodium
Medium Chili with Vegetables
Spicy Chili
Spicy Chili - Light in Sodium

Bashas'
Chili with Beans
Chili with Beans - Hot

Bush's Best
Bush's Best Products (All BUT
Chili Magic Chili Starter Line and
Homestyle Chili Line)

Carroll Shelby Chili
Original Texas Chili Kit
White Chicken Chili

Casa Fiesta
Bean and Green Chili Burrito Filling
Whole Green Chili

Cattle Drive
Cattle Drive Chicken Chili
Cattle Drive Chili with Beans

Del Monte ⓘ
Harvest Selection "Heat & Eat" Chili &
Beans

Eden Foods ⓘ ✓
Black Bean & Quinoa Chili

Fresh & Easy ◐
Chili Beef No Beans
Chili Beef with Beans
Chili Beef with Beans- 99% Fat Free
Chili Chicken with Beans

Frontier Soups ⓘ
  California Gold Rush White Bean Chili
  Michigan Ski Country Chili
  Midwest Weekend Cincinatti Chili
Hormel ⓘ
  Chili Master - Chipotle Chicken No Bean
  Chili Master - Chipotle Chicken with Beans
  Chili Master - White Chicken Chili with Beans
  Chili with Beans (Beef Only) - Chunky
  Chili with Beans (Beef Only) - Hot
  Chili with Beans (Beef Only) - Regular
Hy-Vee
  Chili with Beans
  Hot Chili with Beans
Juanitas
  Juanitas (All BUT Mole, Caldo de Pollo, Chile Colorado, Chicken Veracruz, Chile Verde, and Albondigas Soup)
Meijer
  Chili No Beans (Regular)
  Chili with Beans (Regular)
Shelton's
  Chicken Chili Mild
  Chicken Chili Spicy
  Turkey Chili Mild
  Turkey Chili Spicy
Stagg ⓘ
  Chunkero Chili
  Classic Chili
  Dynamite Hot Chili
  Ranch House Chicken Chili
  Silverado Beef Chili
  Steak House Chili
  Turkey Ranchero Chili
  Vegetable Garden Chili
  White Chicken Chili
Texas Pete
  Chili No Bean ⓘ
  Hot Dog Chili ⓘ
Wick Fowler's
  2-Alarm Chili Kit
  False Alarm Chili Kit
  One Step Wick Fowler Chili Mix
  Wick Fowler Chicken Chili Mix

COCONUT MILK

Let's Do...Organic ✓
  Organic Creamed Coconut
Native Forest ✓
  Organic Coconut Milk
  Organic Light Coconut Milk
Sun Luck
  Coconut Milk
  Coconut Milk - Light
Taste of Thai, A
  Taste of Thai, A (All)

CRANBERRY SAUCE

Great Value (Wal-Mart)
  Jellied Cranberry Sauce
  Whole Berry Cranberry Sauce
Haggen
  Cranberry Sauce - Jelly
  Cranberry Sauce - Whole
Hy-Vee
  Jellied Cranberry Sauce
  Whole Berry Cranberry Sauce
Marzetti
  Homestyle Cooked Cranberries
Ocean Spray
  Sauces (All)
Price Chopper
  Jellied Cranberry Sauce
  Whole Cranberry Sauce
Publix ()
  Whole Cranberry Sauce
Winn-Dixie ()
  Jellied Cranberry Sauce

FRUIT

Bashas'
  Apricot Halves Unpeeled - Heavy Syrup
  Cherries - Red Tart Pitted
  Fruit Cocktail - Heavy Syrup
  Fruit Cocktail Juice - Lite
  Mandarin Oranges in Light Syrup
  Peach Preserves
  Peaches - Cling Halves - Heavy Syrup
  Peaches - Cling Sliced - Heavy Syrup

Peaches - Cling Sliced Juice - Lite
Pears - Halves - Heavy Syrup
Pears - Slices - Heavy Syrup
Pears - Slices Juice
Pineapple Chunk in Juice
Pineapple Crushed in Juice
Pineapple Sliced in Juice

Del Monte ⓘ

Canned/Jarred Fruits (All)

Food Club (Marsh)

Canned Apricot Halves - Unpeeled In Heavy Syrup
Fruit Cocktail - Canned In Heavy Syrup
Fruit Cocktail - Canned In Juice
Fruit Cocktail - Canned with Splenda
Mandarin Oranges Can - Lite Syrup
Mandarin Oranges in Lite Syrup
Maraschino Cherry - Green
Maraschino Cherry - Red
Maraschino Cherry - Red with Stems
Mixed Fruit - Extreme Cherry
Peaches Canned Sliced with Splenda
Peaches Cling Canned Halves Heavy Syrup
Peaches Cling Canned Sliced In Juice
Peaches Diced Bowl In Light Syrup
Pears Bartlett Canned Halves Heavy Syrup
Pears Bartlett Canned Halves Juice
Pineapple Chunks Canned In Juice
Pineapple Crushed Canned In Juice
Pineapple Sliced Canned In Juice
Red Tart Pitted Cherries

Fresh & Easy ⟨⟩

Fruit Salad Tropical
Peaches in Heavy Syrup
Peaches in Pear Juice
Pear Halves in Pear Juice
Pineapple Chunks in Pineapple Juice
Pineapple Crushed in Pineapple Juice
Pineapple Slices in Pineapple Juice

Great Value (Wal-Mart)

Bartlett Pear Halves In Heavy Syrup
Bartlett Sliced Pears In Heavy Syrup
Blackberries
Blueberries
Crushed Pineapple

Fruit Cocktail In Heavy Syrup
Fruit Cocktail Sweetened w/Splenda
Fruit Selections Crushed Pineapple
Fruit Selections Diced Peaches & Pears In Strawberry & Raspberry Light Syrup
Fruit Selections Diced Peaches In Light Syrup
Fruit Selections Diced Peaches In Strawberry & Banana Light Syrup
Fruit Selections Diced Peaches w/ Splenda
Fruit Selections Mandarin Oranges In Light Syrup
Fruit Selections Mixed Fruit In Light Syrup
Fruit Selections Mixed Fruit w/Splenda
Fruit Selections Pineapple Chunks
Fruit Selections Pineapple Slices
Fruit Selections Pineapple Tidbits In Pineapple Juice
Fruit Selections Tropical Fruit Mix In Light Syrup
Fruit Slices
Maraschino Cherries w/Stems
No Sugar Added Bartlett Pear Halves
No Sugar Added Chunky Mixed Fruits
No Sugar Added Fruit Cocktail
No Sugar Added Yellow Cling Peach Halves
No Sugar Added Yellow Cling Sliced Peaches
Peaches & Pears In Cherry Gel
Pineapple Chunks
Pineapple Slices
Red Raspberries
Sliced Peaches
Tidbit Pineapple
Triple Cherry Fruit Mix In Light Syrup
Tropical Fruit Salad
Whole Segment Mandarin Oranges In Light Syrup
Whole Strawberries
Yellow Cling Peach Halves In Heavy Syrup
Yellow Cling Sliced Peaches Sweetened w/Splenda

Haggen
Apricot Halves Unpeeled Heavy Syrup
Fruit - Mixed X-treme Cherry
Fruit Cocktail Heavy Syrup
Fruit Cocktail in Juice
Peaches - Cling Halves Heavy Syrup
Peaches - Cling Sliced Heavy Syrup
Peaches - Cling Sliced in Juice
Pears - Barlett Sliced Heavy Syrup
Pears - Bartlett Halves Heavy Syrup
Pears - Bartlett Halves Juice
Pumpkin

Hy-Vee
Bartlett Pear Halves
Bartlett Pear Slices
Chunk Pineapple
Crushed Pineapple
Fruit Cocktail
Lite Bartlett Pear Halves
Lite Chunk Mixed Fruit
Lite Fruit Cocktail
Lite Unpeeled Apricot Halves Sweetened
   with Splenda
Lite Yellow Cling Peach Halves
Lite Yellow Cling Peach Slices
Mandarin Oranges
Mandarin Oranges in Light Syrup
Pumpkin
Purple Plums
Unpeeled Apricot Halves
Yellow Cling Peach Halves
Yellow Cling Peach Slices

Kroger ⓘ
Fruit - Canned

Libby's ⓘ
Libby's 100% Pure Pumpkin

Meijer
Apricot Halves in Pear Juice
Fruit Cocktail in Heavy Syrup
Fruit Cocktail in Pear Juice Lite
Fruit Cocktail Juice
Fruit Cocktail Juice Easy Open
Fruit Mix Juice
Fruit Salad Tropical
Grapefruit Sections in Juice
Grapefruit Sections in Syrup
Mandarin Oranges Light Syrup

Peaches - Cling Halves Heavy Syrup
Peaches - Cling Halves Juice Lite
Peaches - Cling Halves Pear Juice
Peaches - Cling Sliced Heavy Syrup
Peaches - Cling Sliced in Juice
Peaches - Cling Slices Pear Juice
Peaches - Yellow Sliced Heavy Syrup
Pear - Sliced Heavy Syrup
Pear Halves - Lite
Pears - Halves Heavy Syrup
Pears - Halves Juice Easy Open
Pears - Slices in Juice Lite
Pineapple - Crushed Heavy Syrup
Pineapple - Crushed in Juice
Pineapple - Sliced Heavy Syrup
Pineapple - Sliced in Juice
Pineapple Chunks - Heavy Syrup
Pineapple Chunks in Juice
Pineapple Juice
Pumpkin

Midwest Country Fare (Hy-Vee)
Bartlett Pear Halves in Light Syrup
Crushed Pineapple in Natural Juice
Fruit Cocktail in Heavy Syrup
Pineapple Chunks In Natural Juice
Pineapple Slices In Natural Juice
Pineapple Tidbits In Natural Juice
Yellow Cling Peach Halves in Light
   Syrup
Yellow Cling Peach Slices in Heavy
   Syrup
Yellow Cling Peach Slices in Light Syrup

Native Forest ✓
Mangosteen
Organic Mango Chunks
Organic Papaya Chunks
Organic Pineapple Chunks
Organic Pineapple Crushed
Organic Pineapple Slices
Organic Sliced Asian Pears
Organic Sliced Peaches
Organic Tropical Fruit Salad
Rambutan

Oregon Fruit Products
Canned Fruit (All)

Publix ()
- Apricot Halves - Unpeeled in Heavy Syrup
- Bartlett Pears in Heavy Syrup (Halves and Slices)
- Chunky Mixed Fruit in Heavy Syrup
- Fruit Cocktail in Heavy Syrup
- Lite Bartlett Pear Halves in Pear Juice
- Lite Chunky Mixed Fruit in Pear Juice
- Lite Fruit Cocktail in Pear Juice
- Lite Yellow Cling Peaches in Pear Juice (Halves and Slices)
- Mandarin Oranges in Light Syrup
- Pineapple (All Styles)
- Yellow Cling Peaches in Heavy Syrup (Halves and Slices)

Raley's
- Chunk Pineapple
- Crushed Pineapple
- Sliced Pineapple

S&W Fine Foods ⓘ
- Canned/Jarred Fruits (All)

Thrifty Maid (Winn-Dixie) ()
- Bartlett Pears - Halves and Slices
- Yellow Cling Peaches - Halves and Slices

Valu Time (Marsh)
- Fruit Cocktail Light Syrup
- Peaches Cling Canned Halves Light
- Peaches Sliced Light Syrup
- Pears Halves Canned Light Syrup

White House
- White House (All)

Winn-Dixie ()
- Apricots - Halves Unpeeled
- Bartlett Pears - Halves and Slices
- Chunky Mixed Fruit
- Fruit Cocktail
- Fruit Cups - Mandarin Oranges
- Fruit Cups - Mixed Fruit
- Fruit Cups - Peaches
- Fruit Cups - Pears
- Mandarin Orange Segments
- Pineapple - Chunks
- Pineapple - Crushed
- Pineapple - Sliced
- Pineapple - Tidbits
- Yellow Cling Peaches - Halves and Slices

Wyman's
- Wyman's (All)

MEALS & MEAL STARTERS

Annie's Homegrown ⓘ ✓
- Gluten Free Deluxe Rice Pasta and Cheddar
- Gluten Free Rice Pasta & Cheddar

Asian Helper ✓
- Beef Fried Rice Skillet Meal
- Chicken Fried Rice Skillet Meal

Caesar's Pasta ⓘ ✓
- Gluten-Free Cheese Lasagna in Marinara Sauce
- Gluten-Free Manicotti in Marinara Sauce
- Gluten-Free Potato Gnocchi without Sauce
- Gluten-Free Spinach & Potato Gnocchi without Sauce
- Gluten-Free Stuffed Shells in Marinara Sauce
- Gluten-Free Vegetable Lasagna in Marinara Sauce

Chi-Chi's ⓘ
- Fiesta Plates Creamy Chipotle Chicken
- Fiesta Plates Salsa Chicken
- Fiesta Plates Savory Garlic Chicken

DeBoles
- Gluten Free Rice Elbow Style Pasta & Cheese
- Gluten Free Rice Shells & Cheddar

Del Monte ⓘ
- Harvest Selections "Heat & Eat" Santa Fe Style Rice & Beans

Dinty Moore ⓘ
- Microwaveable Cups - Beef Stew
- Microwaveable Cups - Rice with Chicken
- Microwaveable Cups - Scalloped Potatoes & Ham

Empire Kosher
- Fully Cooked Barbecue Chicken - Fresh
- Fully Cooked Barbecue Turkey - Fresh

Food Club (Marsh)
- Beef Stew

Foods by George ♂
Cheese Lasagna

Fresh & Easy ◐
Cooked Organic Brown Rice Bowls
Cooked Organic Medley with Wild Rice
Bowls
Cooked Organic White Jasmine Rice
Bowls
Cooked Organic White Rice Bowls

Gluten Free & FABULOUS ✓
Bon Appetit! Quinoa with Marinara

Hamburger Helper ✓
Cheesy Hashbrowns Skillet Meal

Hormel ⓘ
Compleats Microwave Meals - Chicken
& Rice
Refrigerated Entrées - Beef Roast Au Jus
Refrigerated Entrées - Chipotle Chicken
Refrigerated Entrées - Italian Style Beef
Roast
Refrigerated Entrées - Pork Loin with
Honey Mustard
Refrigerated Entrées - Pork Roast Au Jus
Refrigerated Entrées - Turkey Breast
Roast
Refrigerated Entrées - Turkey Stroganoff

Juanitas
Juanitas (All BUT Mole, Caldo de Pollo,
Chile Colorado, Chicken Veracruz,
Chile Verde, and Albondigas Soup)

Luzianne
Creole Dinner Kit

Nueva Cocina ⓘ
Black Beans and Rice Mix
Chicken Rice Mix
Mexican Rice Mix
Seafood Rice Mix

Orgran ✓
Canned Pasta Range (All)
Falafel Mix
Pasta & Sauce Tomato & Basil
Ready Meal Pasta - Tomato & Basil
Spirals
Ready Meal Pasta - Vegetable Bolognese
Spirals

Ortega
Pizza Grande Dinner Kit

Sponge Bob Dinner Kit
Taco Kit (12-count and 18-count)

Oscar Mayer Lunchables ∾
Cheese Dip & Salsa Cracker Stackers/
Nachos

Road's End Organics ✓
GF Alfredo Chreese Mix
GF Cheddar Chreese Mix
Organic GF Alfredo Mac & Chreese
Organic GF Cheddar Penne & Chreese

Simply Potatoes
Simply Potatoes (All BUT Macaroni and
Cheese)

St. Dalfour ⓘ
Gourmet on the Go - Three Beans
Gourmet on the Go - Wild Salmon

Taco Bell ∾
Sauce & Taco Shells 12 Ct Taco Dinner

Taste of China, A
Taste of China, A (All)

Taste of Thai, A
Taste of Thai, A (All)

Tastee Choice
Shrimp Biryani Meal

Tasty Bite
Agra Peas & Greens
Aloo Palak
Bengal Lentils
Bombay Potatoes
Channa Masala
Chunky Chickpeas
Jaipur Vegetables
Jodhpur Lentils
Kashmir Spinach
Kerala Vegetables
Lentil Magic
Madras Lentils
Mushroom Takatak
Paneer Makhani
Peas Paneer
Punjab Eggplant
Snappy Soya
Spinach Dal
Vegetable Korma
Zesty Lentils & Peas

Meat

Armour
Corned Beef
Corned Beef Hash
Vienna Sausages (All BUT Cajun flavor)

Bashas'
Corned Beef Hash

Food Club (Marsh)
Canned Chicken, Chunk White - 98%
Fat Free

Fresh & Easy ()
Canned Chicken Breast
Canned Roast Beef
Canned Turkey Breast

Great Value (Wal-Mart)
Potted Meat Product
Vienna Sausage

Hormel ⓘ
Black Label - Canned Hams
Breast of Chicken Chunk Meats
Chicken Chunk Meats
Corned Beef
Corned Beef Hash
Dried Beef
Ham Chunk Meats
Turkey Chunk Meats

Hy-Vee
98% Fat Free Breast of Chicken
Spiced Luncheon Loaf

Kroger ⓘ
Chicken - Canned
Chicken - Pouch
Vienna Sausage - Canned

Meijer
Chicken Chunk White
Corned Beef Hash

Plumrose
Plumrose (All)

SPAM ⓘ
Classic
Less Sodium
Lite
Oven Roasted Turkey
Smoke Flavored

Thrifty Maid (Winn-Dixie) ()
Chicken Vienna Sausage

Underwood
Deviled Ham Spread

Valley Fresh ⓘ
Chicken
Turkey

Valu Time (Marsh)
Chicken Chunk White-In Water

Pie Fillings

Baker
Dessert Fillings (All Flavors)
Pie Fillings (All Flavors)

Bashas'
Pie Filling - Apple
Pie Filling - Blueberry
Pie Filling - Cherry

Comstock
Pie Fillings

Fischer & Wieser
Fredericksburg Golden Peach Pie Filling
Harvest Apple & Brandy Pie Filling

Food Club (Marsh)
Pie Filling Apple
Pie Filling Blueberry
Pie Filling Cherry
Pie Filling Cherry Lite
Pie Filling Peach

Grainless Baker, The
The Grainless Baker (All)

Grandmother's
Apple
Blueberry
Cherry Pie Filling
Fig Pastry Filling
Lemon Pie & Pastry Filling
Red Raspberry Pie & Pastry Filling
Rum Flavored Mincemeat
Traditional Mincemeat

Great Value (Wal-Mart)
Apple Pie Filling
Blueberry Pie Filling
Cherry Pie Filling

No Sugar Added Apple Pie Filling w/ Splenda

No Sugar Added Cherry Pie Filling w/ Splenda

Hy-Vee

More Fruit Apple Pie Filling Or Topping

More Fruit Cherry Pie Filling Or Topping

Kroger ⓘ

Canned Pie Filling

Libby's ⓘ

Libby's Easy Pumpkin Pie Mix

Meijer

Pie Filling - Apple

Pie Filling - Blueberry

Pie Filling - Cherry

Pie Filling - Cherry Lite

Pie Filling - Peach

Midwest Country Fare (Hy-Vee)

Apple Pie Filling

Cherry Pie Filling

Solo

Cake & Pastry Fillings (All Flavors)

Wilderness

Pie Fillings

Winn-Dixie ()

Pie Filling - Apple

Pie Filling - Blueberry

Pie Filling - Cherry

SEAFOOD, OTHER

Bar Harbor ⓘ

Cherrystone Clams

Chopped Clams

Clam Juice

Herring with Cracked Pepper

Smoked Kippers

Smoked Mackerel

Whole Lobster

Beach Cliff

Sardines (All)

Bumble Bee

Canned Seafood Products (All BUT Teriyaki Salmon Steak & Crackers in Ready-To-Eat Salads & Crackers)

Chicken of the Sea

Chicken of The Sea (All BUT Tuna Salad Kit)

Crown Prince

Canned Seafood Products (All)

Faust

Canned Salmon (All)

Fresh & Easy ()

Canned Salmon

Great Value (Wal-Mart)

Crab Meat

Lightly Smoked Sardines In Oil

Naturally Smoked Kipper Snacks

Smoked Oysters (China)

Smoked Oysters (South Korea)

Tiny Shrimp

Hy-Vee

Alaska Pink Salmon

Alaska Red Salmon

Kroger ⓘ

Salmon - Canned

Sardines - Canned

Lily

Lily (All)

Meijer

Salmon - Pink

Salmon - Sockeye Red

Pastene

Anchovy Fillets - Wild Caught

Phillips

Crab Meat

Pink Pride

Canned Salmon (All)

Royal Pink

Canned Salmon (All)

Royal Red

Canned Salmon (All)

Rubenstein

Canned Salmon (All)

Sea Alaska

Canned Salmon (All)

Sno Tip

Canned Salmon (All)

Wild Planet

Wild Planet (All)

SEAFOOD, TUNA

Bumble Bee
Canned Seafood Products (All BUT Teriyaki Salmon Steak & Crackers in Ready-To-Eat Salads & Crackers)
Mesquite Albacore Tuna Steak (All BUT Teriyaki Salmon Steak & Crackers in Ready-To-Eat Salads & Crackers)

Chicken of the Sea
Chicken of The Sea (All BUT Tuna Salad Kit)

Fresh & Easy ()
Canned Tuna

Great Value (Wal-Mart)
Chunk Light Tuna In Water
Premium Chunk Light Tuna In Water
Solid White Albacore Tuna In Water

Kroger ⓘ
Tuna - Canned
Tuna - Pouch

Pastene
Tonno
Tuna with Fresh Ginger
Tuna with Hot Chili Pepper

StarKist Tuna
Starkist Canned Tuna (All BUT Crackers in Lunch To-Go and Charlie's Lunch Kit)
Starkist Tuna Creations (All BUT Herb & Garlic and Tomato Pesto Albacore)
Starkist Tuna Fillets (All BUT Teriyaki)
Starkist Tuna Salad

Wild Planet
Wild Planet (All)

SOUPS & SOUP MIXES

4C
Dehydrated Onion Soup Mix

Amy's Kitchen ⓘ ✔
Black Bean Vegetable Soup
Chunky Tomato Bisque
Chunky Tomato Bisque - Light in Sodium
Chunky Vegetable Soup
Corn Chowder
Cream of Tomato Soup
Cream of Tomato Soup - Light in Sodium
Fire Roasted Southwestern Vegetable Soup
Lentil Soup
Lentil Soup - Light in Sodium
Lentil Vegetable Soup
Lentil Vegetable Soup - Light in Sodium
Potato Leek Soup
Split Pea Soup
Split Pea Soup - Light in Sodium
Thai Coconut Soup
Tuscan Bean & Rice Soup

Bashas'
Soup - Chicken with Rice
Soup - New England Style Clam Chowder RTS

Bear Creek
Cheddar Broccoli
Cheddar Potato
Chili
Clam Chowder
Creamy Potato
Creamy Wild Rice
Navy Bean
Split Pea
Tortilla

Casa Fiesta
Gazpacho Soup Mix

Eden Foods ⓘ ✔
Genmai (Brown Rice) Miso - Organic

Fantastic World Foods
Blarney Stone Simmer Soup
Creamy Potato Simmer Soup

Food Club (Marsh)
Soup Condensed Chicken Rice Ezo

Frontier Soups ⓘ
Carolina Springtime Asparagus Almond Soup
Chicago Bistro French Onion Soup
Far East Ginger Beef Bowl
Florida Sunshine Red Pepper Corn Chowder
Holiday Gathering Cranberry Bean Soup
Idaho Outpost Potato Leek Soup

Illinios Prairie Corn Chowder
Indiana Harvest Sausage Lentil Soup
Ivory Coast Chai Chocolate Dessert
 Soup
Kansas Sunflower Yellow Pea Soup
Louisiana Red Bean Gumbo
Minnesota Heartland 11-Bean Soup
Mississippi Delta Tomato Basil Soup
Missouri Homestead Garden Gazpacho
 Soup
Nebraska Barnraising Green Split Pea
 Soup
New Mexico Mesa Spicy Fiesta Soup
New Orleans Jambalaya Soup
Oregon Lakes Wild Rice & Mushroom
 Soup
San Francisco Thai Golden Peanut Soup
South of the Border Tortilla Soup
Texas Wrangler Black Bean Soup
Virginia Blue Ridge Brocoli Cheddar
 Soup

Gold's
Borscht
Lo-Calorie Borscht
Russian Style Borscht
Schav
Unsalted Borscht

Haggen
Chunky Soup w/Vegetables
Homestyle Roast Chicken w/Rice Soup

Hormel ⓘ
Microwaveable Cup Bean & Ham Soup
Microwaveable Cup Chicken with
 Vegetables & Rice Soup

Imagine
Creamy Portobello Mushroom Soup
Creamy Sweet Corn & Lemongrass Soup
Organic Creamy Acorn Squash &
 Mango Soup
Organic Creamy Broccoli Soup
Organic Creamy Butternut Squash Soup
Organic Creamy Potato Leek Soup
Organic Creamy Sweet Pea Soup
Organic Creamy Tomato Basil Soup
Organic Creamy Tomato Soup

Juanitas
Juanitas (All BUT Mole, Caldo de Pollo,
 Chile Colorado, Chicken Veracruz,
 Chile Verde, and Albondigas Soup)

Lucini Italia () ✓
Lucini Italia (All BUT Russian Tomato
 Vodka Sauce and Minestrone Soup)

Manischewitz
Borscht (All)

Meijer
Chicken (Aseptic)
Condensed Chicken with Rice Soup
Homestyle Chicken with Rice Soup

Midwest Country Fare (Hy-Vee)
Onion Soup

Miso-Cup ✓
Japanese Restaurant Style
Original Golden Vegetable
Reduced Sodium
Savory Seaweed
Traditional with Tofu

Nueva Cocina ⓘ
Black Bean Soup with Chipotle
Cuban Black Bean Soup
Red Bean Soup

Orgran ✓
Tomato Soup
Vegetable Soup

Pacific Natural Foods ⓘ
All Natural Rosemary Potato Chowder
Cashew Carrot Ginger
Curried Red Lentil
Organic Cream of Celery Condensed
 Soup
Organic Cream of Chicken Condensed
 Soup
Organic Cream of Mushroom
 Condensed Soup
Organic Creamy Butternut Squash
Organic Creamy Roasted Red Pepper &
 Tomato
Organic Creamy Tomato
Organic French Onion
Organic Light Sodium Creamy
 Butternut Squash
Organic Light Sodium Creamy Tomato

Organic Light Sodium Roasted Red
Pepper & Tomato
Organic Savory Chicken & Wild Rice
Organic Savory White Bean with Bacon
Organic Spicy Chicken Fajita
Organic Split Pea with Bacon & Swiss
Spicy Black Bean Soup

Progresso ✓
Reduced Sodium Garden Vegetable
Soup
Rich & Hearty Chicken Corn Chowder
Rich & Hearty New England Clam
Chowder
Traditional 99% Fat Free New England
Clam Chowder
Traditional Chicken Cheese Enchilada
Traditional Chicken Rice with Vegetable
Traditional Manhattan Clam Chowder
Traditional New England Clam
Chowder
Traditional Potato Broccoli Cheese
Chowder
Traditional Southwestern Style Chicken
Traditional Split Pea with Ham
Vegetable Classics 99% Fat Free Lentil
Vegetable Classics Creamy Mushroom
Vegetable Classics French Onion
Vegetable Classics Garden Vegetable
Vegetable Classics Hearty Black Bean
Vegetable Classics Lentil

Shelton's
Black Bean & Chicken Soup
Chicken Corn Chowder
Chicken Rice Soup
Chicken Tortilla Soup

Simply Asia
Rice Noodle Soup Bowls - Garlic
Sesame
Rice Noodle Soup Bowls - Sesame
Chicken
Rice Noodle Soup Bowls - Spring
Vegetable

Taste of Thai, A
Taste of Thai, A (All)

STEWS

Bashas'
Beef Stew
Dinty Moore ⓘ
Beef Stew
Chicken Stew
Frontier Soups ⓘ
Hungarian Goulash
New England Seaport Fisherman's Stew
Juanitas
Juanitas (All BUT Mole, Caldo de Pollo,
Chile Colorado, Chicken Veracruz,
Chile Verde, and Albondigas Soup)

TOMATO PASTE

Amore
Amore (All)
Bashas'
Tomato Paste Domestic
Contadina ⓘ
Flavored Tomato Paste (All BUT Italian
Tomato Paste with Italian Seasonings)
Tomato Paste
Del Monte ⓘ
Tomatoes & Tomato Products (All BUT
Spaghetti Sauce Flavored with Meat)
Food Club (Marsh)
Tomato Paste
Fresh & Easy ()
Tomato Paste
Great Value (Wal-Mart)
Tomato Paste
Haggen
Tomato Paste - Domestic
Hy-Vee
Tomato Paste
Meijer
Tomato Paste Domestic
Tomato Paste Organic
Pastene
Tomato Paste
Publix ()
GreenWise Market Organic Tomato
Paste

Tomato Paste

Redpack
Tomato Products (All)

S&W Fine Foods ⓘ
Tomato & Tomato Products

Winn-Dixie ◌
Tomato Paste

TOMATOES

Bashas'
Diced Tomatoes
Diced Tomatoes in Juice
Diced Tomatoes Italian
Diced Tomatoes Mexican
Stewed Tomatoes
Tomato Clam Juice Cocktail - Spicy Picante (bi-lingual)
Tomato Crushed in Puree
Tomato Sauce
Tomatoes - Diced - Petite
Tomatoes - Diced - Petite - Chipotle
Tomatoes - Diced - Petite with Sweet Onion
Tomatoes Diced Peeled with Green Chilies
Tomatoes Diced Petite
Tomatoes Diced Southwestern
Tomatoes Diced with Roasted Garlic & Onion
Tomatoes Whole Peeled

Bionaturae
Canned Tomatoes ☒

Bubbies ☒
Pickled Green Tomatoes

Cara Mia
Cara Mia Products (All)

Contadina ⓘ
Crushed Tomatoes (All)
Diced Tomatoes (All)
Stewed Tomatoes (All)
Tomato Puree
Tomato Sauces (All)
Whole Tomatoes

Dei Fratelli
Dei Fratelli (All BUT Tomato Soup)

Del Fuerte ⓘ
Tomato Sauce

Del Monte ⓘ
Tomatoes & Tomato Products (All BUT Spaghetti Sauce Flavored with Meat)

Eden Foods ⓘ ✓
Crushed Tomatoes - Organic
Crushed Tomatoes with Basil - Organic
Crushed Tomatoes with Onion & Garlic - Organic
Diced Tomatoes - Organic
Diced Tomatoes with Basil - Organic
Diced Tomatoes with Green Chilies - Organic
Diced Tomatoes with Roasted Onion - Organic
Whole Tomatoes - Organic
Whole Tomatoes with Basil - Organic

Food Club (Marsh)
Tomato Puree
Tomato Sauce
Tomatoes Crushed
Tomatoes Crushed In Puree
Tomatoes Diced
Tomatoes Diced - Chili Ready
Tomatoes Diced & Green Chilies
Tomatoes Diced & Green Chilies - Milder
Tomatoes Diced In Juice
Tomatoes Diced In Juice No Salt Added
Tomatoes Diced Petite
Tomatoes Diced with Onion - Chili Ready
Tomatoes Diced with Roasted Garlic & Onion
Tomatoes Petite Dice Peeled with Green Chilies
Tomatoes Stewed
Tomatoes Stewed Italian
Tomatoes Stewed Mexican
Tomatoes Whole Peeled

Fresh & Easy ◌
Crushed Tomatoes with Basil
Diced & Fire Roasted Tomatoes
Diced Tomatoes - No Salt Added
Diced Tomatoes - Organic
Diced Tomatoes - Regular

Diced Tomatoes with Garlic & Olive Oil
Diced Tomatoes with Jalapeno Peppers
Organic Italian Style Tomatoes
Stewed Tomatoes - Italian Style
Stewed Tomatoes - Regular
Sun Dried Tomatoes in Olive Oil
Sun Dried Tomatoes in Pesto
Tomato Sauce - Organic
Tomato Sauce - Regular
Whole Peeled Round Tomatoes - No Salt Added
Whole Peeled Round Tomatoes - Regular

Furmano's
Furmano's (All)

Great Value (Wal-Mart)
Chili Ready Tomatoes
Concentrated Crushed Tomatoes
Crushed Tomatoes In Puree
Diced No Salt Added Tomatoes
Diced Tomatoes In Tomato Juice
Italian Diced Tomatoes
Italian Stewed Tomatoes
Italian Stewed Tomatoes w/Basil, Garlic, & Oregano
Mexican Hot Style Tomato Sauce, Bilingual
No Salt Added Diced Tomatoes
No Salt Added Tomato Sauce
Pear Tomato Strips
Pear Tomato Strips w/Basil In Puree
Petite Diced Tomatoes
Sliced Stewed Tomatoes In Tomato Juice
Tomato Puree
Tomato Sauce
Whole Peeled Pear Tomatoes
Whole Tomatoes
Whole Tomatoes In Tomato Juice

Haggen
Tomato Juice
Tomato Sauce
Tomato Sauce - No Salt Added
Tomatoes - Crushed in Puree
Tomatoes - Diced
Tomatoes - Diced Italian
Tomatoes - Diced No Salt

Tomatoes - Diced Peeled w/Green Chilies
Tomatoes - Diced Petite
Tomatoes - Stewed
Tomatoes - Stewed Italian
Tomatoes - Stewed Mexican
Tomatoes - Whole Peeled
Tomatoes - Whole Peeled No Salt
Tomatos - Diced Juice

Hanover Foods ⓘ
Superfine Tomatoes w/Okra
Tomato Juice
Tomato Puree
Tomato Sauce

Hy-Vee
Crushed Italian Style Tomatoes
Diced Tomatoes
Diced Tomatoes - Chili Ready
Diced Tomatoes with Chilies
Diced Tomatoes with Roasted Garlic & Onions
Italian Style Diced Tomatoes
Italian Style Stewed Tomatoes
Original Diced Tomatoes & Green Chilies
Petite Cut Diced Tomatoes
Petite Cut Diced Tomatoes with Garlic & Olive Oil
Petite Cut Diced Tomatoes with Sweet Onion
Petite Diced Tomatoes
Stewed Tomatoes
Tomato Sauce
Whole Peeled Tomatoes

L'Esprit de Campagne
Dried Tomato Products

Lucini Italia () ✔
Lucini Italia (All BUT Russian Tomato Vodka Sauce and Minestrone Soup)

Meijer
Diced Tomatoes
Diced Tomatoes Chili Ready
Diced Tomatoes in Italian
Diced Tomatoes in Juice
Diced Tomatoes Organic
Stewed Tomatoes
Stewed Tomatoes Italian

Stewed Tomatoes Mexican
Tomato Puree
Tomato Sauce
Tomato Sauce - Organic
Tomatoes - Diced with Green Chiles
Tomatoes - Petite Diced
Tomatoes - Whole Peeled
Tomatoes - Whole Peeled No Salt
Tomatoes - Whole Peeled Organic
Tomatoes Crushed in Puree
Tomatoes with Basil, Organic

Midwest Country Fare (Hy-Vee)
Tomato Sauce

Pastene
California Tomatoes - Whole Peeled
  with Basil
Chateau Tomato Sauce
Diced Tomatoes with Green Chilis
Italian Tomatoes
Kitchen Ready
Kitchen Ready - Chunky
Kitchen Ready - No Salt
San Marzano Tomatoes
Sun Dried Tomato Halves
Sun Dried Tomato Pesto
Sun Dried Tomatoes - Julienne Cut

Publix ()
GreenWise Market Organic Crushed
  Tomatoes
GreenWise Market Organic Diced
  Tomatoes, Basil, Garlic, and Oregano
GreenWise Market Organic Diced
  Tomatoes, Regular
GreenWise Market Organic Tomato
  Sauce
Tomato Sauce
Tomatoes - Crushed
Tomatoes - Diced with Green Chilies
Tomatoes - Diced with Roasted Garlic
  & Onion
Tomatoes - Peeled Whole
Tomatoes - Sliced, Stewed

Raley's
Diced Tomatoes

Rao's Homemade ()
Rao's Homemade (All)

Red Gold
Tomato Products (All)

Redpack
Tomato Products (All)

S&W Fine Foods ⓘ
Tomato & Tomato Products (All)

Strub's
Strub's (All)

Tuttorosso
Tomato Products

Valu Time (Marsh)
Tomato Sauce

Winn-Dixie ()
Tomato Puree
Tomato Sauce
Tomatoes, Crushed
Tomatoes, Diced
Tomatoes, Diced with Green Chilies
Tomatoes, Italian Style Stewed
Tomatoes, Mexican Style Stewed
Tomatoes, Petite Diced
Tomatoes, Sliced Stewed
Tomatoes, Whole Peeled

VEGETABLES

Allens ⓘ
Canned Products (All)

Bashas'
Asparagus - Cut
Carrots - Sliced
Corn Cream Style
Corn Whole Kernel
Green Beans - Blue Lake Cut
Green Beans, Blue Lake French Style
Hominy Gold
Hominy White
Mushroom Stems & Pieces - No Salt
  Added
Mushrooms Sliced (Jar)
Mushrooms Stems & Pieces
Mushrooms Whole
Peas - Sweet Ungraded
Spinach, Cut Leaf
White Potatoes Sliced

Bruce Foods
Bruce's Cut Okra

Bruce's Cut Okra and Tomatoes
Bruce's Okra, Tomatoes, and Corn
Cut Yams
Whole Yams

Bush's Best
Bush's Best Products (All BUT
Chili Magic Chili Starter Line and
Homestyle Chili Line)

Cara Mia
Cara Mia Products (All)

Central Market Classics (Price Chopper)
Green Asparagus

Colavita
Vegetables in Oil (All)

Del Monte ⓘ
Canned Vegetables (All)

Embasa ⓘ
Sliced Carrots
Sliced Nopalitos
Whole Tomatillos

Food Club (Marsh)
Canned Asparagus Spears
Canned Beets - Sliced
Canned Corn - Crisp & Sweet
Canned Corn - Gold Cream Style
Canned Corn - Gold Whole Kernel
Canned Corn - Gold Whole Kernel, No Salt
Canned Corn - Whole Kernel, Gold & White
Canned Cut Green Beans
Canned Cut Green Beans - No Salt
Canned Cut Green Beans - Veri Green
Canned French Style Green Beans - Veri Green
Canned Green Beans - French Style - No Salt
Canned Mixed Vegetables
Canned Mixed Vegetables - No Salt
Canned Mushrooms - Stems & Pieces
Canned Mushrooms - Stems & Pieces, No Salt
Canned Peas & Sliced Carrots
Canned Potatoes - Sweet Cut (Yams)
Canned Potatoes - White, Sliced
Canned Sliced Carrots

Canned Spinach
Canned Whole Beets - Small
Canned Whole Potatoes - White, Small
Mushrooms Whole Jar
Mushrooms Whole Sliced Jar
Sliced, Pickled Beets (Glass)
Whole, Pickled Beets (Glass)

Fresh & Easy ⓞ
Artichoke Antipasta
Cut Green Beans - No Salt Added
Cut Green Beans - Regular
French-Style Green Beans
Mixed Vegetables
Sliced Beets
Sweet Peas - Organic
Sweet Peas - Regular
White Potatoes - Diced
White Potatoes - Whole
Whole Green Beans
Whole Kernel Corn

Freshlike ⓘ ✓
Canned Items (All)

Furmano's
Furmano's (All)

Glory Foods
Canned Vegetables (All)

Grand Selections (Hy-Vee)
Fancy Cut Green Beans
Fancy Whole Green Beans
Young, Early June Premium Peas

Great Value (Wal-Mart)
Asparagus Cut Spears
Asparagus Cuts & Tips
Blackeye Peas
Collard Greens
Cream Style Corn
Cream Style Sweet Corn
Crinkle Cut Carrots
Diced Potatoes
French Style Green Beans
Golden Sweet Whole Kernel Corn
Green Beans
Green Split Peas
Italian Cut Green Beans
Minced Garlic
Mustard Greens
No Salt Added Cut Green Beans

No Salt Added French Style Green Beans
No Salt Added Golden Sweet Whole Kernel Corn
No Salt Added Sweet Peas
Nopalitos Sliced Tender Cactus, Bilingual
Peas & Carrots
Pieces & Stems Mushrooms
Sliced Beets
Sliced Carrots
Sliced Mushrooms
Sliced New Potatoes
Sliced Pickled Beets
Sweet Corn
Sweet Peas
Turnip Greens
White Hominy
Whole Green Beans
Whole Kernel Golden Corn
Whole Leaf Spinach
Whole New Potatoes
Whole Spear Asparagus
Yellow Hominy

Haggen
Beets Whole
Carrots Sliced
Corn Gold Cream Style
Corn Gold Whole Kernel
Corn Super Sweet
Cut Green Beans
Cut Green Beans No Salt
French Style Green Beans
Peas - Blended No Salt
Peas - Sweet
Potatoes - Whole Small
Sliced Beets
Sliced Pickled Beets
Spinach
Vegetables Mixed
Wax Cut Beans

Hanover Foods ⓘ
Blue Lake Cut Green Beans
Blue Lake Cut Green Beans and Whole Potatoes (in Ham Flavored Sauce)
Sliced White Potatoes
Small Whole White Potatoes

Superfine Triple Succotash
Vegetable Salad
Whole Boiled Onions

HealthMarket (Hy-Vee)
Organic Cut Green Beans
Organic French Cut Green Beans
Organic Sweet Peas
Organic Whole Kernel Corn

Hy-Vee
Cut Green Beans
Fancy Diced Beets
Fancy Sliced Beets
French Style Green Beans
Green Split Peas
Mixed Vegetables
Mushrooms Stems & Pieces
Sliced Carrots
Sliced Mushrooms
Sliced Water Chestnuts
Sweet Peas
Whole Green Beans
Whole Kernel Golden Corn
Whole Kernel White Sweet Corn

Juanitas
Juanitas (All BUT Mole, Caldo de Pollo, Chile Colorado, Chicken Veracruz, Chile Verde, and Albondigas Soup)

Kroger ⓘ
Plain Canned Vegetables

Las Palmas
Crushed Tomatillos

Litehouse
Freeze-Dried Mushrooms

Meijer
Asparagus Cuts & Tips
Beets - Harvard Sweet Sour
Beets - Sliced
Beets - Sliced, No Salt
Beets - Sliced, Pickled
Beets - Whole Medium
Beets - Whole Pickled
Carrots - Sliced
Carrots - Sliced, No Salt
Chilies - Diced Mild Mexican Style
Corn - Cream Style
Corn - Golden Sweet Organic
Corn - Whole Kernel Crisp and Sweet

Corn - Whole Kernel Golden
Corn - Whole Kernel Golden No Salt
Corn - Whole Kernel White
Green Beans - Cut
Green Beans - Cut Blue Lake
Green Beans - Cut No Salt
Green Beans - Cut Organic
Green Beans - Cut Veri Green
Green Beans - French Blue Lake
Green Beans - French No Salt
Green Beans - French Organic
Green Beans - French Style
Green Beans - French Veri Green
Green Beans - Whole
Hominy - White
Kale Greens - Chopped
Mixed Vegetables
Mushrooms - Sliced
Mushrooms - Stems & Pieces
Mushrooms - Stems & Pieces No Salt
Mushrooms - Whole
Mustard Greens - Chopped
Peas & Sliced Carrots
Pimentos - Pieces
Pimentos - Sliced
Spinach
Spinach - Cut Leaf
Spinach - No Salt
Sweet Peas
Sweet Peas - No Salt
Sweet Peas - Organic
Sweet Potatoes Cut
Turnip Greens, Chopped
Wax Beans Cut
White Potatoes - Sliced
White Potatoes - Whole

Midwest Country Fare (Hy-Vee)
Cream Style Golden Corn
Cut Green Beans
French Style Green Beans
Mushrooms No Salt Added Stems &
   Pieces
Mushrooms Stems & Pieces
Sweet Peas
Whole Kernel Golden Corn

Native Forest ✓
Artichoke Hearts - Marinated

Artichoke Hearts - Quartered
Artichoke Hearts - Whole
Green Asparagus Cuts & Tips
Green Asparagus Spears
Organic Baby Corn
Organic Bamboo Shoots
Organic Hearts of Palm
Organic Mushroom Pieces & Stems

Pastene
Marinated Mushrooms

Princella Sweet Potatoes ⓘ ✓
Canned Items (All)

Publix ⟨⟩
Beets
Carrots
Corn - Cream Style Golden
Corn - Whole Kernel Golden Sweet
Green Beans
Green Beans - Veggi-Green
GreenWise Market Organic Green
   Beans
GreenWise Market Organic Sweet Peas
GreenWise Market Organic Whole
   Kernel Corn
Mixed Vegetables
Potatoes - White
Spinach
Sweet Peas
Sweet Peas - Small

Raley's
Artichoke Hearts
Cut Spinach
Peas & Diced Carrots
Whole Asparagus Spears
Whole Kernel Corn

Rao's Homemade ⟨⟩
Rao's Homemade (All)

Royal Prince Sweet Potatoes ⓘ ✓
Canned Items (All)

S&W Fine Foods ⓘ
Canned Vegetables (All)
Pickled Beets

Sabrett
Onions

Santa Barbara Olive Co.
Santa Barbara Olive Co. (All BUT Pasta
   Sauce and Salsa)

Sun Luck
- Baby Corn - Cut - Stir Fry
- Baby Corn - Whole

Teasdale
- Hominy (All)

Trappey
- Okra

Trappey's ⓘ ✓
- Canned Items (All)

Valu Time (Marsh)
- Canned - Cut Green Beans
- Canned - French Style Cut Green Beans
- Canned - Short Cut Green Beans
- Canned Beans - Hominy-White
- Canned Beans - Hominy-Yellow
- Canned Carrots - Sliced
- Canned Gold Corn - Cream Style
- Canned Gold Corn - Whole Kernel
- Canned Potatoes White Small Whole
- Canned Sweet Peas
- Canned Turnip Greens Chopped
- Canned Vegetables Mixed

Veg-All ⓘ ✓
- Canned Items (All)

Winn-Dixie ()
- Beets
- Carrots - Length Cut
- Carrots - Sliced
- Corn - White Whole Kernel
- Corn - Yellow Whole Kernel
- Corn - Yellow Whole Kernel - No Salt Added
- Green Beans - Cut
- Green Beans - French Style Sliced
- Green Beans - Whole
- Mixed Vegetables
- Mixed Vegetables - No Salt Added
- Peas - Green
- Peas - No Salt Added
- Spinach
- Spinach - No Salt Added
- White Potatoes - No Salt Added (Whole)
- White Potatoes (Dried, Sliced, & Diced)

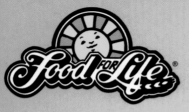

Start your day with

GLUTEN FREE
ENGLISH MUFFINS

Made with Organic Brown Rice

- Fork Split
- No Added Oil

Available at natural & specialty food stores in the frozen section.

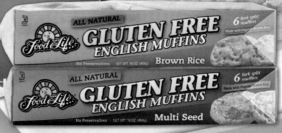

ALL NATURAL
GLUTEN FREE ENGLISH MUFFINS
6 fork split muffins
Made with Organic Brown Rice
No Preservatives   NET WT. 16 OZ (454g)
Brown Rice

ALL NATURAL
GLUTEN FREE ENGLISH MUFFINS
6 fork split muffins
Made with Organic Brown Rice
No Preservatives   NET WT. 16 OZ (454g)
Multi Seed

(800) 797-5090
www.foodforlife.com

Food For Life Baking Co., Inc. • P.O. Box 1434 • Corona, CA 92878-1434

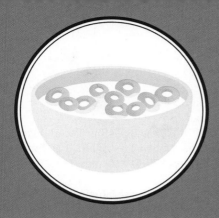

BREAD, CEREAL, PASTA, etc.

BREAD

Against the Grain
Against the Grain (All)

Bi Aglut
Bi Aglut (All)

Ener-G
Brown Rice English Muffins with Flax
Brown Rice Hamburger Buns
Brown Rice Loaf
Corn Loaf

- Egg Free Raisin Loaf
- English Muffins
- Four Flour Loaf
- Hi Fiber Loaf
- Light Brown Rice Loaf
- Light Tapioca Loaf
- Light White Rice Flax Loaf
- Light White Rice Loaf
- Papas Loaf
- Rice Starch Loaf
- Seattle Brown Loaf

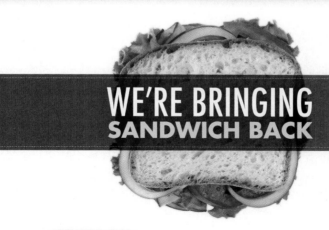

Seattle Hamburger Buns
Seattle Hot Dog Buns
Tapioca Dinner Rolls
Tapioca Hamburger Buns
Tapioca Hot Dog Bun
Tapioca Loaf
White Rice Flax Loaf
White Rice Hamburger Buns
White Rice Loaf
Yeast Free Brown Rice Loaf
Yeast Free White Rice Loaf

Enjoy Life Foods
Cinnamon Raisin Bagels
Classic Original Bagels

Food for Life
Gluten-Free English Muffins
Wheat & Gluten-Free Bhutanese Red
Rice Bread
Wheat & Gluten-Free Brown Rice Bread
Wheat & Gluten-Free China Black Rice
Bread
Wheat & Gluten-Free Millet Bread

Wheat & Gluten-Free Raisin Pecan
Bread
Wheat & Gluten-Free Rice Almond
Bread
Wheat & Gluten-Free Rice Pecan Bread
Wheat & Gluten-Free White Rice Bread
Yeast-Free, Wheat & Gluten-Free Brown
Rice Bread
Yeast-Free, Wheat & Gluten-Free Fruit
& Seed Medley Rice Bread
Yeast-Free, Wheat & Gluten-Free Multi
Seed Rice Bread

Foods by George
English Muffins - Cinnamon Currant
English Muffins - No-Rye Rye
English Muffins - Plain

French Meadow Bakery
Gluten-Free Cinnamon Raisin Bread
Gluten-Free Honey Multigrain Bread
Gluten-Free Italian Baked Roll
Gluten-Free Sandwich Bread

Gillian's Foods
Cinnamon Raisin Loaf

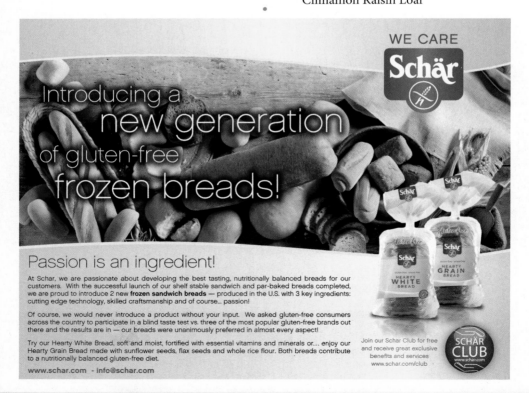

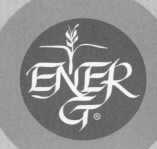
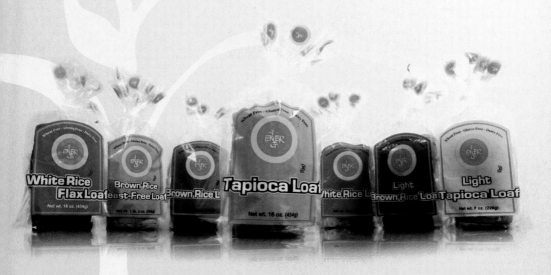

Gluten Free, Goodness Loaded

Rudi's Gluten-free Bakery bread is certified GF but very worthy of your ♡.

Each delicious slice has real fresh-bread taste to make the whole ✲✲ happy,

bring a ☺ to your day and add ☼ to your life.

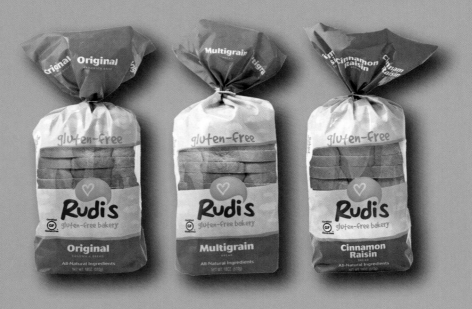

All-natural and organic ingredients.   ♡   No artificial chemicals or preservatives.

Tastes like real bread because it is real bread.

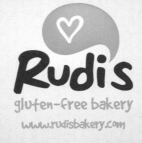

gluten-free bakery

www.rudisbakery.com

Certified
GF
Gluten-Free

French Loaf
Rye No Rye Loaf
Sandwich Loaf

Glutino

Premium Cinnamon & Raisin Bread
Premium Cinnamon 'n Raisin Bagels
Premium Cornbread
Premium English Muffins
Premium Fiber Bread
Premium Flax Seed Bread
Premium Multigrain Bagels
Premium Plain Bagels
Premium Poppy Seed Bagels
Premium Sesame Bagels

Grainless Baker, The

The Grainless Baker (All)

Joan's GF Great Bakes

Joan's Corn Bread
Joan's Italian Bread
Joan's Pumpernickel Raisin Rolls
Joan's Sandwich Rolls

Katz Gluten Free

Gluten Free Dinner Rolls (Small Challah)
Gluten Free Kaiser Rolls (Large Challah)
Gluten Free Oat Challah Rolls
Gluten Free Round Challah
Gluten Free Round Raisin Challah
Gluten Free Sandwich Rolls
Gluten Free Sliced Challah Bread
Gluten Free White Bread
Gluten Free Whole Grain Bread
Gluten Free Wholesome Bread

Kinnikinnick Foods

Brown Sandwich Bread
Cheese Tapioca Rice Bread
Italian White Tapioca Rice Bread
Many Wonder Multigrain Rice Bread
Raisin Tapioca Rice Bread
Robins Honey Brown Rice Bread
Sunflower Flax Rice Bread
Tapioca Rice Bread
White Sandwich Bread

Lydia's Organics

Lydia's Organics (All)

Mariposa Baking Company

Bagels - Plain
Bagels - Sesame
Focaccia
Multi-Grain Bread
Rosemary Rolls
Sandwich Bread

Nature's Own

Gluten Free Extra Fiber White
Gluten Free Healthy Multi-Grain

Orgran

Crispibread Range (All)
Multigrain Crispibread with Quinoa

Outside the Breadbox

Outside the Breadbox (All)

Rudi's Gluten-Free Bakery

Gluten-Free Cinnamon Raisin
Gluten-Free Multigrain
Gluten-Free Original

Schar

Baguettes Par-Baked
Ciabatta Par-Baked Rolls
Classic White Bread (Shelf stable)
Classic White Rolls (Shelf stable)
Hearty Grain Bread (Frozen)
Hearty White Bread (Frozen)
Italian Breadsticks
Multigrain Bread (Shelf stable)
Sub Sandwich Par-Baked Rolls

Smart Treat

Smart Treat (All)

Udi's Gluten Free Foods

Plain Bagels
White Sandwich Bread Loaf
Whole Grain Bread Loaf

Whole Foods Gluten-Free Bakehouse

Cinnamon Raisin Bread
Cornbread
Hamburger Buns
Honey Oat Bread
Light White Bread
Prairie Bread
Sandwich Bread
Sundried Tomato & Roasted Garlic Bread

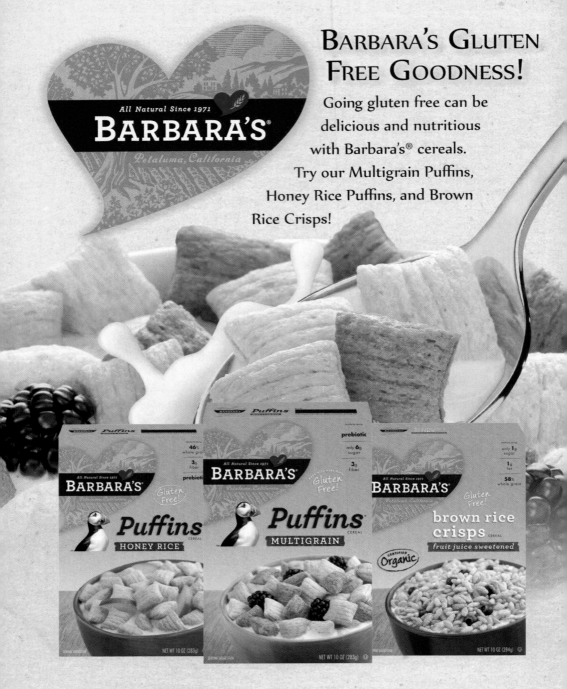

BARBARA'S GLUTEN FREE GOODNESS!

Going gluten free can be delicious and nutritious with Barbara's® cereals. Try our Multigrain Puffins, Honey Rice Puffins, and Brown Rice Crisps!

Since 1971, we've been making great tasting 100% natural foods – free of artificial colors, preservatives or additives. Because that's Barbara's way.

Find us in the natural aisle at your local store and online at BarbarasBakery.com

Cereal & Granola

Arrowhead Mills ✓
- Maple Buckwheat Flakes Cereal
- Rice & Shine Hot Cereal
- Rice Flakes Sweetened Cereal
- Yellow Corn Grits

Bakery on Main ✓
- Apple Raisin Walnut Snack Size Gluten-Free Granola
- Cinnamon Raisin Fiber Power Gluten-Free Granola
- Extreme Fruit & Nut Family Size Gluten-Free Granola
- Extreme Fruit & Nut Snack Size Gluten-Free Granola
- Gluten-Free Apple Raisin Walnut
- Gluten-Free Cranberry Orange Cashew Granola
- Gluten-Free Extreme Fruit & Nut
- Gluten-Free Nutty Maple Cranberry Granola
- Gluten-Free Rainforest Granola
- Nutty Cranberry Maple Family Size Gluten-Free Granola
- Nutty Cranberry Maple Snack Size Gluten-Free Granola
- Triple Berry Fiber Power Gluten-Free Granola

Barbara's Bakery ⓘ ✓
- Brown Rice Crisps
- Honey Rice Puffins Cereal
- Multigrain Puffins

Bashas'
- Grits Quick

Bob's Red Mill 🍴 ✓
- Creamy Brown Rice Farina
- GF Mighty Tasty Hot Cereal
- Organic Brown Rice Farina
- Organic Creamy Buckwheat
- Soy Grits

Chex ✓
- Chocolate Chex
- Cinnamon Chex
- Corn Chex
- Honey Nut Chex

TO TRY IT IS TO LOVE IT

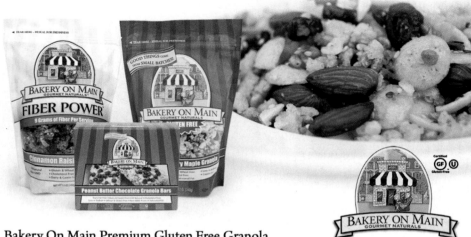

Bakery On Main Premium Gluten Free Granola

Delightfully Addictive • Certified Gluten Free • Kosher OU Parve • All Natural • Non GMO
Free from Wheat, Gluten, Dairy, Casein, Trans Fat & Cholesterol • Low in Sodium & Saturated fat

SAVE $1.50 when you join the club at www.bakeryonmain.com & LOVE IT MORE

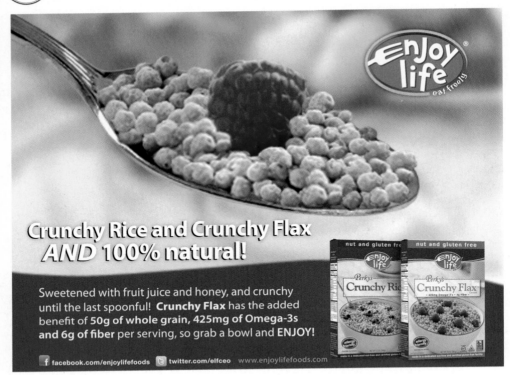

Crunchy Rice and Crunchy Flax AND 100% natural!

Sweetened with fruit juice and honey, and crunchy until the last spoonful! **Crunchy Flax** has the added benefit of **50g of whole grain, 425mg of Omega-3s and 6g of fiber** per serving, so grab a bowl and **ENJOY!**

f facebook.com/enjoylifefoods t twitter.com/elfceo www.enjoylifefoods.com

Rice Chex

Cocoa Pebbles ⓘ ♈
Cocoa Pebbles

Cream of Rice
Cream of Rice

Eco-Planet ♈
Hot Cereals (All)

Enjoy Life Foods ♈ ✓
Cinnamon Crunch Granola
Cranapple Crunch Granola
Crunchy Flax Cereal
Crunchy Rice Cereal
Very Berry Crunch Granola

EnviroKidz ⓘ ✓
Amazon Frosted Flakes
Gorilla Munch
Koala Crisp
Leapin Lemurs
Peanut Butter Panda Puffs

Erewhon ⓘ ✓
Cocoa Crispy Brown Rice
Corn Flakes
Crispy Brown Rice - Gluten-Free

Crispy Brown Rice with Mixed Berries
Rice Twice
Strawberry Crisp

Fruity Pebbles ⓘ ♈
Fruity Pebbles

Glutenfreeda ♈
Granola (All)
Oatmeal (All)

Glutino
Apple Cinnamon Cereal
Berry Sensible Beginnings
Frosted Sensible Beginnings
Honey Nut Cereal
Sensible Beginnings

Hodgson Mill ♈
Buckwheat Hot Cereal with Milled Flax
Seed ✓

Kinnikinnick Foods ♈
Kinnikinnick Foods (All)

Lundberg Family Farms ♈ ✓
Purely Organic Hot Cereal

Lydia's Organics ♈
Lydia's Organics (All)

You'd be amazed how tasty gluten free can be after 25 years of practice.

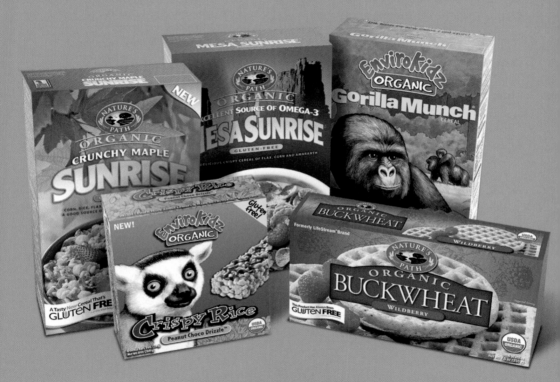

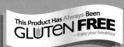
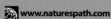 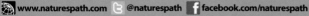

Malt-O-Meal ()
Fruity Dyno-Bites

Meijer
Grits Buttered Flavored Instant
Grits Quick

Nature's Path ⓘ ✓
Crispy Rice
Crunchy Maple Sunrise
Crunchy Vanilla Sunrise
Fruit Juice Cornflakes
Honey'd Cornflakes
Mesa Sunrise Flakes
Whole O's

Orgran ✓
100% Amaranth Puffed Breakfast Cereal
Multigrain Breakfast O's with Quinoa

Post ⓘ ⚱
Cupcake Pebbles Cereal

Smart Treat ⚱
Smart Treat (All)

Udi's Gluten Free Foods ⚱
Gluten Free Au Naturel Granola

Gluten Free Cranberry Granola
Gluten Free Original Granola
Gluten Free Vanilla Granola

Wolff's Kasha
Cream of Buckwheat

PASTA & NOODLES

Ancient Harvest
Gluten-Free Pasta ⚱

Andean Dream ⚱
Quinoa Pasta - Fusilli
Quinoa Pasta - Macaroni
Quinoa Pasta - Spaghetti

Annie Chun's
Pad Thai Rice Noodles - Original
Rice Noodles - Original

Bi Aglut
Bi Aglut (All)

Bionaturae
Gluten Free Elbows ⚱
Gluten Free Fusilli ⚱

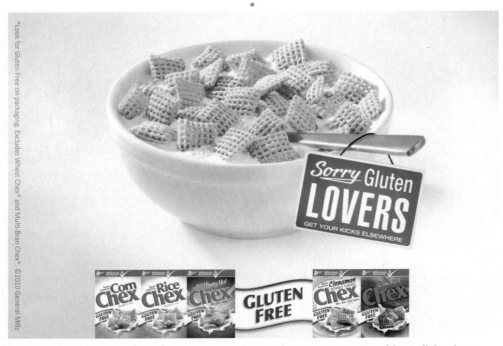

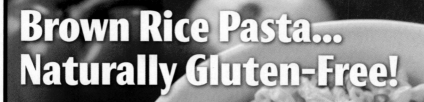

Brown Rice Pasta... Naturally Gluten-Free!

- 100% Organic

- 55g of Whole Grains per Serving

- Good Source of Fiber, 4g per Serving

- Made in a Gluten-Free Facility

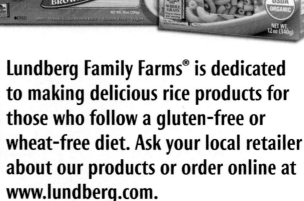

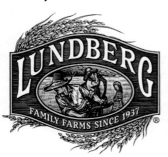

Lundberg Family Farms® is dedicated to making delicious rice products for those who follow a gluten-free or wheat-free diet. Ask your local retailer about our products or order online at www.lundberg.com.

Gluten Free Linguine 🙂
Gluten Free Rigatoni 🙂
Gluten Free Spaghetti 🙂
Gluten-Free Penne 🙂

DeBoles
Rice Angel Hair
Rice Fettuccine
Rice Lasagna
Rice Penne
Rice Spaghetti Style Pasta
Rice Spirals
Wheat Free Corn Elbow Style Pasta
Wheat Free Corn Spaghetti Style Pasta

Eden Foods ⓘ ✔
Bifun (Rice) Pasta
Kuzu Pasta
Mung Bean Pasta (Harusame)

Ener-G 🙂 ✔
White Rice Lasagna
White Rice Macaroni
White Rice Small Shells
White Rice Spaghetti
White Rice Vermicelli

Food for Life ✔
Wheat & Gluten-Free Rice Elbow Pasta

Fresh & Easy ()
Brown Rice Spaghetti
Brown Rice Spiral Rotini

Gillian's Foods 🙂
Gillian's Foods (All)

Gluten Free & FABULOUS ✔
Macaroni & Cheese

Heartland ⓘ ✔
Gluten-Free Fusilli
Gluten-Free Penne
Gluten-Free Spaghetti

Hodgson Mill 🙂
Gluten-Free Brown Rice Angel Hair
  with Milled Flaxseed ✔
Gluten-Free Brown Rice Elbows with
  Milled Flaxseed ✔
Gluten-Free Brown Rice Linguine with
  Milled Flaxseed ✔
Gluten-Free Brown Rice Penne with
  Milled Flaxseed ✔
Gluten-Free Brown Rice Spaghetti with
  Milled Flaxseed ✔

Lundberg Family Farms 🙂 ✔
Organic Elbow Pasta
Organic Penne Pasta
Organic Rotini Pasta
Organic Spaghetti Pasta

Manischewitz
Passover Noodles

Mrs. Leeper's
Mrs. Leeper's (All)

Namaste Foods 🙂
Pastas (All)

Notta Pasta
Notta Pasta (All)

Orgran ✔
Essential Fibre Lasagnette
Essential Fibre Pasta Range (All)
Gourmet Pasta Range (All)
Rice & Corn Pasta Range (All)
Stoneground Pasta Range (All)
Supergrains Pasta Range (All)

Schar 🙂 ✔
Anellini
Fusilli
Multigrain Penne Rigate
Penne
Spaghetti
Tagliatelle

Taste of Thai, A
Taste of Thai, A (All)

Tinkyada
Gluten-Free Rice Pasta (All)

PIZZA CRUST

Against the Grain 🙂
Against the Grain (All)

Ener-G 🙂 ✔
Rice Pizza Shells
Yeast Free Rice Pizza Shells

French Meadow Bakery
Gluten-Free Pizza Crust

Gillian's Foods 🙂
Gillian's Foods (All)

Glutino
Premium Pizza Crusts

Grainless Baker, The ⛊
   The Grainless Baker (All)
Joan's GF Great Bakes ⛊
   Joan's GF Great Bakes (All)
Katz Gluten Free ⛊
   Katz Gluten Free (All)
Kinnikinnick Foods ⛊
   Kinnikinnick Foods (All)
Mariposa Baking Company ⛊ ✓
   10" Pizza Crusts
Namaste Foods ⛊
   Pizza Crust
Outside the Breadbox ⛊
   Outside the Breadbox (All)
Rustic Crust ✓
   Napoli Herb Gluten-Free Crust
Schar ⛊ ✓
   Pizza Crusts

POLENTA

Bob's Red Mill ⛊ ✓
   GF Corn Grits/Polenta
De La Estancia
   Polenta
Fresh & Easy ()
   Organic Polenta
Pastene
   Instant Polenta

POTATO, INSTANT & MIXES

Bashas'
   Potatoes - Instant Mashed
Edward & Sons ✓
   Cheesy Mashed Potato Mix
   Organic Home Style Mashed Potato Mix
   Organic Roasted Garlic Mashed Potato
      Mix
Food Club (Marsh)
   Potatoes Dried Hash Browns
   Potatoes Instant Mashed
Great Value (Wal-Mart)
   Au Gratin Potatoes
   Instant Mashed Potatoes
   Scalloped Potatoes In Creamy Sauce

Haggen
   Potatoes - Instant Mashed
Honest Earth
   Baby Reds
   Creamy Mashed
   Yukon Golds
Hy-Vee
   Four Cheese Mashed Potatoes
   Mashed Potatoes Real Russet Potatoes
   Roasted Garlic Mashed Potatoes
   Sour Cream & Chive Mashed Potatoes
Idahoan
   Au Gratin
   Baby Reds
   Baby Reds Garlic & Parmesan
   Butter & Herb
   Creamy Home Style
   Four Cheese
   Original Flakes
   Real
   Roasted Garlic
   Romano Cheese
   Scalloped
   Southwest
   Yukon Golds
Kroger ⓘ
   Plain Instant Potatoes
Meijer
   Potatoes - Hash Browns
   Potatoes - Instant Mashed
Potato Buds ✓
   Mashed Potatoes

RICE & RICE MIXES

AA Rice
   Plain Brown
   Plain Parboiled
   Plain White
Alter Eco Fair Trade
   Alter Eco Fair Trade (All) ⓘ
Annie Chun's
   Sprouted Brown Rice
   Sticky White Rice
Arrowhead Mills ✓
   Brown Rice, Basmati
   Brown Rice, Long Grain

Bashas'
- Rice - Brown Long Grain
- Rice - Calrose Medium Grain
- Rice - Instant
- Rice - Instant Brown

Blue Ribbon Golden
- Plain Rice

Blue Ribbon Rice
- Plain Rice

Carolina Rice
- Authentic Spanish Rice
- Basmati Rice
- Broccoli Cheese Rice
- Brown Rice (Whole Grain)
- Gold (Parboiled)
- Jasmine Rice
- Long Grain & Wild Rice
- Saffron Yellow Rice
- White Rice

Casa Fiesta
- Mexican Style Rice
- Mexican Style Rice Style Mix

Colusa Rose Rice
- Plain Rice

Comet Rice
- Plain Rice

Dragon Rice
- Plain Rice

Eden Foods ⓘ ✔
- Brown Rice & Mugwort Mochi
- Sprouted Brown Rice Mochi
- Sweet Brown Rice Mochi
- Wild Rice

Fantastic World Foods
- Arborio Rice
- Basmati Rice
- Jasmine Rice

Food Club (Marsh)
- Rice Instant
- Rice Instant Brown

Fresh & Easy ()
- Arborio Rice
- Calrose Rice
- Instant Boil-In Bag Brown Rice
- Instant Brown Rice
- Instant Rice

- Jasmine Rice
- Long Grain Brown Rice
- Long Grain White Rice
- Medley Rice

Glutino
- Whole Grain Brown Rice with Prebiotics
- Whole Grain Brown Rice with Prebiotics HOMESTYLE

GoGo Rice
- Organic Brown Rice
- Organic Quinoa
- Organic Rice Medley
- Organic White Rice
- Sprouted Brown Rice

Great Value (Wal-Mart)
- Brown Rice
- Enriched Long Grain Rice, Extra Fancy
- Parboiled Rice

Green Peacock Rice
- Plain Rice

Haggen
- Bagged Brown Rice
- Long Grain Brown Rice
- Long Grain Rice
- Rice - Instant
- Rice - Instant Brown

Hy-Vee
- Boil-In-Bag Rice
- Enriched Extra Long Grain Rice
- Enriched Long Grain Instant Rice
- Extra Long Grain Rice
- Instant Brown Rice
- Natural Long Grain Brown Rice
- Spanish Rice - Canned

Konriko
- Aix En Provence Brown Rice (Box)
- Artichoke Brown Rice Mix (Box)
- Hot 'n Spicy Brown Rice Pilaf (Box)
- Original Brown Rice
- Wild Pecan Rice

Lotus Foods
- Rice (All)

Louisiana Fish Fry ()
- Dirty Rice Mix
- Jambalaya Mix

Lundberg Family Farms ⛟ ✓

    Heat & Eat Organic Bowls - Country Wild

    Heat & Eat Organic Bowls - Long Grain

    Heat & Eat Organic Bowls - Short Grain

    Olde World Pilaf

    Risotto - Butternut Squash

    Risotto - Cheddar Broccoli

    Risotto - Creamy Parmesan

    Risotto - Garlic Primavera

    Risotto - Italian Herb

    Risotto - Organic Alfredo

    Risotto - Organic Florentine

    Risotto - Organic Tuscan

    Risotto - Organic Wild Porcini Mushroom

    Roasted Brown Rice CousCous - Mediterranean Curry

    Roasted Brown Rice CousCous - Plain Original

    Roasted Brown Rice CousCous - Roasted Garlic and Olive Oil

    Roasted Brown Rice CousCous - Savory Herb

Luzianne

    Jambalaya Dinner Kit

Mahatma

    Authentic Spanish Rice

    Basmati Rice

    Broccoli Cheese Rice

    Gold (Parboiled) Rice

    Jasmine Rice

    Long Grain & Wild Rice

    Valencia (Short Grain) Rice

    White Rice

    Whole Grain Brown Rice

    Yellow Rice

Meijer

    Rice - Brown

    Rice - Instant

    Rice - Instant Boil in a Bag

    Rice - Instant Brown

    Rice - Long Grain

    Rice - Medium Grain

Midwest Country Fare (Hy-Vee)

    Pre-Cooked Instant Rice

Minute Rice

    Brown Rice

    Premium White Rice

    Ready to Serve Brown & Wild Rice

    Ready to Serve Brown Rice

    Ready to Serve Chicken Rice Mix

    Ready to Serve Spanish Rice Mix

    Ready to Serve White Rice

    Ready to Serve Yellow Rice Mix

    White Rice

Ortega

    Saffron Yellow Rice

    Spanish Rice

Pastene

    Italian Arborio Rice

Publix ⟨⟩

    Long Grain Brown Rice

    Long Grain Enriched Rice

    Medium Grain White Rice

    Precooked Instant Boil in Bag

    Precooked Instant Brown Rice

    Precooked Instant White Rice

    Yellow Rice Mix

Success Rice

    Jasmine Rice

    White Rice

    Whole Grain Brown Rice

Sun Luck

    Jasmine Rice

    Long Grain Rice

    Niko Niko Brown Rice

    Niko Niko Calrose Rice

Taste of China, A

    Taste of China, A (All)

Taste of India, A

    Taste of India, A (All)

Taste of Thai, A

    Taste of Thai, A (All)

Tasty Bite

    Basmati Rice

    Brown Rice

    Jasmine Rice

    Long Grain Rice

    Mexican Fiesta Pilaf

    Pesto Pilaf

    Tandoori Pilaf

Uncle Ben's
Boil-In-Bag Whole Grain Brown Rice
Fast & Natural Whole Grain Instant
 Brown Rice
Natural Whole Grain Brown Rice
Ready Rice - Whole Grain Brown

TACO SHELLS

Bashas'
Taco Shells
Casa Fiesta
Taco Shells
Taco Shells, Jumbo
Taco Trays
Food Club (Marsh)
Taco Shells
Haggen
Taco Shells
Hy-Vee
Taco Shells
Meijer
Taco Shells
Mission Foods ☷
Corn Taco Shells (All)
Ortega
Hard Shells - Yellow & White
Tostada Shells
Whole Grain Taco Shells
Taco Bell ∿
Taco Shells

TORTILLAS & WRAPS

Chi-Chi's ⓘ
Corn Tortillas
Food for Life ✓
Wheat & Gluten Free Sprouted Corn
 Tortillas
Wheat & Gluten-Free Brown Rice
 Tortillas
French Meadow Bakery
Gluten-Free Tortilla
Fresh & Easy ⟨⟩
Corn Tortillas
Tostada Shells

Great Value (Wal-Mart)
Corn Tortillas
La Tortilla Factory ⓘ ✓
Smart & Delicious Teff Wraps
Sonoma Organic & All Natural Ivory
 Teff Wraps
Mission Foods ☷
Corn Gorditas (All)
Corn Sopes (All)
Corn Tortillas (All)
Corn Tostadas (All)
V & V Supremo
Sopes
Winn-Dixie ⟨⟩
Corn Tortillas

MISCELLANEOUS

Ener-G ☷ ✓
Communion Wafers

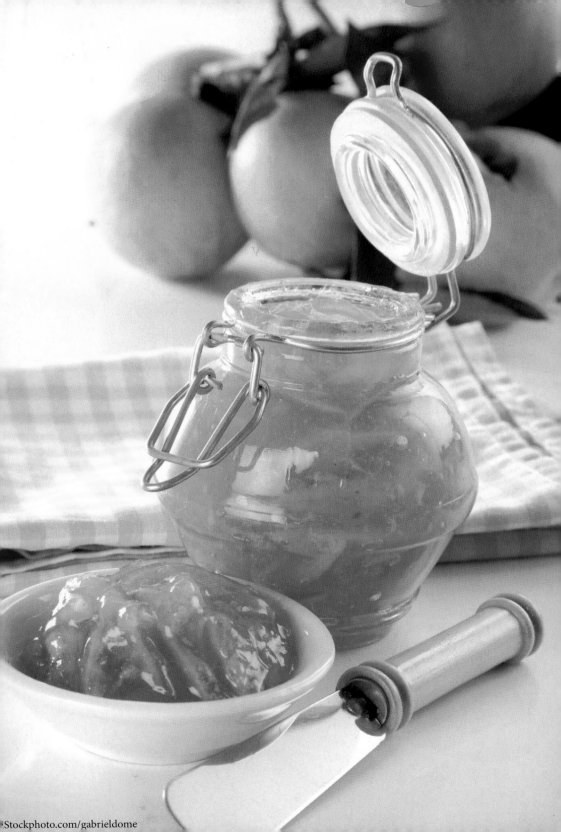

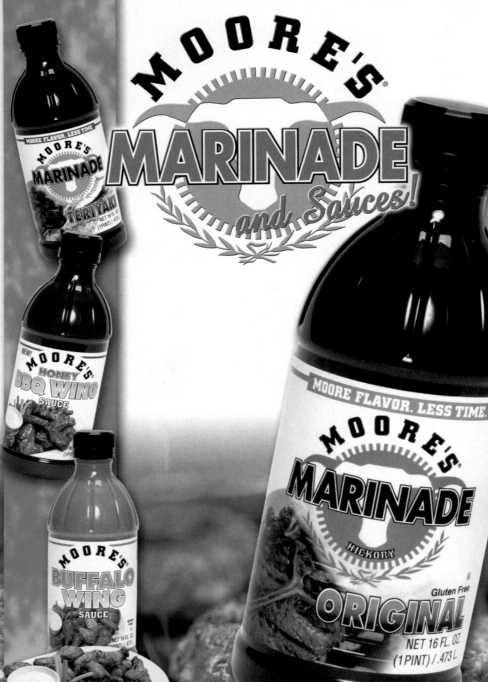

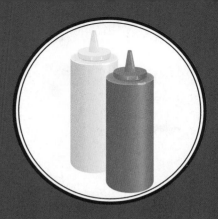

CONDIMENTS, SAUCES & DRESSINGS

ASIAN SAUCES, MISC.

Ah So Sauces
Chinese Rib Sauce
Chinese Style BBQ Squeeze
Duck Sauce
Mandarin Duck Sauce
Sweet & Sour Sauce

Bashas'
Teriyaki Sauce

China Pride
Duck Sauce

Chun's
Chili Lemongrass Sauce
Chili Vinegar Sauce
Fish Sauce
Sweet and Sour Sauce

Crystal
Teriyaki Sauce

Dai-Day Oriental Sauces
Duck Sauce
Garlic Sparerib Sauce
Hunan Hot Duck Sauce

Eden Foods ⓘ ✔
Dulse Flakes, Organic
Mirin (Rice Cooking Wine)
Ume Plum Vinegar

Fischer & Wieser
Asian Wasabi Plum Dipping Sauce

Fresh & Easy ⟨⟩
Spicy Stir Fry Sauce
Sweet & Sour Sauce

Gold's
Hot & Spicy Duck Sauce
Oriental Garlic Duck Sauce

Squeeze Wasabi Sauce
Sweet and Sour Duck Sauce

Jack Daniel's Sauces ⓘ
EZ Marinader - Teriyaki

Lee Kum Kee
Chili Garlic (All Sizes)
Choy Sun Oyster Flavored Sauce (In
Glass Bottles or Metal Cans)
Duck Sauce (All Sizes)
Gold Label Plum Sauce (All Sizes)
Plum Stir-Fry & Dipping Sauce (All
Sizes)

Mee Tu Oriental Sauces
BBQ Hoisin Sauce
Chinese Marinade
Duck Sauce
Light Teri-Yaki Sauce
Sparerib Sauce
Teri-Yaki Sauce

Moore's ⛾
Moore's Teriyaki Marinade

Organicville
Organicville (All)

Polynesian Sauces
Hoisin Sauce
Oyster Sauce

Premier Japan ✔
Organic Wheat-Free Hoisin
Organic Wheat-Free Teriyaki

San-J ⓘ ✔
Gluten Free Sweet and Tangy Sauce
Gluten Free Szechuan Sauce
Gluten Free Teriyaki Sauce
Gluten Free Thai Peanut Sauce

Saucy Susan
Peking Duck

Silver Spring ⓘ
Silver Spring (All)

Sun Luck
Black Bean Garlic Sauce
Mirin Sweet Cooking Wine
Plum Sauce
Sweet & Sour Sauce

Taste of Thai, A
Taste of Thai, A (All)

TryMe
Oyster & Shrimp Sauce

Asian, Soy & Tamari Sauces

Bashas'
Soy Sauce

Crystal
Soy Sauce

Eden Foods ⓘ ✓
Tamari Soy Sauce - Brewed in U.S. -
Organic
Tamari Soy Sauce - Imported - Organic

Fresh & Easy ⟨⟩
Organic Tamari Sauce

Hy-Vee
Soy Sauce

Mee Tu Oriental Sauces
Light Soy Sauce
Soy Sauce

San-J ⓘ ✓
Organic Gluten Free Reduced Sodium
Tamari Soy Sauce
Organic Gluten Free Tamari Soy Sauce

Bacon Bits

Great Value (Wal-Mart)
Imitation Bacon Bits

Hormel ⓘ
Bacon Bits, Pieces & Crumbles

Barbeque Sauce

Annie's Naturals ⓘ ✓
Organic Hot Chipotle
Organic Original Recipe
Organic Smokey Maple
Organic Sweet & Spicy

Bashas'
Barbecue Sauce - Hickory
Barbecue Sauce - Honey
Barbecue Sauce - Mesquite
Barbecue Sauce - Regular

Beano's ⟨⟩
Condiments (All)

Beverly Hillbillies, The
Elly May's Wild Mountain Honey BBQ
Sauce

Bone Suckin' Sauce ✓
Bone Suckin' Sauce - Hiccuppin' Hot
Bone Suckin' Sauce - Hot
Bone Suckin' Sauce - Hot Thicker Style
Bone Suckin' Sauce - Regular
Bone Suckin' Sauce - Thicker Style

Bull's-Eye ✍
Brown Sugar & Hickory Barbecue Sauce
Hickory Smoke Barbecue Sauce
Original Barbecue Sauce
Regional Carolina Style Barbecue Sauce
Regional Kansas City Style Barbecue
Sauce
Regional Memphis Style Barbecue Sauce
Regional Texas Style Barbecue Sauce
Sweet & Tangy Barbecue Sauce

Busha Browne ⚉
Busha Browne Products (All)

Cattlemen's Barbecue
Barbecue Sauce (All BUT Honey Flavor
& Southern Gold)

Dinosaur BBQ
Devil's Duel
Garlic Chipotle
Roasted Garlic Honey
Sensuous Slathering Sauce
Wango Tango

Follow Your Heart ⓘ ⚉ ✓
Unforgettable Balsamic Barbecue Sauce
- Mild

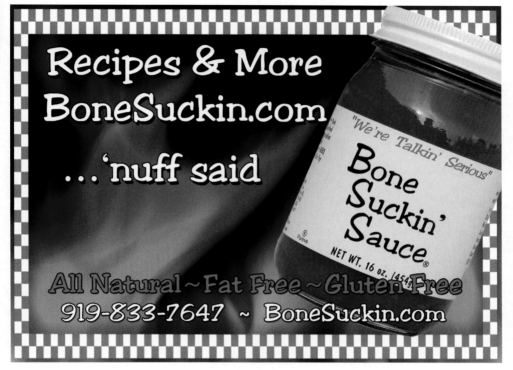

Unforgettable Balsamic Barbecue Sauce
- Spicy

Food Club (Marsh)
Hickory Bbq Sauce
Honey Bbq Sauce
Regular Bbq Sauce

Frank's
Mississippi BBQ Sauce

Fresh & Easy ()
Hickory BBQ Sauce
Honey BBQ Sauce
Hot & Spicy BBQ Sauce
Original BBQ Sauce
Whiskey BBQ Sauce

Golding Farms ()
Lexington Style Barbeque Dip

Gold's
Barbecue Sauce with Horseradish
New England Barbecue Sauce
Saucy Rib Sauce

Heinz ⓘ
Chicken & Rib BBQ Sauce
Garlic BBQ Sauce

Honey Garlic BBQ Sauce
Original BBQ Sauce

Hy-Vee
Hickory BBQ Sauce
Honey Smoke BBQ Sauce
Original BBQ Sauce

Jack Daniel's Sauces ⓘ
Hickory Brown Sugar BBQ Sauce
Honey Smokehouse BBQ Sauce
Original #7 BBQ Sauce
Spicy BBQ Sauce

Kraft Barbecue Sauce ⌇
Brown Sugar
Char-Grill
Hickory Smoke
Honey
Honey Hickory Smoke
Honey Mustard
Honey Roasted Garlic
Hot
Light Original
Mesquite Smoke
Original

Spicy Honey

Midwest Country Fare (Hy-Vee)
Hickory BBQ Sauce
Honey BBQ Sauce
Original BBQ Sauce

Nash Brothers
Organic Barbeque Sauce

Naturally Delicious ⓘ
Barbeque Sauce

Open Pit ⓘ
Original Char-Grill
Original Honey
Thick & Tangy Sweet

Organicville
Organicville (All)

Polynesian Sauces
Sparerib Sauce

Publix ()
Hickory BBQ Sauce
Honey BBQ Sauce
Original BBQ Sauce

Rio Grande
Steaksauce

San-J ⓘ ✓
Gluten Free Asian BBQ

Stubb's ⓘ ✓
Hickory Bourbon Bar-B-Q Sauce
Honey Pecan Bar-B-Q Sauce
Mild Bar-B-Q Sauce
Moppin' Sauce
Original Bar-B-Q Sauce
Smokey Mesquite Bar-B-Q Sauce
Spicy Bar-B-Q Sauce

Sweet Baby Ray's ()
Sweet Baby Ray's Barbeque Sauce (All)

CHOCOLATE SYRUP

Bashas'
Syrup - Chocolate

Bosco
Bosco Products (All)

Hershey's
Chocolate Syrup

Hy-Vee
Chocolate Flavored Syrup

Chocolate Syrup

Meijer
Syrup - Chocolate

Midwest Country Fare (Hy-Vee)
Chocolate Flavored Syrup

Nesquik ⓘ
Syrup (All Flavors)

Publix ()
Chocolate Syrup

CHUTNEYS

Busha Browne ♟
Busha Browne Products (All)

Crosse & Blackwell
Crosse & Blackwell (All BUT Plum
Pudding and Branston Pickle Relish)

COCKTAIL & SEAFOOD SAUCE

Cains ⓘ
Cocktail Sauce

Cajun's Choice
Cajun's Choice (All BUT Seasoned Fish
Fry and Creole Mustard)

Crosse & Blackwell
Crosse & Blackwell (All BUT Plum
Pudding and Branston Pickle Relish)

Food Club (Marsh)
Sauce Seafood Cocktail

Fresh & Easy ()
Cocktail Sauce

Golding Farms ()
Cocktail Sauce

Gold's
Cocktail Sauce

Heinz ⓘ
Cocktail Sauce (All Varieties)

Heluva Good
Cocktail Sauce

Hy-Vee
Cocktail Sauce For Seafood

Ken's Steak House Salad Dressing ()
Blue Label Cocktail Sauce
Green Label Cocktail Sauce

Little River ()
Cocktail Sauce
Louisiana Fish Fry ()
Cocktail Sauce
Seafood Sauce
Naturally Fresh ()
Seafood Cocktail
Seafood Dipping Sauce
Silver Spring ⓘ
Silver Spring (All)
Texas Pete
Seafood Sauce ⵑ
Woeber
Woeber (All)

CROUTONS

Ener-G ⵑ ✓
Plain Croutons
Gillian's Foods ⵑ
Gillian's Foods (All)

DESSERT SYRUPS, SAUCES & GLAZES

Hy-Vee
Strawberry Syrup
Litehouse
Peach Glaze
Strawberry Glaze
Sugar Free Strawberry Glaze
Marzetti
Blueberry Glaze
Glaze for Strawberries
Peach Glaze
Sugar Free Strawberry Glaze
Mrs. Richardson's
Toppings (All)
Sweet'N Low
Sweet'N Low (All)

DIP & DIP MIXES - SAVORY

Axelrod
Sour Cream with Onion Dip
Bashas'
Mix - Ranch Party Dip

Cabot
Cabot Products (All)
Casa Fiesta
Black Bean Dip
Jalapeno Beans Dip
Jalapeno Cheese Dip
Mexican Style Cheese Sauce
Cheez Whiz ⌇
Original Cheese Dip
Chi-Chi's ⓘ
Con Queso
Nacho Cheese Snackers
Crowley Foods
Sour Cream with Onion Dip
Emeril's
Classic Onion Dip
Guacamole Dip
Veggie Ranch Dip
Fischer & Wieser
Cilantro Pepito Pesto Appetizer Spread
Guacamole Starter - Just Add
Guacamole
Queso Starter - Just Add Cheese
Fresh & Easy ()
Antipasto Pesto Genovese
Black Bean & Corn Dip
Cuban Black Bean Dip
Fritos ⓘ
Bean Dip
Chili Cheese Dip
Hot Bean Dip
Jalapeno & Cheddar Flavored Cheese
Dip
Mild Cheddar Flavor Cheese Dip
Southwest Enchilada Black Bean
Flavored Dip
Great Value (Wal-Mart)
Homestyle Pimento Spread
Guiltless Gourmet
Bean Dips (All) ⵑ
Haggen
Medium Heat Bean Dip
Heluva Good
Bacon Horseradish
Bodacious Onion
Buttermilk Ranch

Fat Free French Onion
Fiesta Salsa
French Onion
Garlic Parmesan
Jalapeno Cheddar
Ranch
White Cheddar Bacon

Herr's
Bean Dip
Jalapeno Cheddar Dip
Mild Cheddar Dip
Salsa & Cheese Dip

Hy-Vee
Bacon & Cheddar Sour Cream Dip
French Onion Sour Cream Dip
Ranch & Dill Sour Cream Dip
Salsa Sour Cream Dip
Toasted Onion Sour Cream Dip
Vegetable Party Sour Cream Dip

Juanitas
Juanitas (All BUT Mole, Caldo de Pollo, Chile Colorado, Chicken Veracruz, Chile Verde, and Albondigas Soup)

Kraft Dips ⌒
Bacon & Cheddar
Creamy Ranch
French Onion
Green Onion
Guacamole Flavor

Lay's ⓘ
Creamy Ranch Dip
French Onion Dip
French Onion Flavored Dry Dip Mix
Green Onion Flavored Dry Dip Mix
Heavenly Baked Potato Flavored Dip
Ranch Flavored Dry Dip Mix

Litehouse
Avocado Dip
Dilly Dip
French Onion Dip
Garden Ranch Dip
Lite Dilly Dip
Ranch Dip
Ranch Veggie Dippers
Southwest Ranch Dip

Marzetti
Blue Cheese Veggie Dip

Dill Veggie Dip
Fat Free Dill Veggie Dip
Fat Free Ranch Veggie Dip
French Onion Veggie Dip
Guacamole Veggie Dip
Horseradish Veggie Dip
Light Dill Veggie Dip
Light French Onion Veggie Dip
Light Ranch Veggie Dip
Organic Ranch Veggie Dip
Ranch Veggie Dip
Spinach Veggie Dip

Naturally Fresh ()
Ranch Veggie Dip

Oberweis Dairy
Roasted Pepper Dip

Ortega
Nacho Cheese Sauce (Pouch)

Penn Maid
Creamy Salsa Dip
French Onion Dip
Ranch Dip
Southwestern Ranch

Prairie Farms
French Onion Dip

Publix ()
French Onion Dip
Green Onion Dip
Guacamole Dip

Ricos ✓
Cheese (All)

Road's End Organics ✓
Mild Nacho Chreese Dip
Spicy Nacho Chreese Dip

Sabra ()
Sabra (All)

Santa Barbara Salsa
Santa Barbara Salsa (All)

Tostitos ⓘ
Creamy Southwestern Ranch Dip
Creamy Spinach Dip
Monterey Jack Queso
Smooth & Cheesy Dip
Spicy Nacho Dip
Spicy Queso Supreme
Zesty Bean & Cheese Dip

Utz ⓘ
Cheddar & Jalapeno Dip
Mild Cheddar Cheese Dip
Wholly Guacamole ⅄
Guacamole (All)

DIP & DIP MIXES - SWEET

Litehouse
Chocolate Caramel
Cinnamon Caramel
Low Fat Caramel
Original Caramel
Reduced Sugar Caramel
Strawberry Yogurt Fruit Dip
Vanilla Yogurt Fruit Dip
Marzetti
Chocolate Fruit Dip
Cinnamon Caramel Apple Dip
Cream Cheese Fruit Dip
Fat Free Caramel Apple Dip
Light French Vanilla Yogurt Fruit Dip
Original Caramel Apple Dip
Peanut Butter Caramel Apple Dip
Strawberry Cream Cheese Fruit Dip
Saco
Saco (All)

FRUIT BUTTERS & CURDS

Bashas'
Apple Butter
Dickinson's
Dickinson's (All)
Eden Foods ⓘ ✓
Apple Butter - Organic
Apple Cherry Butter - Organic
Cherry Butter, Montmorency Tart - Organic
Fischer & Wieser
Peach Pecan Butter
Pecan Apple Butter
Great Value (Wal-Mart)
Spiced Apple Butter
MacKays
Curds (All BUT Picallili and Plum Chutney With Ale)

Manischewitz
Apple Butter
Simon Fischer
Apricot Butter
Prune Lekvar
Vermont Village ⅄
Apple Butter (All)
White House
White House (All)

GRAVY & GRAVY MIXES

Orgran ✓
Gravy Mix
Road's End Organics ✓
Organic Golden Gravy Mix
Organic Savory Herb Gravy Mix
Organic Shiitake Gravy Mix

HORSERADISH

Beano's ⟨⟩
Condiments (All)
Boar's Head
Condiments (All)
Bubbies ⅄
Beet Horseradish
Prepared Horseradish
Di Lusso ⓘ
Horseradish Sauce
Gold's
Hot Horseradish
Red Horseradish
Squeeze Horseradish Sauce
White Horseradish
Heinz ⓘ
Horseradish Sauce
Hellmann's
Spreads (All)
Heluva Good
Horseradish
Hy-Vee
Prepared Horseradish
Louisiana Hot Sauce
Chipotle Flavor Hot Sauce
Jalapeno Flavor Hot Sauce

Manischewitz
Horseradish (All)

Naturally Fresh ()
Dijon Horseradish

Penn Maid
Bacon Horseradish

Price Chopper
Beet Horseradish
White Horseradish

Saag's
Saag's (All BUT British Bangers)

Silver Spring ⓘ
Silver Spring (All)

Strub's
Strub's (All)

Thumann's ✓
Condiments (All BUT Deep Fry Hot Dogs)

Woeber
Woeber (All)

HOT SAUCE

Beano's ()
Condiments (All)

Buckeye Mustard Inc.
Buckeye Buffalo Wing Sauce

Busha Browne ♨
Busha Browne Products (All)

Cholula Hot Sauce
Cholula Hot Sauce (All)

Crystal
Hot Sauce
Wing Sauce

El Pinto ♨
El Pinto (All)

Fischer & Wieser
Four Star Black Raspberry Chipotle Sauce
Mango Ginger Habanero Sauce
Original Roasted Raspberry Chipotle Sauce, The
Papaya Lime Serrano Sauce
Pomegranate & Mango Chipotle Sauce
Roasted Blackberry Chipotle Sauce
Roasted Blueberry Chipotle Sauce

Food Club (Marsh)
Chili Sauce
Louisiana Hot Sauce

Frank's RedHot
Buffalo Wings Sauce
Chile 'n Lime Hot Sauce
HOT Wings Sauce
Original RedHot Sauce
Sweet Chili Sauce
Sweet Heat BBQ Wings Sauce
Xtra Hot RedHot Sauce

Ginger People, The
Ginger Wasabi Sauce
Hot Ginger Jalapeno Sauce
Sweet Ginger Chili Sauce
Thai Green Curry Sauce

Great Value (Wal-Mart)
Chili Sauce
Louisiana Hot Sauce

Heinz ⓘ
Chili Sauce (All Varieties)

Huy Fong
Chili Garlic Sauce
Sambal Oelek
Sriracha Chili Sauce

Hy-Vee
Chili Sauce

Juanitas
Juanitas (All BUT Mole, Caldo de Pollo, Chile Colorado, Chicken Veracruz, Chile Verde, and Albondigas Soup)

Ken's Steak House Salad Dressing ()
Buffalo Wing Sauce Marinade

Kunzler
Hot Dog Chili Sauce

La Costena
La Costena (All BUT Jalapeno Hot Sauce)

La Victoria ⓘ
Jalapeno Hot Sauce
Salsa Brava Hot Sauce

Lee Kum Kee
Sambal Oelek Chili Sauce (All Sizes)
Sriracha Chili Sauce (All Sizes)
Sweet & Sour Sauce (All Sizes)

Louisiana Fish Fry ()
Hot Sauce

Louisiana Hot Sauce
Habanero Flavor Hot Sauce
LA Gold Hot Sauce
Louisiana Hot Sauce
Red Chili Flavor Hot Sauce
Roasted Garlic Flavor Hot Sauce

Meijer
Chili Sauce
Hot Dog Chili Sauce

Moore's
Moore's Buffalo Wing Sauce
Moore's Honey BBQ Wing Sauce

Nance's
Chili Sauce
Hot Wing Sauce
Mild Wing Sauce

Price Chopper
Hot Sauce

Santa Barbara Salsa
Santa Barbara Salsa (All)

Strub's
Strub's (All)

Stubb's
Original Wing Sauce

Sun Luck
Chili Garlic Sauce
Chili Sauce, Hot
Chili Sauce, Sweet

Tabasco
Chipotle Pepper Sauce
Garlic Basting Sauce
Garlic Pepper Sauce
Green Pepper Sauce
Habanero Pepper Sauce
New Orleans Style Sauce
Pepper Sauce

Taco Bell
Hot Sauce
Mild Hot Sauce

Tapatio
Tapatio Hot Sauce

Texas Pete
Buffalo Chicken Wing Sauce - Extra
Mild

Buffalo Chicken Wing Sauce - Hot
Buffalo Chicken Wing Sauce - Mild
Green Pepper Sauce
Hot Sauce - Garlic
Hot Sauce - Hotter
Hot Sauce - Original

Thumann's
Condiments (All BUT Deep Fry Hot
Dogs)

Trappey
Hot Sauces

TryMe
Yucatan Sunshine Habanero Sauce

Wizard's, The
Organic Hot Stuff

JAMS, JELLIES & PRESERVES

Bashas'
Concord Grape Jelly
Jelly - Apple
Jelly - Grape
Preserves - Apricot
Preserves - Blackberry Seedless
Preserves - Marmalade Orange
Red Raspberry Preserves
Strawberry Preserves

Bionaturae
Spreads (All)

Busha Browne
Busha Browne Products (All)

Crofter's
Crofter's (All)

Crosse & Blackwell
Crosse & Blackwell (All BUT Plum
Pudding and Branston Pickle Relish)

Dickinson's
Dickinson's (All)

Fischer & Wieser
Amaretto Peach Pecan Preserves
Apricot Orange Marmalade
Jalapeno Peach Preserves
Mild Green Jalapeno Jelly
Old Fashioned Peach Preserves
Red Hot Jalapeno Jelly
Southern Style Preserves

Strawberry Rhubarb Preserves
Whole Lemon & Fig Marmalade

Food Club (Marsh)
Grape Jam
Grape Jelly
Grape Jelly - Squeezable
Preserves Apricot
Preserves Marmalade Orange
Preserves Strawberry
Spread Strawberry Squeezable

Fragata
Fragata (All BUT Imitation Bacon Bits)

Fresh & Easy ()
Fig Spread

Ginger People, The
Ginger Spread

Hy-Vee
Apple Jelly
Apricot Preserves
Blackberry Jelly
Cherry Jelly
Cherry Preserves
Concord Grape Jelly
Concord Grape Preserves
Grape Jelly
Orange Marmalade
Peach Preserves
Red Plum Jelly
Red Raspberry Jelly
Red Raspberry Preserves
Strawberry Jelly
Strawberry Preserves

Knott's Berry Farms
Fruit Spreads

Kroger ⓘ
Jams
Jellies
Preserves

MacKays
Jams (All BUT Picallili and Plum
   Chutney With Ale)
Marmalades (All BUT Picallili and Plum
   Chutney With Ale)

Marsh
Jam Grape Concord

Meijer
Apple Jelly

Fruit Spread - Apricot
Fruit Spread - Blackberry
Fruit Spread - Red Raspberry
Fruit Spread - Strawberry
Grape Jam
Grape Jelly
Preserves - Apricot
Preserves - Blackberry Seedless
Preserves - Marmalade Orange
Preserves - Peach
Preserves - Red Raspberry
Preserves - Red Raspberry with Seeds
Preserves - Strawberry

Nash Brothers
Organic Jelly

Polaner
All Fruit
Sugar Free

Publix ()
Jams (All Flavors)
Jellies (All Flavors)
Preserves (All Flavors)

Smucker's
Fruit Spreads

Sorrell Ridge
100% Specialty Flavors - Black Cherry
100% Specialty Flavors - Black
   Raspberry
100% Specialty Flavors - Blackberry
100% Specialty Flavors - Cherry
100% Specialty Flavors - Plum Good
100% Specialty Flavors - Strawberry
   Rhubarb
100% Specialty Flavors - Wild Blueberry
100% Spreadable Fruit - Apricot
100% Spreadable Fruit - Boysenberry
100% Spreadable Fruit - Concord Grape
100% Spreadable Fruit - Orange
   Marmelade
100% Spreadable Fruit - Peach
100% Spreadable Fruit - Raspberry
100% Spreadable Fruit - Seedless
   Raspberry
100% Spreadable Fruit - Seedless
   Strawberry
100% Spreadable Fruit - Strawberry
Organic Apricot Fruit Spread

Organic Blueberry Fruit Spread
Organic Orange Marmelade Fruit
  Spread
Organic Raspberry Fruit Spread
Organic Strawberry Fruit Spread
St. Dalfour ⓘ
Fruit Conserves (All)
Valu Time (Marsh)
Jelly Grape
Preserves Strawberry
Welch's
Welch's (All)

KETCHUP

Annie's Naturals ⓘ ✓
Organic Ketchup
Bashas'
Ketchup
Ketchup - Squeeze
Ketchup Squeeze Upside Down Bottle
Sauce - Picante Medium
Del Monte ⓘ
Tomatoes & Tomato Products (All BUT
  Spaghetti Sauce Flavored with Meat)
Food Club (Marsh)
Ketchup
Ketchup Squeeze
Ketchup Squeeze Upside Down Bottle
Frank's
Frank's Ketchup
French's
Fancy Tomato Ketchup
Fresh & Easy ◌
Ketchup - Organic
Ketchup - Regular
Gold's
Ketchup with Horseradish
Great Value (Wal-Mart)
Ketchup
Haggen
Squeeze Ketchup (Upside Down &
  Regular)
Hanover Foods ⓘ
Catsup (Ketchup)

Heinz ⓘ
Hot Ketchup
Ketchup
No Sodium Added Ketchup
Organic Ketchup
Reduced Sugar Ketchup
Hy-Vee
Ketchup
Squeezable Thick & Rich Tomato
  Ketchup
Thick & Rich Tomato Ketchup
Meijer
Ketchup
Ketchup Squeeze
Tomato Ketchup - Organic
Midwest Country Fare (Hy-Vee)
Tomato Ketchup
Nature's Basket (Giant Eagle)
Organic Tomato Ketchup USDA
Organicville
Organicville (All)
Publix ◌
GreenWise Market Organic Ketchup
Ketchup
Red Gold
Tomato Products (All)
Valu Time (Marsh)
Ketchup Squeeze
Winn-Dixie ◌
Ketchup

MARASCHINO CHERRIES

Bashas'
Maraschino Cherry Red
Whole Maraschino Cherries with Stems
Fragata
Fragata (All BUT Imitation Bacon Bits)
Great Value (Wal-Mart)
Maraschino Cherries
Haggen
Maraschino Cherry - Red Plain
Maraschino Cherry - Red w/Stems
Hy-Vee
Red Maraschino Cherries
Red Maraschino Cherries with Stems

Mario
Mario (All BUT Imitation Bacon Bits)

Meijer
Maraschino Cherry Red
Maraschino Cherry Red with Stems

Midwest Country Fare (Hy-Vee)
Maraschino Cherries

Price Chopper
Cherries with Stems
Maraschino Cherries

Publix ()
Maraschino Cherries

Santa Barbara Olive Co.
Santa Barbara Olive Co. (All BUT Pasta Sauce and Salsa)

Thrifty Maid (Winn-Dixie) ()
Maraschino Cherries

Winn-Dixie ()
Maraschino Cherries

MARINADES & COOKING SAUCES

Annie's Naturals ⓘ ✓
Baja Lime Marinade
Roasted Garlic & Balsamic Marinade

Beverly Hillbillies, The
Granny's Peach 'n' Pepper Pourin' Sauce

Cains ⓘ
Franklin Italian Marinade

Central Market Classics (Price Chopper)
Burgundy Cooking Wine
Sherry Cooking Wine

Chun's
Sweet Chili Marinade

Contadina ⓘ
Sweet & Sour Sauce

Crosse & Blackwell
Crosse & Blackwell (All BUT Plum Pudding and Branston Pickle Relish)

Fischer & Wieser
!Especial! Pasilla Chile Finishing Sauce
All Purpose Vegetable & Meat Marinade
Charred Pineapple Bourbon Sauce
Plum Chipotle Grilling Sauce
Sweet & Savory Onion Glaze

Traditional Steak & Grilling Sauce

Follow Your Heart ⓘ ⓧ ✓
Unforgettable Balsamic Vinaigrette Sauce
Unforgettable Balsamic Vinaigrette Sauce - Lowfat

Fresh & Easy ()
Balsamic Vinegar Glaze
Chipotle Glaze Grill Sauce
Chop & Steak Marinade
Garlic & Herb Marinade
Lemon Pepper Marinade
Mesquite Marinade
Mojo Criollo Marinade
Raspberry Chipotle Grill Sauce
Rosemary & Oil Marinade
Tequila Lime Marinade
Thai Chili Lime Grill Sauce

Ginger People, The
Ginger Juice
Ginger Lemon Grass Sauce

Golding Farms ()
Chipotle Ranch Sauce

Gold's
Saucy Chicken Sauce

Holland House ⓘ
Cooking Wines

Howard's
Howard's (All)

Hy-Vee
Citrus Grill Marinade
Herb & Garlic Marinade
Lemon Pepper Marinade
Mesquite Marinade

Jack Daniel's Sauces ⓘ
EZ Marinader - Garlic & Herb
EZ Marinader - Steakhouse

Johnny's Fine Foods ⓘ
Jamaica Me Sweet Hot & Crazy Dressing/Marinade
Jamaica Mistake Dressing/Marinade
Jamaica Mistake Lite Dressing/Marinade
Salmon Sauce

Kitchen Bouquet ()
Kitchen Bouquet

Lea & Perrins ⓘ
White Wine Marinade

Maya Kaimal ⓘ
Butter Masala Fresh Sauce
Classic Korma Fresh Sauce
Coconut Curry Fresh Sauce
Tamarind Curry Fresh Sauce
Tikki Masala Fresh Sauce
Vindaloo Fresh Sauce

Meijer
Marinade - Garlic and Herb
Marinade - Lemon Pepper
Marinade - Mesquite

Moore's ⚇
Moore's Original Marinade

Mrs. Dash ⓘ ⚇
Mrs. Dash (All)

Newman's Own ⓘ
Herb & Roasted Garlic Marinade
Lemon Pepper Marinade
Mesquite with Lime Marinade

Olde Cape Cod ⓘ
Chipotle Grilling Sauce
Cranberry Grilling Sauce
Honey Orange Grilling Sauce
Lemon Ginger Grilling Sauce
Sweet & Bold Grilling Sauce

Polynesian Sauces
Chicken Nugget Sauce
Ham Glaze

Rao's Homemade ⟨⟩
Rao's Homemade (All)

Regina
Cooking Wines (All)

Saucy Susan
Ham Glaze
Peach Apricot - Original
Peach Apricot - Spicy

Seeds of Change ⓘ
Jalfrezi Simmer Sauce
Korma Simmer Sauce
Madras Simmer Sauce
Tikka Masala Simmer Sauce

Soy Vay ⓘ
Toasted Sesame Dressing and Marinade

Stubb's ⓘ ✓
Beef Marinade
Burger Rub
Chicken Marinade
Pork Marinade
Texas Steakhouse Marinade

Tasty Bite
Good Korma Simmer Sauce
Pad Thai Simmer Sauce
Rogan Josh Simmer Sauce
Satay Partay Simmer Sauce
Tikka Masala Simmer Sauce

TryMe
Cajun Sunshine
Tennessee Sunshine
TryMe Tiger Sauce

Weber
Black Peppercorn Marinade
Chipotle Marinade
Italian Herb Marinade
Tequila Lime Marinade
White Wine and Herb Marinade

MAYONNAISE

Bashas'
Mayonnaise
Mayonnaise, with Lime Juice

Best Foods
Mayonnaise Products and Spreads (All)

Blue Plate
Low Fat Mayonnaise ⚇
Mayonnaise ⚇
Sandwich Spread ⚇
Sugar Free Mayonnaise ⚇

Boar's Head
Condiments (All)

C. F. Sauer Company, The ⟨⟩
Mayonnaise (All)

Cains ⓘ
All-Natural Mayonnaise
Fat Free Mayonnaise
Kitchen Recipe Mayonnaise
Light Mayonnaise

Food Club (Marsh)
Mayonnaise

Mayonnaise - Light
Mayonnaise Squeeze - Inverted
Roasting Bag Pot Roast
Salad Dressing
Salad Dressing Lite Whipped

Fresh & Easy ()
Lite Mayonnaise
Mayonnaise

Haggen
Mayonnaise
Mayonnaise - Lite

Hellmann's
Mayonnaise Products (All)

J&D's
Baconnaise ()
Lite Baconnaise ()

JFG Mayonnaise
Mayonnaise
Reduced Fat Mayonnaise
Sandwich Spread
Squeeze Mayonnaise

Kraft Mayonnaise ⌒
Fat Free
Light Mayo
Real Mayo
Sandwich Shop Chipotle
Sandwich Shop Garlic & Herb
Sandwich Shop Horseradish-Dijon
Sandwich Shop Hot & Spicy
with Olive Oil

Meijer
Mayonnaise
Mayonnaise Lite

Miracle Whip ⌒
Fat Free Dressing
Light Dressing
Original Dressing

Naturally Delicious ⓘ
Mayonnaise

Naturally Fresh ()
Lite Mayonnaise

Olde Cape Cod ⓘ
Mayonnaise

Publix ()
Mayonnaise

Valu Time (Marsh)
Mayonnaise

Vegenaise ⓘ ⛾ ✓
Expeller
Grapeseed
Organic
Original

Woeber
Woeber (All)

MEXICAN, MISC.

Casa Fiesta
Enchilada Sauce
Habanero Sauce
Hot Pepper Sauce

Hy-Vee
Mild Diced Tomatoes & Green Chilies
Mild Enchilada Sauce

La Victoria ⓘ
Green Enchilada Sauce - Mild
Red Chili Sauce
Red Enchilada Sauce - Hot
Red Enchilada Sauce - Mild

Las Palmas
Red Chile Sauce
Red Enchilada Sauce

Taco Bell ⌒
Home Originals Bean Con Queso
Home Originals with Meat Chili Con
Queso

MUSTARD

Annie's Naturals ⓘ ✓
Organic Dijon Mustard
Organic Honey Mustard
Organic Horseradish Mustard
Organic Yellow Mustard

Bashas'
Mustard Salad Squeeze
Mustard Spicy Brown Squeeze

Beano's ()
Condiments (All)

Boar's Head
Condiments (All)

Bone Suckin' Sauce ✓
Mustard

Buckeye Mustard Inc.
Buckeye Fresh Horseradish Mustard

Cajun's Choice
Cajun's Choice (All BUT Seasoned Fish
Fry and Creole Mustard)

Di Lusso ⓘ
Chipotle Mustard
Cranberry Honey Mustard
Deli Style Mustard
Dijon Mustard
Honey Mustard
Jalapeno Mustard

Eden Foods ⓘ ✓
Brown Mustard - Organic
Yellow Mustard - Organic

Emeril's
Dijon Mustard
Kicked Up Horseradish Mustard
NY Deli Style Mustard
Smooth Honey Mustard
Yellow Mustard

Fischer & Wieser
Smokey Mesquite Mustard
Sweet Heat Mustard
Sweet, Sour & Smokey Mustard Sauce

Food Club (Marsh)
Mustard Dijon
Mustard Honey Squeeze
Mustard Salad Squeeze
Mustard Spicy Brown Squeeze

French's
Honey Mustard
Prepared Mustards (All)

Fresh & Easy ⟨⟩
Dijon Mustard
Spicy Brown Mustard
Stoneground Horseradish Mustard
Sweet & Hot Mustard
Wholegrain Mustard
Yellow Mustard

Golding Farms ⟨⟩
Dijon Gourmet Mustard
Honey Dijon Mustard
Honey Mustard

Horseradish Gourmet Mustard
Three Pepper Mustard

Gold's
Deli Mustard
Dijon Mustard
Honey Mustard Sauce
Mustard with Horseradish
Squeeze Honey Mustard

Great Value (Wal-Mart)
Course Ground Mustard
Honey Mustard
Prepared Dijon Mustard
Prepared Mustard
Southwest Spicy Sweet, Hot Mustard
Spicy Brown Mustard
Squeeze Prepared Mustard

Grey Poupon ✐
Country Dijon Mustard
Deli Mustard
Dijon Mustard
Harvest Coarse Ground Mustard
Hearty Spicy Brown Mustard
Honey Mustard
Savory Honey Mustard
Spicy Brown Mustard

Haggen
Mustard - Dijon
Mustard - Salad Squeeze
Mustard - Spicy Brown Squeeze

Heinz ⓘ
Mustard (All Varieties)

Hellmann's
Spreads (All)

Hy-Vee
Dijon Mustard
Honey Mustard
Mustard
Spicy Brown Mustard

Jack Daniel's Mustards ⓘ
Hickory Smoke Mustard
Honey Dijon Mustard
Horseradish Mustard
Old No. 7 Mustard
Spicy Southwest Mustard
Stone Ground Dijon Mustard

Koops'
Koops' Mustards (All)

Meijer
Mustard - Dijon Squeeze
Mustard - Honey Squeeze
Mustard - Horseradish Squeeze
Mustard - Hot & Spicy
Mustard - Salad
Mustard - Salad Squeeze
Mustard - Spicy Brown Squeeze

Midwest Country Fare (Hy-Vee)
Yellow Mustard

Morehouse
Mustard Products (All)

Nathan's
Deli Mustard

Olde Cape Cod ⓘ
Mustards

Organicville
Organicville (All)

Publix ()
Classic Yellow Mustard
Dijon Mustard
GreenWise Market Organic Creamy
    Yellow Mustard
GreenWise Market Organic Spicy
    Brown Mustard
GreenWise Market Organic Tangy Dijon
Honey Mustard
Spicy Brown Mustard

Raley's
Dijon Mustard
Yellow Mustard

Saag's
Saag's (All BUT British Bangers)

Sabrett
Mustard

Silver Spring ⓘ
Silver Spring (All)

Texas Pete
Honey Mustard Sauce ⚇

Thumann's ✓
Condiments (All BUT Deep Fry Hot
    Dogs)

Valu Time (Marsh)
Mustard - Salad Squeeze

Winn-Dixie ()
Dijon Mustard

Honey Mustard
Horseradish Mustard
Spicy Brown Mustard
Yellow Mustard

Woeber
Woeber (All)

NUT BUTTERS

Adam's Peanut Butter
Adam's Peanut Butter

Arrowhead Mills ✓
Creamy Almond Butter
Creamy Cashew Butter
Creamy Valencia Peanut Butter
Crunchy Valencia Peanut Butter
Organic Creamy Valencia Peanut Butter
Organic Crunchy Valencia Peanut
    Butter
Organic Sesame Tahini

Bashas'
Fun Stripes Peanut Butter & Grape Jelly
Fun Stripes Peanut Butter & Strawberry
    Jelly
Peanut Butter - Creamy
Peanut Butter - Creamy Reduced Fat
Peanut Butter - Crunchy

Blue Diamond Growers ✓
Almond Butter (All)

Earth Balance
Earth Balance (All)

Fisher Nuts ()
Peanut Butter - Chunky
Peanut Butter - Creamy

Food Club (Marsh)
Peanut Butter Creamy
Peanut Butter Crunchy

Fragata
Fragata (All BUT Imitation Bacon Bits)

Fresh & Easy ()
Almond Butter
Cashew Butter
Peanut Butter

Great Value (Wal-Mart)
Creamy Peanut Butter
Crunchy Peanut Butter

Peanut Free Smooth Soy Butter

Hy-Vee
Creamy Peanut Butter
Crunchy Peanut Butter
Reduced Fat Creamy Peanut Butter

I.M. Healthy ⅛
SoyNut Butter

Jif
Peanut Butters (All)

Kroger ⓘ
Creamy Peanut Butter
Crunchy Peanut Butter
Natural Creamy Peanut Butter
Natural Crunchy Peanut Butter
Reduced Fat Creamy Peanut Butter
Reduced Fat Crunchy Peanut Butter

Laura Scudder's
Laura Scudder's Smooth Peanut Butter

Maple Grove Farms
Peanut Butter (All Varieties)

Meijer
Peanut Butter - Creamy
Peanut Butter - Crunchy
Peanut Butter - Natural Creamy
Peanut Butter - Natural Crunchy

Midwest Country Fare (Hy-Vee)
Creamy Peanut Butter
Crunchy Peanut Butter

Nash Brothers
Organic Peanut Butter

Nature's Basket (Giant Eagle)
Organic Creamy Peanut Butter - No Salt
Organic Creamy Peanut Butter (Nutco)
Organic Crunchy Peanut Butter (Nutco)

Publix ()
Creamy Peanut Butter
Crunchy Peanut Butter
Old Fashioned Creamy Peanut Butter
Old Fashioned Crunchy Peanut Butter
Reduced Fat Spread Creamy Peanut
    Butter
Reduced Fat Spread Crunchy Peanut
    Butter

Skippy
Skippy (All)

Smucker's
Peanut Butter

SunButter
Sunflower Seed Spreads

Valu Time (Marsh)
Peanut Butter Creamy
Peanut Butter Crunchy

OLIVES

B&G Foods
Black Olives
Green Olives

Bashas'
Olives - Ripe Large
Olives - Ripe Medium
Olives - Ripe Sliced
Olives - Ripe Sliced Buffet
Olives Manzanilla Queen Stuffed
    Thrown
Olives Manzanilla Stuffed Thrown
Olives Ripe Pitted Small

Central Market Classics (Price Chopper)
Pitted Queen Olives
Stuffed Garlic Olives
Stuffed Jalapeno Olives

Di Lusso ⓘ
Green Ionian Olives
Mediterranean Mixed Olives

Food Club (Marsh)
Olives Manzanilla Stuffed Thrown
Olives Ripe Pitted Large
Olives Ripe Pitted Medium
Olives Ripe Sliced Buffet

Fresh & Easy ()
Black Olive Tapenade
Olives

Great Value (Wal-Mart)
Chopped Ripe Olives
Jumbo Pitted Ripe Olives
Large Pitted Ripe Olives
Medium Pitted Ripe Olives
Minced Pimento Stuffed Manzanilla
    Olives
Minced Pimento Stuffed Queen Olives
Sliced Ripe Olives

Sliced Salad Olives

Haggen
Manzanilla Stuffed Thrown Olives
Queen Stuffed Thrown Olives
Ripe Chopped Olives
Ripe Pitted Jumbo Olives
Ripe Pitted Large Olives
Ripe Pitted Medium Olives
Ripe Sliced Olives
Salad Olives
Salad Sliced Olives

Hy-Vee
Chopped Ripe Olives
Large Ripe Black Olives
Manzanilla Olives
Medium Ripe Black Olives
Queen Olives
Sliced Ripe Black Olives
Sliced Salad Olives

Kroger ⓘ
Black Olives - Not Stuffed
Green Olives - Not Stuffed
Green Olives - Pimento Stuffed

Lindsay Olives
Olives (All)

Mario
Mario (All BUT Imitation Bacon Bits)

Meijer
Olives - Manzanilla Stuffed Placed
Olives - Manzanilla Stuffed Thrown
Olives - Manzanilla Stuffed Tree
Olives - Queen Stuffed Placed
Olives - Queen Whole Thrown
Olives - Ripe Large
Olives - Ripe Medium
Olives - Ripe Pitted Jumbo
Olives - Ripe Pitted Small
Olives - Ripe Sliced
Olives - Salad
Olives - Salad Sliced

Midwest Country Fare (Hy-Vee)
Large Ripe Black Olives
Sliced Ripe Black Olives

Musco Family Olive Co.
Black Ripe Olives

Pastene
Black Greek Olives

Extra Large Pitted Olives
Gaeta Olives
Kalamata Olives
Oil Cured Olives
Sicilian Olives
Sliced Ripe Olives

Peloponnese ⓘ
Kalamata Olive Spread
Kalamata Olives

Price Chopper
Sliced Spanish Olives
Stuffed Manzanilla Olives
Stuffed Spanish Olives

Publix ()
Colossal Olives
Green Olives (All Sizes & Styles)
Large Olives
Ripe Olives
Small Olives

Raley's
Pimento Stuffed Olives
Sliced Olives

Santa Barbara Olive Co.
Santa Barbara Olive Co. (All BUT Pasta
Sauce and Salsa)

Valu Time (Marsh)
Olives Salad
Olives Stuffed

Winn-Dixie ()
Green Olives (All)
Ripe Olives (All)

PASTA & PIZZA SAUCE

Amy's Kitchen ⓘ ✓
Family Marinara Pasta Sauce
Garlic Mushroom Pasta Sauce
Low Sodium Marinara Sauce
Puttanesca Pasta Sauce
Roasted Garlic Pasta Sauce
Tomato Basil Pasta Sauce

Bove's of Vermont ♘
Sauces (All)

Classico ⓘ
Alfredo Sauces (All)
Bruschetta Toppings (All)
Pesto Sauces (All)

Red Sauces   (All)

Colavita
Sauce (All)

Contadina ⓘ
Pizza Sauces (All)

Pizza Squeeze

Dei Fratelli
Dei Fratelli (All BUT Tomato Soup)

Del Monte ⓘ
Tomatoes & Tomato Products (All BUT
Spaghetti Sauce Flavored with Meat)

Eden Foods ⓘ ✓
Pizza Pasta Sauce - Organic

Spaghetti Sauce - No Salt Added,
Organic

Spaghetti Sauce - Organic

Emeril's
Cacciatore Dinner Sauce

Eggplant & Gaaahlic

Home Style Marinara Pasta Sauce

Italian Style Tomato and Basil

Kicked Up Tomato Pasta Sauce

Roasted Gaaahlic Pasta Sauce

Roasted Red Pepper Pasta Sauce

Sicilian Gravy Pasta Sauce

Three Cheeses

Vodka Pasta Sauce

Food Club (Marsh)
Sauce Pizza

Francesco Rinaldi ()
Garden Style Sauces (All)

Hearty Sauces (All)

Traditional Sauces (All)

Fresh & Easy ()
Arrabiata Pasta Sauce

Chunky Vegetable Pasta Sauce

Organic Marinara Pasta Sauce

Organic Marinara with Eggplant Pasta
Sauce

Puttanesca Pasta Sauce

Roasted Garlic Pasta Sauce

Three Cheese Pasta Sauce

Tomato Basil Marinara Pasta Sauce

Tomato Bruschetta (Glass Jar)

Vodka Cream Sauce

Furmano's
Furmano's (All)

Great Value (Wal-Mart)
Italian Garden Combination Chunky
Pasta Sauce

Mushrooms & Green Peppers Spaghetti
Sauce

Onions & Garlic Chunky Pasta Sauce

Pizza Sauce

Traditional Spaghetti Sauce

Hanover Foods ⓘ
Spaghetti Sauce

HealthMarket (Hy-Vee)
Tomato Basil Sauce

Hy-Vee
3 Cheese Spaghetti Sauce

Garden Spaghetti Sauce

Mushroom Spaghetti Sauce

Pizza Sauce

Spaghetti Sauce with Meat

Traditional Spaghetti Sauce

Lucini Italia () ✓
Lucini Italia (All BUT Russian Tomato
Vodka Sauce and Minestrone Soup)

Meijer
Pasta Sauce Four Cheese - Select

Pasta Sauce Marinara - Select

Pasta Sauce Mushroom and Olive -
Select

Pasta Sauce Onion and Garlic - Select

Pizza Sauce

Spaghetti Extra Chunk Garden

Spaghetti Sauce Extra Chunk 3 Cheese

Spaghetti Sauce Extra Chunk Garlic and
Cheese

Spaghetti Sauce Extra Chunk
Mushroom/Green Pepper

Spaghetti Sauce Plain

Spaghetti Sauce with Meat

Spaghetti Sauce with Mushroom

Midwest Country Fare (Hy-Vee)
All Natural Garlic & Onion Spaghetti
Sauce

Four Cheese Spaghetti Sauce

Garden Vegetable Spaghetti Sauce

Garlic & Herb Spaghetti Sauce

Meat Flavor Spaghetti Sauce

Mushroom Spaghetti Sauce

Traditional Spaghetti Sauce

Mom's
- Artichoke Heart & Asiago Cheese Pasta Sauce
- Garlic & Basil Spaghetti Sauce
- Martini Pasta Sauce
- Organic Roasted Pepper Pasta Sauce
- Organic Traditional Pasta Sauce
- Puttanesca Spaghetti Sauce
- Special Marinara Spaghetti Sauce
- Spicy Arrabbiata

Nash Brothers
- Organic Pasta Sauce

Naturally Fresh ()
- Marinara Sauce

Nature's Basket (Giant Eagle)
- Organic Marinara Sauce
- Organic Roasted Garlic Pasta Sauce
- Organic Three Cheese Pasta Sauce
- Organic Tomato Basil Pasta Sauce
- Organic Vodka Cream Pasta Sauce

Newman's Own ⓘ
- Alfredo
- Bombolina (Basil)
- Diavolo (Spicy Simmer Sauce)
- Five Cheese
- Italian Sausage & Peppers
- Marinara (Venetian)
- Marinara with Mushrooms
- Organic Marinara Sauce
- Organic Tomato Basil Sauce
- Organic Traditional Herb Sauce
- Pesto and Tomato
- Roasted Garlic and Peppers
- Sockarooni (Mushrooms, Onions, Peppers)
- Sweet Onion and Roasted Garlic
- Tomato and Roasted Garlic
- Vodka Sauce

Organicville
- Organicville (All)

Pastene
- Arrabbiata Sauce
- Chateau Marinara Sauce
- Italian (Basil) Pesto
- Pizza Sauce
- Puttanesca Sauce
- Tomato with Basil Sauce

- Vodka Sauce
- White Clam Sauce

Prego ⓘ
- Chunky Garden Combo
- Chunky Garden Mushroom & Green Pepper
- Chunky Garden Mushroom Supreme with Baby Portobello
- Chunky Garden Tomato Onion & Garlic
- Flavored with Meat
- Fresh Mushroom
- Heart Smart Mushroom
- Heart Smart Onion & Garlic
- Heart Smart Ricotta Parmesan
- Heart Smart Roasted Red Pepper & Garlic
- Heart Smart Traditional
- Italian Sausage & Garlic
- Marinara
- Mushroom & Garlic
- Roasted Garlic & Herb
- Roasted Garlic Parmesan
- Three Cheese
- Tomato Basil Garlic
- Traditional

Rao's Homemade ()
- Rao's Homemade (All)

Red Gold
- Tomato Products (All)

Redpack
- Tomato Products (All)

Santa Barbara Salsa
- Santa Barbara Salsa (All)

Sauces 'n Love
- Sauces 'n Love (All)

Seeds of Change ⓘ
- Arrabiatta di Roma
- Marinara di Venzia
- Romagna Three Cheese
- Tomato Basil Genovese
- Tuscan Roasted Tomato & Garlic
- Vodka Americano

Taste of Thai, A
- Taste of Thai, A (All)

Tuttorosso
- Tomato Products

Valu Time (Marsh)
- Pasta Sauce - Original
- Pasta Sauce Meat - Can
- Pasta Sauce Mushroom - Can

Vino de Milo ⓘ
- Bruschettas (All)
- Wine-Based Pasta Sauces (All)

Winn-Dixie ⓘ
- Classic Fra Diavolo Pasta Sauce
- Classic Home Style Pasta Sauce
- Classic Marinara
- Classic Peppers & Onions Pasta Sauce
- Classic Style Double Garlic Pasta Sauce
- Classic Style Fat Free Pasta Sauce
- Classic Tomato Basil Pasta Sauce
- Garden Vegetable Combination Pasta Sauce
- Garlic & Onion Pasta Sauce
- Meat Pasta Sauce
- Mushroom Pasta Sauce
- Parmesan & Romano Pasta Sauce
- Pizza Sauce
- Traditional Pasta Sauce

PEPPERS

B&G Foods
- Peppers

Bashas'
- Chilies Diced Mild
- Green Chilies, Diced
- Pepper Rings - Banana Mild
- Pepperoncini

Casa Fiesta
- Diced Green Chili Peppers
- Diced Jalapeno Peppers
- Nacho Sliced Jalapeno Peppers
- Whole Chipotle Peppers

Chi-Chi's ⓘ
- Green Chilis
- Red Jalapenos

Di Lusso ⓘ
- Roasted Red Peppers

Embasa ⓘ
- Chiles Gueritos
- Chipotle Peppers
- Nacho Sliced Jalapenos

- Sliced Jalapenos
- Whole Jalapenos

Food Club (Marsh)
- Diced Chilies - Mild
- Pepper Rings Banana Hot
- Pepper Rings Banana Mild
- Pepperocini
- Peppers Jalepenos Sliced

Fragata
- Fragata (All BUT Imitation Bacon Bits)

Fresh & Easy ⓘ
- Cherry Peppers
- Nacho Jalapeno Peppers
- Pepperocini Peppers

Great Value (Wal-Mart)
- Fire Roasted Green Chiles, Bilingual
- Nacho Sliced Jalapenos, Bilingual
- Sliced Jalapenos
- Whole Jalapenos, Bilingual

Heinz ⓘ
- Peppers (All Varieties)

Hy-Vee
- Diced Green Chilies
- Green Salad Pepperoncini
- Hot Banana Peppers
- Mild Banana Peppers
- Sliced Hot Jalapenos
- Whole Green Chilies

La Costena
- La Costena (All BUT Jalapeno Hot Sauce)

La Victoria ⓘ
- Green Chiles - Diced & Whole
- Jalapeno Peppers - Diced
- Jalapeno Peppers - Sliced

Mario
- Mario (All BUT Imitation Bacon Bits)

Meijer
- Hot Pepper Rings
- Mild Pepper Rings
- Pepper Ring - Banana Hot
- Pepper Rings - Banana Mild
- Pepperoncini

Mount Olive Pickle Company
- Mount Olive Pickle Company (All)

Ortega
Chiles & Jalapenos

Pastene
Giardiniera
Gourmet Peppers
Green Vinegar Peppers
Hot Cherry Peppers
Hot Crushed Peppers
Hot Finger Peppers
Hot Garden Salad
Hot Pepper Rings
Jalapeno Peppers
Pepper Salad
Pepperoncini
Sliced Hot Peppers in Oil
Sliced Red Peppers
Sweet Banana Peppers
Sweet Cherry Peppers
Sweet Garlic Peppers

Peloponnese ⓘ
Roasted Sweet Peppers

Strub's
Strub's (All)

Thumann's ✓
Condiments (All BUT Deep Fry Hot Dogs)

Trappey
Peppers

Winn-Dixie ⟨⟩
Jalapenos
Pepperoncini
Sliced Banana Peppers - Hot
Sliced Banana Peppers - Mild

PICANTE SAUCE

Bashas'
Picante Sauce - Mild

Casa Fiesta
Salsa Picante

Chi-Chi's ⓘ
Picante

Fresh & Easy ⟨⟩
Salsa Picante

Haggen
Sauce - Picante Medium

Sauce - Picante Mild

Hy-Vee
Hot Picante Sauce
Medium Picante Sauce
Mild Picante Sauce

Kroger ⓘ
Picante Sauce Salsa - Hot
Picante Sauce Salsa - Medium
Picante Sauce Salsa - Mild

Ortega
Picante - Hot
Picante - Medium
Picante - Mild

Pace ⓘ
Picante Sauce - Extra Mild
Picante Sauce - Hot
Picante Sauce - Medium
Picante Sauce - Mild

Tostitos ⓘ
All Natural Medium Picante Sauce
All Natural Mild Picante Sauce

PICKLES

B&G Foods
Capers
Pickles

Bashas'
Pickle Bread & Butter Chips FP
Pickle Bread & Butter Slickles FP
Pickle Dill Hamburger Slices - Processed
Pickle Dill Kosher Baby FP
Pickle Dill Kosher Sandwich Slickles
Pickle Dill Kosher Spears FP
Pickle Dill Kosher Whole FP
Pickle Dill Polish FP
Pickle Sweet Whole - Processed

Bubbies ⚇
Pure Kosher Dills

Claussen ⌇
Pickles - Bread 'n Butter Chips
Pickles - Bread 'n Butter Sandwich Slices
Pickles - Deli Style Kosher Dill Halves
Pickles - Deli Style Kosher Dill Spears
Pickles - Half Sours New York Deli Style Wholes

Pickles - Hearty Garlic Deli Style
Sandwich Slices
Pickles - Hearty Garlic Deli Style
Wholes
Pickles - Kosher Dill Halves
Pickles - Kosher Dill Sandwich Slices
Pickles - Kosher Dill Spears
Pickles - Kosher Dill Wholes
Pickles - Kosher Dills Mini
Pickles Kosher Dill - Burger Slices

Food Club (Marsh)

Pickle Bread & Butter Chips
Pickle Bread & Butter Slickles
Pickle Bread & Butter Sticks Fresh Pack
Pickle Dill Hamburger Slices
Pickle Dill Kosher Sandwich Slickles
Pickle Dill Kosher Spears
Pickle Dill Kosher Whole
Pickle Dill Polish Spears
Pickle Sweet Gherkin Whole
Pickle Sweet Whole

Fresh & Easy ()

Baby Dill Pickles
Capers
Dill Pickles
Pickle Chips
Pickle Spears
Sandwich Pickles

Gedney

Pickles (All)

Great Value (Wal-Mart)

Baby Dill Pickles
Bread & Butter Pickles
Dill Spears Pickles
Garlic Dill Slicers Pickles
Hamburger Dill Chips Pickles
Kosher Baby Dill Pickles
Kosher Dill Spears Pickles
Kosher Whole Dill Pickles
Sweet Gherkin Pickles
Sweet Whole Pickles
Whole Dill Pickles

Haggen

Hamburger Slices Pickle Dill
Kosher Baby Pickle Dill
Kosher Whole Pickle Dill
Pickles - Baby Kosher Dills

Pickles - Bread & Butter Sandwich Slices
Pickles - Cucumber Chips
Pickles - Kosher Dill Spears
Pickles - Kosher Sandwich Slices
Pickles - Sweet Whole Processed
Pickles - Zesty Kosher Dills Spears

Heinz ⓘ

Pickles (All Varieties)

Hy-Vee

Bread & Butter Sandwich Slices
Bread & Butter Sweet Chunk Pickles
Bread & Butter Sweet Slices
Fresh Pack Kosher Baby Dills
Hamburger Dill Slices
Kosher Baby Dills
Kosher Cocktail Dills
Kosher Dill Pickles
Kosher Dill Spears
Polish Dill Pickles
Polish Dill Spears
Refrigerated Kosher Dill Halves
Refrigerated Kosher Dill Sandwich
Slices
Refrigerated Kosher Dill Spears
Refrigerated Kosher Dill Whole Pickles
Special Recipe Baby Dills
Special Recipe Bread & Butter Slices
Special Recipe Hot & Spicy Zingers
Special Recipe Hot & Sweet Zinger
Chunks
Special Recipe Jalapeno Baby Dills
Special Recipe Sweet Garden Crunch
Sweet Gherkins
Whole Sweet Pickles
Zesty Kosher Dill Spears
Zesty Sweet Chunks

Meijer

Bread & Butter Chips
Bread & Butter Chips - Sugar Free
Dill Spears - Zesty
Halves - Kosher Dill
Kosher Baby Dills
Kosher Dills
Pickle - Bread & Butter Chips
Pickle - Dill Hamburger Slice
Pickle - Dill Kosher Baby
Pickle - Dill Kosher Spears

Pickle - Dill Kosher Whole
Pickle - Dill Kosher Whole - Processed
Pickle - Dill Polish
Pickle - Dill Polish Spears
Pickle - Dill Whole
Pickle - No Garlic Dill Spears
Pickle - Sweet Gherkin Whole - Processed
Pickle - Sweet Midgets Whole - Processed
Pickle - Sweet Whole - Processed
Pickles - Whole - Refrigerated
Sandwich Slice - Bread & Butter
Sandwich Slice - Kosher Dill
Sandwich Slice - Kosher Dill Zesty
Slickles Sandwich Slice - Kosher Dill
Slickles Sandwich Slice - Polish Dill
Sweet Pickles - Sugar Free
Wholes - Kosher Dill

Midwest Country Fare (Hy-Vee)
Fresh Pack Kosher Dill Whole Pickles
Fresh Pack Whole Dill Pickles
Hamburger Dill Slices
Whole Sweet Pickles

Mount Olive Pickle Company
Mount Olive Pickle Company (All)

Pastene
Imported Capers

Publix ()
Pickles (All Varieties)

Raley's
Kosher Dill Spears
Kosher Whole Dills
Sandwich Kosher Dill

Strub's
Strub's (All)

Thumann's ✔
Condiments (All BUT Deep Fry Hot Dogs)

Valu Time (Marsh)
Pickle Dill Hamburger Slices
Pickle Dill Kosher Whole

Vlasic ()
Pickles (All)

Winn-Dixie ()
Dill Pickles (All)
Sweet Pickles (All)

RELISH

B&G Foods
Relishes

Bashas'
Relish Dill
Relish Sweet
Sweet Pickle Relish

Bubbies ⛎
Pure Kosher Dill Relish

Cains ⓘ
Relishes (All)

Central Market Classics (Price Chopper)
Cranberry-Apple Relish

Claussen ⌒
Sweet Pickle Relish
Sweet Squeeze Pickle Relish

Crosse & Blackwell
Crosse & Blackwell (All BUT Plum Pudding and Branston Pickle Relish)

Dickinson's
Dickinson's (All)

Food Club (Marsh)
Relish Dill
Relish Hot Dog
Relish Sweet

Ginger People, The
Natural Pickled Sushi Ginger

Gold's
Squeeze Hot Dog Relish

Grandmother's
Corn Relish
Hot Pepper Relish
Sweet Pepper Relish

Great Value (Wal-Mart)
Sweet Pickle Relish

Haggen
Dill Relish
Sweet Relish

Heinz ⓘ
Relish (All Varieties)

Howard's
Howard's (All)

Hy-Vee
Dill Relish

Three Cheese Ranch
Tuscan House Italian
Vidalia Onion Vinaigrette with Roasted
  Red Pepper
Zesty Italian

La Martinique
Balsamic Vinaigrette
Blue Cheese Vinaigrette
Original Poppy Seed
True French Vinaigrette

Lily's Gourmet Dressings ()
Balsamic Vinaigrette
Northern Italian
Poppyseed
Raspberry Walnut Vinaigrette

Litehouse
Bacon Bleu Cheese
Balsamic Vinaigrette
Big Bleu
Bleu Cheese Vinaigrette
Buttermilk Ranch
Caesar Caesar
Chunky Bleu Cheese
Chunky Garlic Caesar
Classic Feta
Coleslaw
Coleslaw with Pineapple
Creamy Cilantro
Garden Veggie Ranch Dressing
Garlic Vinaigrette
Greek Feta
Harvest Cranberry Vinaigrette
Homestyle Ranch
Honey Mustard
Huckleberry Vinaigrette
Jalapeno Ranch
Lite 1000 Island
Lite Bleu Cheese
Lite Caesar
Lite Coleslaw
Lite Greek
Lite Honey Dijon Vinaigrette
Lite Ranch
Original Bleu Cheese
Parmesan Caesar
Pear Gorgonzola
Pomegranate Blueberry Vinaigrette

Poppyseed Dressing
Ranch
Raspberry Walnut Vinaigrette
Red Wine Olive Oil Vinaigrette
Romano Caeser
Salsa Ranch
Spinach Salad
Sweet and Sour
Sweet French
Thousand Island
White Balsamic
Zesty Italian Vinaigrette

Lucini Italia () ✓
Lucini Italia (All BUT Russian Tomato
  Vodka Sauce and Minestrone Soup)

Maple Grove Farms
Asiago & Garlic
Asiago with Preservative
Blueberry Pomegranate
Caesar Lite
Champagne Vinaigrette
Fat Free Balsamic Vinaigrette
Fat Free Caesar
Fat Free Cranberry Balsamic
Fat Free Greek
Fat Free Honey Dijon
Fat Free Lime Basil Vinaigrette
Fat Free Poppyseed
Fat Free Raspberry Vinaigrette
Fat Free Vidalia Oinion
Fat Free Wasabi Dijon
Ginger Pear Vinaigrette
Honey Mustard
Honey Mustard, Lite
Maple Balsamic
Maple Fig
Strawberry Balsamic
Sugar Free Balsamic Vinaigrette
Sugar Free Dijon
Sugar Free Italian with with Balsamic
Sugar Free Raspberry Vinaigrette
Sweet & Sour

Marzetti
Aged Parmesan Ranch
Asiago Peppercorn
Balsamic Vinaigrette
Bistro Blue Cheese

Blue Cheese Italian Vinaigrette
Blue Cheese Slaw Dressing
California French
Chunky Blue Cheese
Classic Ranch
Country French
Creamy Caesar
Creamy Italian
Fat Free Honey Dijon
Fat Free Italian
Fat Free Sweet & Sour
French Blue Cheese
Garlic Vinaigrette
Honey Balsamic
Honey Dijon
Honey French
House Italian
Italian
Italian with Blue Cheese Crumbles
Light Ancho Chipotle
Light Balsamic
Light Balsamic Vinaigrette
Light Berry Balsamic
Light Chunky Blue Cheese
Light Citrus Poppyseed
Light Classic Ranch
Light Honey Dijon
Light Honey French
Light Original Slaw
Light Raspberry Cabernet Vinaigrette
Light Supreme Caesar
Lite Slaw Dressing
Low Fat Slaw Dressing
Organic Balsamic Vinaigrette
Organic Blue Cheese
Organic Caesar
Organic Parmesan Ranch
Organic Raspberry Cranberry
Original Slaw
Peppercorn Vinaigrette
Poppyseed
Potato Salad Dressing
Ranch
Refrigerated Premium Dressing - The
    Ultimate Blue Cheese
Refrigerated Premium Dressing - The
    Ultimate Gorgonzola
Roasted Garlic Italian Vinaigrette

Slaw Dressing
Southern Recipe Slaw Dressing
Strawberry Chardonnay Vinaigrette
Supreme Caesar
Sweet & Sour
Sweet Italian
Sweet Vidalia Onion
Thousand Island
Venice Italian
White Balsamic Vinaigrette

Midwest Country Fare (Hy-Vee)
French Dressing
Italian Dressing
Ranch Dressing
Thousand Island Dressing

Mount Olive Pickle Company
Mount Olive Pickle Company (All)

Naturally Delicious ⓘ
Balsamic
Blue Cheese
Chipotle Ranch
French
Honey Mustard
Italian
Light Blush Wine
Light Italian
Light Raspberry
Peppercorn Parmesan

Naturally Fresh ()
Bleu Cheese
Bleu Cheese Vinaigrette
Buttersauce
Caesar Dressing
Classic Caesar
Classic Ranch
Cranberry Walnut
Fat-Free Balsamic Vinaigrette
Fat-Free Italian
Fat-Free Raspberry
Honey French
Honey Mustard
Jalapeno Ranch
Lite Ranch
Olive Oil & Balsamic
Organic Dressings
Poppy Seed
Roasted Garlic Bleu Cheese

Slaw Dressing
Thousand Island
Wine & Cheese

Nature's Basket (Giant Eagle)
Organic Balsamic Dressing
Organic Italian Dressing
Organic Ranch Dressing
Organic Raspberry Vinaigrette
Organic Roasted Red Pepper Dressing
Organic Sesame Ginger Dressing

Newman's Own ⓘ
Balsamic Vinaigrette
Caesar
Creamy Caesar
Greek Vinaigrette
Light Balsamic Vinaigrette
Light Caesar Dressing
Light Cranberry and Walnut
Light Honey Mustard
Light Italian
Light Lime Vinaigrette
Light Raspberry and Walnut
Light Red Wine and Vinegar
Light Roasted Garlic Balsamic
Light Sun Dried Tomato
Olive Oil and Vinegar
Orange Ginger
Organic Creamy Caesar Dressing
Organic Light Balsamic Vinaigrette
    Dressing
Organic Tuscan Italian Dressing
Parmesan and Roasted Garlic
Ranch Dressing
Red Wine and Vinegar
Three Cheese Balsamic Vinaigrette

Olde Cape Cod ⓘ
Balsamic
Balsamic with Olive Oil
Chipotle Ranch
Honey Dijon
Honey French Lite
Lemon and Mint with Green Tea
    Vinaigrette
Lemon Poppyseed
Lite Blush Wine Vinaigrette
Lite Caesar
Lite Raspberry Vinaigrette

Lite Sweet & Sour Poppyseed
Orange Poppyseed
Parmesan & Peppercorn
Sundried Tomato Lite
Zesty Mango Vinaigrette

Organicville
Organicville (All)

Pfeiffer
Balsamic Vinaigrette
Blue Cheese
Caesar
California French
Cole Slaw
Creamy Italian
Fat Free Italian
Fat Free Ranch
French
Garden Ranch
Honey Dijon
Italian
Light Italian
Light Ranch
Light Thousand Island
Peppercorn Ranch
Poppyseed
Ranch
Red Wine Vinaigrette
Roasted Garlic Vinaigrette
Sweet & Sour
Thousand Island
Tuscan Italian
Zesty Garlic Italian

Publix ()
Balsamic Vinaigrette
California French
Chunky Blue Cheese
Creamy Parmesan
Fat Free Italian
Fat Free Thousand Island
Italian
Lite Caesar
Lite Honey Dijon
Lite Ranch
Lite Raspberry Walnut
Ranch
Thousand Island
Zesty Italian

Rao's Homemade ()
Rao's Homemade (All)

San-J ⓘ ✓
Gluten Free Tamari Ginger Dressing
Gluten Free Tamari Peanut Dressing
Gluten Free Tamari Sesame Dressing

Seeds of Change ⓘ
Balsamic Vinaigrette
French Tomato
Greek Feta
Italian Herb
Roasted Red Pepper

Seven Seas Salad Dressing ᘓ
Green Goddess
Red Wine Vinaigrette

Teresa's Select Recipes
Asiago Pepper Crème
Balsamic Vinaigrette
Blackberry Poppyseed
Fat Free Honey Dijon
Raspberry White Balsamic
Roasted Garlic Vinaigrette
Strawberry Chardonnay
Sun Dried Tomato Vinaigrette

Valu Time (Marsh)
Dressing French
Dressing Italian
Dressing Ranch

Vino de Milo ⓘ
Salad Dressings (All)

Winn-Dixie ()
Balsamic Vinaigrette
California French
Chunky Blue Cheese
Creamy French
Creamy Ranch
Fat Free Italian
Fat Free Ranch
Fat Free Thousand Island
Garden Ranch
Honey Dijon
Italian
Lite Italian
Lite Ranch
Robust Italian
Thousand Island
Zesty Italian

SALSA

Amy's Kitchen ⓘ ✓
Black Bean & Corn Salsa
Fire Roasted Vegetable Salsa
Medium Salsa
Mild Salsa
Spicy Chipotle Salsa

Bashas'
Salsa - Medium
Salsa - Mild

Bone Suckin' Sauce ✓
Salsa - Hot
Salsa - Regular

Casa Fiesta
Chili Salsa
Jalapeno Cheese Salsa
Salsa Dip
Thick and Chunky Salsa

Chi-Chi's ⓘ
Fiesta Salsa
Garden Salsa
Natural Salsa
Original Salsa

Dei Fratelli
Dei Fratelli (All BUT Tomato Soup)

El Pinto ⚇
El Pinto (All)

Embasa ⓘ
Salsa Casera - Hot
Salsa Mexicana - Medium

Emeril's
Gaaahlic Lovers Medium Salsa
Kicked Up Chunky Hot Salsa
Original Recipe Medium Salsa
Southwest Style Medium Salsa

Fischer & Wieser
Artichoke & Olive Salsa
Black Bean & Corn Salsa
Chipotle & Corn Salsa
Cilantro & Olive Salsa
Das Peach Haus Peach Salsa
Havana Mojito Salsa
Hot Habanero Salsa
Salsa A La Charra
Salsa Verde Ranchera
Silican Tomato Pesto Salsa

Fresh & Easy ()
New Mexico Style Green Chili Salsa
Roasted Tomato Salsa
Salsa Authentica
Salsa Chipotle
Salsa Verde
Smoky Peach Salsa
Thick & Chunky Salsa - Medium
Thick & Chunky Salsa - Mild

Garden Fresh Gourmet
Salsa

Gold's
Extra Chunky Salsa - Hot
Extra Chunky Salsa - Mild

Great Value (Wal-Mart)
Salsa Con Queso
White Salsa Con Queso

Green Mountain Gringo ⓘ
Salsa - Hot
Salsa - Medium
Salsa - Mild
Salsa - Roasted Chile
Salsa - Roasted Garlic

Haggen
Salsa - Medium
Salsa - Mild

Herdez ⓘ
Salsa Casera

Herr's
Chunky Salsa Medium
Chunky Salsa Mild

Hy-Vee
Thick & Chunky Hot Salsa
Thick & Chunky Medium Salsa
Thick & Chunky Mild Salsa

Kroger ⓘ
Thick & Chunky Salsa - Hot
Thick & Chunky Salsa - Medium
Thick & Chunky Salsa - Mild
Traditional Salsa - Hot
Traditional Salsa - Medium
Traditional Salsa - Mild

La Costena
La Costena (All BUT Jalapeno Hot Sauce)

La Victoria ⓘ
Cilantro - Medium
Cilantro - Mild
Green Salsa Jalapena - Extra Hot
Red Salsa Jalapena - Extra Hot
Salsa Ranchera - Hot
Salsa Suprema - Medium
Salsa Suprema - Mild
Salsa Victoria - Hot
Thick 'N Chunky - Hot
Thick 'N Chunky - Mild
Thick 'N Chunky Verde - Medium
Thick 'N Chunky Verde - Mild

Litehouse
Medium Salsa

Margaritaville Foods
Margaritaville Salsa (All)

Meijer
Salsa - Hot
Salsa - Medium
Salsa - Mild
Salsa - Restaurant Style Hot
Salsa - Restaurant Style Medium
Salsa - Restaurant Style Mild
Salsa - Santa Fe Style Medium
Salsa - Santa Fe Style Mild
Salsa - Thick & Chunky Hot
Salsa - Thick & Chunky Medium
Salsa - Thick & Chunky Mild

Nathan's
Salsa - Hot
Salsa - Mild

Naturally Fresh ()
Medium Salsa
Salsa w/Cilantro

Nature's Basket (Giant Eagle)
Organic Corn & Black Bean Salsa
Organic Hot Salsa
Organic Medium Salsa
Organic Mild Salsa
Organic Pineapple Salsa

Newman's Own ⓘ
Black Bean & Corn Salsa
Farmer's Garden Salsa
Hot Salsa
Mango Salsa
Medium Salsa

Mild Salsa
Peach Salsa
Pineapple Salsa
Roasted Garlic Salsa
Tequila Lime Salsa

Organicville
Organicville (All)

Ortega
Black Bean & Corn (Mexican)
Garden - Medium
Garden - Mild
Original - Medium
Original - Mild
Roasted Garlic
Salsa con Queso
Salsa Verde
Thick & Chunky - Medium
Thick & Chunky - Mild

Pace ⓘ
Black Bean & Roast Corn Salsa
Chunky Salsa - Medium
Chunky Salsa - Mild
Pico de Gallo
Pineapple Mango Chipotle Salsa
Salsa Dip - Medium
Salsa Dip - Mild
Salsa Verde
Thick & Chunky Salsa - Extra Mild
Thick & Chunky Salsa - Hot
Thick & Chunky Salsa - Medium
Thick & Chunky Salsa - Mild

Publix ⓞ
All Natural - Hot Salsa
All Natural - Medium Salsa
All Natural - Mild Salsa
GreenWise Market Organic Medium
   Salsa
GreenWise Market Organic Mild Salsa
Southwestern Black Bean and Corn
   Salsa
Thick & Chunky - Hot Salsa
Thick & Chunky - Medium Salsa
Thick & Chunky - Mild Salsa

Red Gold
Tomato Products (All)

Sally's ⚕
Sally's (All)

Santa Barbara Salsa
Santa Barbara Salsa (All)

Sorrell Ridge
Pineapple Salsa - Medium

Taco Bell ⌇
Home Originals Medium Salsa Con
   Queso
Home Originals Mild Salsa Con Queso
Thick 'n Chunky Medium Salsa
Thick 'n Chunky Mild Salsa

Timpone's
Salsa Muy Rica

Tostitos ⓘ
All Natural Hot Chunky Salsa
All Natural Medium Black Bean & Corn
   Salsa
All Natural Medium Chunky Salsa
All Natural Mild Chunky Salsa
Creamy Salsa
Restaurant Style Salsa
Salsa Con Queso
Sweet & Spicy Summer Salsa

Utz ⓘ
Mt. Misery Mike's Salsa Dip
Sweet Salsa Dip

Valu Time (Marsh)
Salsa Medium
Salsa Mild

Wholly Salsa
Salsa (All BUT Queso)

SAUERKRAUT

B&G Foods
Sauerkraut

Bashas'
Sauerkraut

Bubbies ⚕
Sauerkraut

Claussen ⌇
Crisp Sauerkraut

Dei Fratelli
Dei Fratelli (All BUT Tomato Soup)

Eden Foods ⓘ ✓
Sauerkraut - Organic

Food Club (Marsh)
Canned Sauerkraut

Frank's
Frank's Sauerkraut

Great Value (Wal-Mart)
Sauerkraut

Haggen
Sauerkraut

Hy-Vee
Shredded Kraut

Meijer
Sauerkraut

Price Chopper
Sauerkraut

Sabrett
Sauerkraut

Strub's
Strub's (All)

Thumann's ✓
Condiments (All BUT Deep Fry Hot Dogs)

Sloppy Joe Sauce

Armour
Armour Sloppy Joe Sauce

Bashas'
Sloppy Joe Sauce

Dei Fratelli
Dei Fratelli (All BUT Tomato Soup)

Food Club (Marsh)
Sloppy Joe Sauce

Heinz ⓘ
Sloppy Joe Sauce

Hy-Vee
Sloppy Joe Sauce

Meijer
Sloppy Joe Sauce

Not-So-Sloppy Joe ⓘ
Sloppy Joe Sauce

Steak Sauce

A.1. �
Bold & Spicy with Tabasco Steak Sauce
Carb Well Steak Sauce

Chicago Steakhouse
Jamaican Jerk
New Orleans Cajun
New York Steakhouse
Smoky Mesquite Steak Sauce
Steak House Cracked Peppercorn
Steak Sauce
Supreme Garlic Steak Sauce
Sweet Hickory with Bull's Eye Bbq Sauce
Teriyaki Steak Sauce
Texas Mesquite
Thick & Hearty Steak Sauce

Bashas'
Steak Sauce (Glass)

Beverly Hillbillies, The
Jethro's Heapin' Helping Steak Sauce

Crystal
Steak Sauce

Food Club (Marsh)
Steak Sauce (Glass)

Golding Farms ⟨⟩
Golden Steak Sauce
Premium Steak Sauce
Vidalia Onion Steak Sauce

Gold's
Steak Sauce with Horseradish

Great Value (Wal-Mart)
Steak Sauce

Heinz ⓘ
Traditional Steak Sauce

Hy-Vee
Classic Steak Sauce

Jack Daniel's Sauces ⓘ
Steak Sauce (Both Varieties)

Lea & Perrins ⓘ
Traditional Steak Sauce

Meijer
Steak Sauce

Tabasco ✓
Caribbean Style Steak Sauce

TryMe
Bullfighter Steak & Burger Sauce

SYRUP, PANCAKE & MAPLE

Aunt Jemima ()
Syrups (All)

Bashas'
Lite Syrup
Original Syrup
Syrup - Lite 2% Maple

Central Market Classics (Price Chopper)
Dark Amber Maple Syrup

Eggo ()
Kellogg's Eggo Syrup

Food Club (Marsh)
Syrup - Butter Flavored
Syrup - Chocolate
Syrup - Lite Butter
Syrup - Strawberry

Fresh & Easy ()
Pure Vermont Maple Syrup

Ginger People, The
Ginger Syrup
Stem Ginger in Syrup

Grand Selections (Hy-Vee)
100% Pure Maple Syrup

Haggen
Syrup - Lite Pancake & Waffle

Howard's
Howard's (All)

Hungry Jack
Syrups (All)

Hy-Vee
Artificial Butter Flavored Syrup
Lite Pancake Syrup
Low Calorie Sugar Free Syrup
Pancake & Waffle Syrup

Karo
Karo Syrups (All)

Kellogg's ()
Eggo Syrup

Knott's Berry Farms
Syrups

Log Cabin (i)
Syrup

Maple Grove Farms
Cream - Pure Maple

Honey Maple Spread
Maple Blend Spread
Syrups (All Varieties)

Market District (Giant Eagle)
Pure Maple Syrup

Meijer
Syrup - Butter Flavored
Syrup - Lite
Syrup - Lite Butter
Syrup - Regular

Midwest Country Fare (Hy-Vee)
Pancake & Waffle Syrup

Mrs. Butterworth's (i)
Syrups (All)

Price Chopper
Maple Syrup

Publix ()
Butter Flavor Pancake Syrup
Lite Butter Flavor Pancake Syrup
Lite Maple Flavor Pancake Syrup
Maple Flavor Pancake Syrup

Right Size
Right Size (All)

Smucker's
Breakfast Syrups

Valu Time (Marsh)
Syrup Butter Flavor
Syrup Regular Flavor

Vermont Maid
Vermont Maid Syrup (All Varieties)

Wholesome Sweeteners
Organic Pancake and Waffle Syrup

Winn & Lovette (Winn-Dixie) ()
Maple Syrup (All Varieties)

Winn-Dixie ()
Butter Flavor Syrup
Chocolate Syrup
Lite Syrup
Regular Syrup

TACO SAUCE

Casa Fiesta
Green Taco Sauce
Taco Sauce

Chi-Chi's ⓘ
Taco Sauce

Food Club (Marsh)
Taco Sauce - Mild

Fresh & Easy ()
Green Taco Sauce
Red Taco Sauce - Medium
Red Taco Sauce - Mild

Great Value (Wal-Mart)
Red Taco Sauce

Hy-Vee
Medium Taco Sauce
Mild Taco Sauce

La Victoria ⓘ
Green Taco Sauce - Medium
Green Taco Sauce - Mild
Red Taco Sauce - Medium
Red Taco Sauce - Mild

Ortega
Green Taco Sauce
Taco Sauce - Hot
Taco Sauce - Medium
Taco Sauce - Mild

Pace ⓘ
Taco Sauce - Medium
Taco Sauce - Mild

Taco Bell ⌒
Medium Taco Sauce
Mild Taco Sauce

Tartar Sauce

Best Foods
Mayonnaise Products and Spreads (All)

Cains ⓘ
Tartar Sauce

Cajun's Choice
Cajun's Choice (All BUT Seasoned Fish
Fry and Creole Mustard)

Food Club (Marsh)
Tartar Sauce (Squeeze)

Fresh & Easy ()
Tartar Sauce

Golding Farms ()
Tartar Sauce

Gold's
Squeeze Tartar Sauce

Heinz ⓘ
Tartar Sauce

Little River ()
Tangy Tartar Sauce

Louisiana Fish Fry ()
Remoulade Dressing
Tartar Sauce

Naturally Fresh ()
Tartar Sauce

Silver Spring ⓘ
Silver Spring (All)

Woeber
Woeber (All)

Vinegar

B.R. Cohn ⚱
Wine Vinegars (All)

Bashas'
Vinegar - Cider
Vinegar - White

Bionaturae
Balsamic Vinegar ⚱

Colavita
Vinegar (All)

Eden Foods ⓘ ✓
Apple Cider Vinegar - Organic
Brown Rice Vinegar - Organic
Red Wine Vinegar

Filippo Berio ⚱
Red Wine Vinegar

Food Club (Marsh)
Vinegar Cider
Vinegar White

Grand Selections (Hy-Vee)
Balsamic Vinegar of Modena
Red Wine Vinegar
White Wine Vinegar

Great Value (Wal-Mart)
Apple Cider Vinegar
Balsamic Vinegar
Distilled White Vinegar
Premium Garlic Flavored Red Wine
Vinegar

Premium Red Wine Vinegar

Haggen
Vinegar - Apple Cider
Vinegar - White Distilled

Heinz ⓘ
Apple Cider Flavored Vinegar
Apple Cider Vinegar
Distilled White Vinegar
Garlic Wine Vinegar
Red Wine Vinegar

Holland House ⓘ
Balsamic Vinegar
Red Wine Vinegar
White Wine Vinegar

Hy-Vee
Apple Cider Flavored Distilled Vinegar
White Distilled Vinegar

Lucini Italia () ✓
Lucini Italia (All BUT Russian Tomato
Vodka Sauce and Minestrone Soup)

Marukan
Rice Vinegars (All)
Seasoned Rice Vinegars (All)

Meijer
Vinegar
Vinegar - Balsamic 12 Year Aged
Vinegar - Balsamic 4 Year Old Aged
Vinegar - Cider
Vinegar - Red Wine
Vinegar - White
Vinegar - White Wine

Nakano ⓘ
Rice Vinegars (All)
Seasoned Rice Vinegars (All)

Newman's Own Organics () ⓘ
Balsamic Vinegar

O Olive Oil ⚕
Vinegars (All)

Publix ()
Red Wine Vinegar
White Distilled Vinegar

Rao's Homemade ()
Rao's Homemade (All)

Regina
Vinegars (All)

Sun Luck
Rice Vinegar - Natural
Rice Vinegar - Seasoned

White House
White House (All)

Woeber
Woeber (All)

Worcestershire Sauce

Bashas'
Worcestershire Sauce

Crystal
Worcestershire Sauce

Food Club (Marsh)
Worcestershire Sauce

French's
Worcestershire Sauce

Great Value (Wal-Mart)
Worcestershire Sauce

Heinz ⓘ
Worcestershire Sauce

Hy-Vee
Worcestershire Sauce

Lea & Perrins ⓘ
Worcestershire Sauce (All Varieties)

Meijer
Worcestershire Sauce

TryMe
Wine & Pepper Worcestershire

Wizard's, The ✓
Organic Wheat-Free Vegan
Worcestershire

Miscellaneous

Di Lusso ⓘ
Sweet Onion Sauce

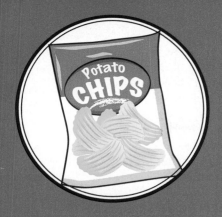

SNACKS & CONVENIENCE FOODS

APPLESAUCE

Bashas'
- Applesauce
- Applesauce - Cinnamon
- Applesauce - Natural (Shelf Stable)
- Applesauce - Unsweetened

Eden Foods ⓘ ✔
- Apple Cherry Sauce - Organic
- Apple Cinnamon Sauce - Organic
- Apple Sauce - Organic
- Apple Strawberry Sauce - Organic

Food Club (Marsh)
- Applesauce
- Chunky Applesauce
- Cinnamon Applesauce
- Natural Applesauce
- Strawberry Applesauce - Single Serve Cup

Fresh & Easy ()
- Applesauce (All Flavors)

Great Value (Wal-Mart)
- Apple Sauce
- Cinnamon Apple Sauce
- Natural Apple Sauce
- No Salt Added Apple Sauce Sweetened w/Splenda
- Strawberry Flavored Apple Sauce
- Unsweetened Apple Sauce

Haggen
- Applesauce - Cinnamon
- Applesauce - Natural
- Applesauce - Regular

Hy-Vee
- Applesauce

- Cinnamon Applesauce
- Natural Applesauce
- Unsweetened Applesauce

Kroger ⓘ
- Applesauce - Flavored
- Applesauce - Plain

Meijer
- Applesauce
- Applesauce Chunky
- Applesauce Cinnamon
- Applesauce Mixed Berry
- Applesauce Natural
- Applesauce Organic Cinnamon
- Applesauce Organic Sweetened
- Applesauce Organic Unsweetened
- Applesauce Original
- Applesauce Regular
- Applesauce Strawberry

Midwest Country Fare (Hy-Vee)
- Applesauce with Cinnamon
- Applesauce with Peaches
- Applesauce with Raspberries
- Applesauce with Strawberries
- Home Style Applesauce
- Natural Applesauce

Nash Brothers
- Organic Applesauce

Publix ()
- Applesauce - Chunky
- Applesauce - Cinnamon
- Applesauce - Old Fashioned
- Applesauce - Unsweetened
- GreenWise Market Organic Unsweetened Apple Sauce

Tree Top
  Applesauce (All)
Vermont Village ⅋
  Applesauce (All)
White House
  White House (All)
Winn-Dixie ()
  Cinnamon Applesauce
  Sweetened Applesauce
  Unsweetened Applesauce

BAKED GOODS

Against the Grain ⅋
  Against the Grain (All)
Bi Aglut
  Bi Aglut (All)
Cookies... for Me? ⅋
  Cookies… For Me? (All)
Ener-G ⅋ ✓
  Brownies
  Chocolate Iced Doughnuts
  Cinnamon Rolls

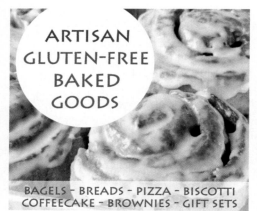

Doughnut Holes - Plain
Doughnuts - Plain
Poundcake
Foods by George ⅋
  Blueberry Muffins
  Brownies
  Corn Muffins
  Crumb Cake
  Pound Cake
Frankly Natural Bakers ✓
  Gluten-Free Carob Almondine Brownie
  Gluten-Free Cherry Berry Brownie
  Gluten-Free Java Jive Brownie
  Gluten-Free Misty Mint Brownie
  Gluten-Free Wacky Walnut Brownie
French Meadow Bakery
  Gluten-Free Apple Cinnamon Muffin
  Gluten-Free Blueberry Muffin
  Gluten-Free Brownie
  Gluten-Free Brownie Bite
  Gluten-Free Chocolate 4" Cake
  Gluten-Free Chocolate Cupcake
  Gluten-Free Fudge Brownie
  Gluten-Free Yellow 4" Cake
  Gluten-Free Yellow Cupcake
Gillian's Foods ⅋
  Gillian's Foods (All)
Gluten Free & FABULOUS ✓
  Brownie Bites
Grainless Baker, The ⅋
  The Grainless Baker (All)
Joan's GF Great Bakes ⅋
  Joan's GF Great Bakes (All)
Katz Gluten Free ⅋
  Katz Gluten Free (All)
Mariposa Baking Company ⅋ ✓
  Almond Biscotti
  Cinnamon Rolls
  Cinnamon Toast Biscotti
  Coconut Lemon Squares
  Cranberry Orange Nut Bread (Seasonal)
  Ginger Spice Biscotti
  Mocha Brownies
  Pumpkin Bread (Seasonal)
  Sour Cream Coffeecake
  Triple Chocolate Brownies
  Walnut Brownies

Outside the Breadbox
Outside the Breadbox (All)

Pamela's Products
Agave Sweetened NY Cheesecake
Chocolate Fudge Cake
Coffee Cake
Hazelnut Cheesecake
New York Cheesecake
White Chocolate Raspberry Cheesecake
Zesty Lemon Cheesecake

Shabtai Gourmet Gluten-Free Bakery

Gluten Free & Egg Free Bon Bons
Gluten Free 7 inch Occasion Layer Cake
Gluten Free Apricot Roll
Gluten Free Brownie Bites
Gluten Free Devils Food Seven Layer
    Cake
Gluten Free Fudge Brownie
Gluten Free Marble Loaf Cake
Gluten Free Raspberry Roll
Gluten Free Ring Ting Cupcakes
Gluten Free Seven Layer Cake - White
    Cake
Gluten Free Sponge Cake Loaf
Gluten Free Swiss Chocolate Roll

Smart Treat
Smart Treat (All)

Udi's Gluten Free Foods
Blueberry Muffins
Cinnamon Rolls
Double Chocolate Muffins
Lemon Streusel Muffins

BARS

ALPSNACK
Alpsnack (All)

ANDI
ANDI Bars

Attune
Almond Milk Chocolate Probiotic Bar
Blueberry Vanilla White Chocolate
    Probiotic Bar
Coffee Bean Dark Chocolate Probiotic
    Bar
Dark Chocolate Probiotic Bar

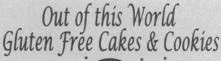
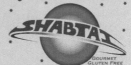
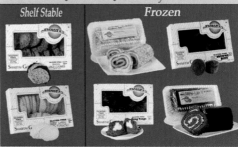

Milk Chocolate Crisp Probiotic Bar
Mint Chocolate Probiotic Bar
Raspberry Dark Chocolate Probiotic Bar

Bakery on Main
Cranberry Maple Nut Gluten-Free
    Granola Bars
Extreme Trail Mix Gluten-Free Granola
    Bars
Peanut Butter Chocolate Chip Gluten-
    Free Granola Bars

Balance Bar
Balance Pure: Berry Berry Chia
Balance Pure: Cherry Pecan
Balance Pure: Chocolate Cashew

Betty Lou's
Almond Butter Ball
Apple Cinnamon Fruit Bar
Apricot Fruit Bar
Blueberry Fruit Bar
Cashew Pecan Ball
Cherry Fruit Bar
Chocolate Walnut Balls
Coconut Macadamia Balls

High Protein Almond Butter Ball
Organic Cacao Acai Bar
Organic Chocolate Dreams Greens Bar
Organic Fruit and Veggie Bar
Organic Krispy Bites
Organic Superberry Acai
Peanut Butter Balls
Spirulina Ginseng Ball
Strawberry Fruit Bar

Bi Aglut
Bi Aglut (All)

BoomiBar ♀
Boomi Bar (All)

Cascade Fresh
Cascade Fresh (All)

Ener-G ♀ ✓
Chocolate Chip Snack Bars

Enjoy Life Foods ♀ ✓
Caramel Apple Chewy On-The-Go Bars
Cocoa Loco Chewy On-The-Go Bars
Sunbutter Crunch Chewy On-The-Go Bars
Very Berry Chewy On-The-Go Bars

EnviroKidz ⓘ ✓
Crispy Rice Bars - Cheetah Berry
Crispy Rice Bars - Koala Chocolate
Crispy Rice Bars - Lemur Choco Drizzle
Crispy Rice Bars - Panda Peanut Butter
Crispy Rice Bars - Penguin Fruity Burst

Figamajigs ⓘ
Figamajigs (All)

Frankly Natural Bakers ✓
Gluten-Free Apricot Energy Bar
Gluten-Free Date Nut Energy Bar
Gluten-Free Raisin Energy Bar
Gluten-Free Tropical Energy Bar

Glucerna
Caramel Nut Glucerna Snack Bar
Lemon Crunch Glucerna Snack Bar

Gluten Free Café ✓
Chocolate Sesame Bar
Cinnamon Sesame Bar
Lemon Sesame Bar

Glutino
Breakfast Bars Apple
Breakfast Bars Blueberry

Breakfast Bars Cherry
Organic Bar - Chocolate & Peanut Butter
Organic Bar - Chocolate Banana
Organic Bar - Wildberry

Greens +
Chia Bar Natural
Energy Bar Berry
Energy Bar Natural
Protein Bar Natural
Whey Krisp

KIND ♀ ✓
KIND Snacks (All)

Lärabar ✓
Apple Pie
Banana Bread
Carrot Cake
Cashew Cookie
Cherry Pie
Chocolate Chip Brownie
Chocolate Chip Cookie Dough
Chocolate Coconut Chew
Cinnamon Roll
Coconut Cream Pie
Ginger Snap
Jŏcalat Chocolate
Jŏcalat Chocolate Cherry
Jŏcalat Chocolate Coffee
Jŏcalat Chocolate Hazelnut
Jŏcalat Chocolate Mint
Key Lime Pie
Lemon Bar
Minis Variety Pack (Apple, Cherry, Cashew)
Peanut Butter & Jelly
Peanut Butter Chocolate Chip
Peanut Butter Cookie
Pecan Pie
Tropical Fruit Tart

Lydia's Organics ♀
Lydia's Organics (All)

Manischewitz
Raspberry Jell Bars

Meijer
Xtreme Snack Bars

Mrs. May's Naturals ✓
Mrs. May's Naturals (All)

Nature Valley Roasted Nut Crunch Bars ✓
- Almond Crunch
- Peanut Crunch

Nugo Nutrition
- Nugo 10 Line
- Nugo Dark Mint Chocolate Chip
- NuGo Free Line

Omega Smart Bar
- Omega Smart Bar (All)

Orgran ✓
- Fruit Bars (All)
- Fruit Filled Bar Range (All)

Planters Carb Well ⌇
- Carb Well Caramel Chocolate Crunch Nut Bar
- Carb Well Peanut Butter Crunch Nut Bar

Planters ⌇
- Original Peanut Bar

POM Wonderful ⚱
- POM Wonderful (All)

PowerBar ⟨⟩
- PowerBar Gels

PranaBar
- PranaBar (All)

Publix ⟨⟩
- Peanut Butter Bars

PureFit
- PureFit (All)

Raw Revolution ✓
- Raw Revolution (All)

Schar ⚱ ✓
- Chocolate Hazelnut Bars

South Beach Living ⌇
- Chocolate Peanut Butter Meal Replacement Bar
- Chocolate Raspberry Snack Bars
- Peanut Butter Snack Bars

SoyJoy
- SoyJoy (All)

Tiger's Milk ⟨⟩
- Peanut Butter
- Peanut Butter & Honey
- Protein Rich

Zing ✓
- Zing Bars (All)

ZonePerfect ⟨⟩
- Chocolate Almond Raisin
- Chocolate Caramel Cluster
- Chocolate Coconut Crunch
- Chocolate Peanut Butter
- Chocolate Raspberry
- Dark Chocolate Caramel Pecan
- Dark Chocolate Mocha
- Double Dark Chocolate
- Fructified: Banana Nut
- Fructified: Blueberry
- Fudge Graham
- Indulgence Bar: Caramel Toffee
- Indulgence Bar: Chocolate Peanut Butter Mousse
- Indulgence Bar: German Chocolate Cheesecake
- Peanut Toffee

BEEF JERKY & OTHER MEAT SNACKS

Bridgford
- Original Beef Jerky
- Peppered Beef Jerky
- Sweet & Hot Beef Jerky

Golden Valley Natural
- Organic Beef Jerky (All)

Haggen
- Peppered Beef Jerky (Open Stock)

Hy-Vee
- Beef Summer Sausage
- Original Beef Jerky
- Summer Sausage

Old Wisconsin ⓘ
- Beef Summer Sausage
- Original Summer Sausage
- Snack Bites - Beef
- Snack Bites - Pepperoni
- Snack Bites - Turkey
- Snack Sticks - Beef
- Snack Sticks - Pepperoni
- Snack Sticks - Spicy Beef
- Snack Sticks - Turkey

Organic Prairie
- Prairie Classic Beef Jerky

Smoky Chipotle Beef Jerky
Spicy Hickory Beef Jerky

Oscar Mayer ～
Spicy Snackers Hot Shots Pepper Cheese
Nuts Picante Snak Saks
Summer Sausage

Shelton's
Beef Jerky
Pepperoni Turkey Sticks
Regular Turkey Sticks
Turkey Jerky Hot
Turkey Jerky Regular

CANDY & CHOCOLATE

3 Musketeers
3 Musketeers Mint
3 Musketeers Original

Altoids
Altoids (All BUT Altoids Chocolate
Dipped Mints)
Altoids Chocolate Dipped Mints ()

Andes
Andes (All)

Atomic FireBall
Atomic Fireball (All)

Baby Bottle Pop ✓
Baby Bottle Pop (All)

Baby Ruth ⓘ
Baby Ruth

Before & After Candy
Mints (All)

Big Hunk
Big Hunk Candy Bar (2 oz. size only)

Bit-O-Honey ⓘ
Bit-O-Honey

Black Forest Gummies
Black Forest Gummies (All)
Fruit Snacks (All)

Boston Baked Beans
Boston Baked Beans

Butterfinger ⓘ
Butterfinger (All BUT Butterfinger Crisp
& Butterfinger Stixx)

Canada Mints ⛑
Mint Lozenges

Wintergreen Lozenges

Candy Carnival
Candy Carnival (All)

Caramel Apple Pops
Caramel Apple Pops (All)

Cella Cherries
Cella Cherries (All)

Charleston Chew
Charleston Chew (All)

Charms Blow Pops
Charms Blow Pops (All)

Charms Flat Pops
Charms Flat Pops (All)

Child's Play
Child's Play (All)

Clark Bar ⛑
Clark Bar

Crispy Cat Candy Bars
Crispy Cat Candy Bar (All)

Crows
Crows (All)

Cry Baby
Cry Baby (All)

Dots
Dots (All)

Dove
Dove Chocolate Products (All)

Endangered Species Chocolate
Chocolate Bars (All)

Enjoy Life Foods ⛑ ✓
Boom CHOCO Boom Dairy Free Rice
Milk Bar
Boom CHOCO Boom Dairy Free Rice
Milk with Crispy Rice Bar
Boom CHOCO Boom Dark Chocolate
Bar

Equal Exchange
Chocolate Bars (All) ⓘ ✓

Fannie May
Apricot Bon Bon
Apricot Cream
Candy Bars (All)
Chocolate & Pastel Meltaways
Chocolate Toffee
Chocolate Wafers
Citrus Peel

Dark Filbert Cluster
English Toffee
Hostess Mints
Irish Toffee
Ivory & Chocolate Bark
Milk & Dark Almond Clusters
Milk & Dark Walnut Clusters
Milk Peanut Butter Crunch Bar
Pastel Toffee
Pastel Wafers
Peanut Cluster
Solid Chocolate Novelties (All)

Ferrara Pan Candy Company
Ferrara Pan Candy (All)

Figamajigs ⓘ
Figamajigs (All)

Fluffy Stuff Cotton Candy
Fluffy Stuff (All)

Fresh & Easy ⟨⟩
Chocolate Bars
Chocolate Covered Almonds
Chocolate Covered Espresso Beans
Chocolate Covered Macadamia Nuts
Chocolate Covered Raisins
Chocolate Covered Raspberries
Chocolate Covered Tart Cherries
Huge Hunk Chocolates (All BUT Pecans
   & Fruit Pieces Variety)
Sweet Boutique Swiss Chocolates
Yogurt Covered Raisins

Frooties
Frooties (All)

Gimbal's Fine Candies
Gimbal's (All)

Ginger People, The
Crystallized Ginger Candy
Crystallized Ginger Chunk
Gin Gins Hard Candy
Ginger Delight
Gin-Gins Boost - Ultra Strength Ginger
   Candy
Hot Coffee Ginger Chews
Original Ginger Chews
Peanut Ginger Chews
Spicy Apple Ginger Chews

Glutino
Chocolate Peanut Butter Candy Bar

Dark Chocolate Candy Bar
Milk Chocolate Candy Bar

GoLightly ✓
Sugar Free Candy (All)

GoNaturally ✓
Organic Candy (All)

Goobers ⓘ
Goobers

Great Value (Wal-Mart)
Assorted Flavors Jelly Beans
Butterscotch Discs
Candy Cinnamon Discs
Candy Corn
Candy Gummy Worms
Cinnamon Disc
Fruit Smiles (Sour Apple, Watermelon,
   Blue Raspberry, Tropical Punch)
Fruit Smiles (Strawberry, Grape,
   Orange, Lemon)
Gummy Bears
Gummy Worms
Jelly Beans
Orange Slices
Peppermint Starlight Mints
Spearmint Starlight Mints
Spice Drops
Starlight Mints

Guittard
Chocolate Products (All)

Haviland
Peppermint & Wintergreen Patties
Thin Mints (All) ⸸

Hawaiian Host ⓘ ⸸
Chocolate Covered Macadamia Nuts
   (All)
Maui and Kona Caramacs (All)

Hershey's
Milk Chocolate Bar
Milk Chocolate Bar with Almonds
Milk Chocolate Kisses

Hint Mint
Hint Mint (All)
Petit Hint Mint (All)

Honees Candies
Honees (All)

Hot Tamales
  Hot Tamales
Hy-Vee
  Chocolate Caramel Clusters
  Chocolate Stars
  Double Dipped Chocolate Covered
    Peanuts
  Milk Chocolate Caramel Cups
  Milk Chocolate Peanut Butter Cups
  Tootsie Pops
JawBreakers
  JawBreakers
Juicy Drop Pop
  Juicy Drop Pop (All)
Junior Mints
  Junior Mints (All)
Just Born
  Just Born Candies (All)
Kellogg's ()
  Yogos
Kroger ⓘ
  Hard Candy
Laffy Taffy ⓘ
  Laffy Taffy Fruitarts Chews
  Laffy Taffy Rope
Lemonhead & Friends
  Lemonhead & Friends (All)
Let's Do…Organic ✔
  Organic Classic Gummi Bears
  Organic Jelly Gummi Bears
  Organic Super Sour Gummi Bears
LifeSavers
  LifeSavers (All)
M&M'S
  M&M's Products (All BUT M&Ms
    Pretzels)
Manischewitz
  Caramel Cashew Patties
  Chocolate Frolic Bears
  Fruit Slices
  Hazelnut Truffles
  Max's Magic Lollycones
  Mini Sour Fruit Slices
  Peppermint Patties
  Swiss Chocolate Mints
  Viennese Crunch

Maple Grove Farms
  Candy (All Varieties)
Mary Janes ⑧
  Mary Jane Peanut Butter Kisses
  Mary Janes
Meijer
  Peanuts - Butter Toffee
Mike and Ike
  Mike and Ike
Milka Chocolate ⌒
  Alpine Milk Chocolate Confection
Milky Way
  Milky Way Products (All BUT Milky
    Way Bar)
Munch Bar
  Munch Bar
Necco
  Banana Split Chews
  Candy Buttons ⑧
  Mint Julep Chews
  Necco Wafers ⑧
  Peach Blossoms
  Squirrel Nut Caramels
  Squirrel Nut Zippers
Nestlé ⓘ
  Milk Chocolate
Newman's Own Organics () ⓘ
  Chocolate Bars (All)
  Chocolate Cups (All)
  Mint Rolls
  Mints in Tins
Nik-L-Nip
  Nik-L-Nip (All)
Nips ⓘ
  Regular
  Sugar Free
Oh Henry! ⓘ
  Oh Henry!
Orgran ✔
  Molasses Licorice
Peanut Chews
  Peanut Chews
Peeps
  Marshmallow Peeps
PEZ
  PEZ Candy

Piedmont Candy Co. ♟
  Piedmont Candy (All)
Pixy Stix ⓘ
  Pixy Stix
Pop Rocks
  Pop Rocks
Publix ()
  Butterscotch Discs
  Chocolate Covered Peanut Brittle
  Double Dipped Chocolate Covered
    Peanuts
  Gummi Worms
  Lollipops
  Pixy Stick Candy
  Smarties Candy
  Sour Worms
  Spearmint Starlight Mints
  Starlight Mints Candy
  Strawberry Bon Bons
Push Pop ✓
  Push Pop (All)
Raisinets ⓘ
  Raisinets
Razzles
  Razzles (All)
Red Bird ♟
  Red Bird (All)
Red Hots
  Red Hots
Reese's
  Reese's Peanut Butter Cups
  Reese's Pieces
Ring Pop ✓
  Ring Pop (All)
Runts ⓘ
  Runts
Skittles
  Skittles (All)
Skybar
  Skybars
Smarties
  Smarties (All)
Snickers
  Snickers
  Snickers Dark

Sno-Caps ⓘ
  Sno-Caps
Sour Patch Kids
  Sour Patch Kids
Spangler Candy Company ♟
  Candy Canes (All)
  Dum Dums (All)
  Marshmallow Products (All)
  Saf-T-Pops (All)
Starburst
  Starburst (All)
Sugar Babies
  Sugar Babies (All)
Sugar Daddy
  Sugar Daddy (All)
Surf Sweets ♟
  Surf Sweets (All)
Swedish Fish
  Swedish Fish
Sweethearts ♟
  Sweethearts Conversation Hearts
    (Valentines Only)
Sweet'N Low
  Sweet'N Low (All)
Teenee Beanee
  Teenee Beanee (All)
Terrys ᕔ
  Orange Dark Chocolate
  Orange Milk Chocolate
  Pure Milk Chocolate
Toblerone ᕔ
  Minis Swiss Chocolate with Honey &
    Almond Nougat
  Minis Swiss Milk Chocolate with Honey
    & Almond Nougat
  Minis White Confection with Honey &
    Almond Nougat
  Swiss Bittersweet with Honey & Almond
    Nougat
  Swiss Milk Chocolate with Honey &
    Almond Nougat
  Swiss White Confection with Honey &
    Almond Nougat
  Truffle Peaks
Tootsie Pops
  Tootsie Pops (All)

Tootsie Rolls
Tootsie Rolls (All)
Topps Company, The ✓
Topps
Tropical Source ✓
Mint Crunch Dark Chocolate Bar
Raspberry Dark Chocolate Bar
Rice Crisp Dark Chocolate Bar
Rich Dark Chocolate Bar
Toasted Almond Dark Chocolate Bar
VerMints ☕
VerMints (All)
Wack-O-Wax
Wack-O-Wax (All)
Zours
Zours

CHEESE PUFFS & CURLS

Baked! Cheetos ⓘ
Crunchy Cheese Flavored Snacks
Flamin' Hot Cheese Flavored Snacks
Bashas'
Cheese Puffs
Crazy Curls Cheese Puffs
Crunchy Cheese Sacks
Cheetos ⓘ
Crunchy Cheddar Jalapeno Cheese
Flavored Snacks
Crunchy Cheese Flavored Snacks
Crunchy Chile Limon Flavored Snacks
Crunchy Flamin' Hot Cheese Flavored
Snacks
Crunchy Flamin' Hot Limon Cheese
Flavored Snacks
Crunchy Wild Habanero Cheese
Flavored Snacks
Giant Puffs Cheese Flavored Snacks
Giant Puffs Flamin' Hot Cheese Flavored
Snacks
Jumbo Puffs Flamin' Hot Cheese
Flavored Snacks
Mighty Zingers Ragin' Cajun & Tangy
Ranch Cheese Flavored Snacks
Mighty Zingers Sharp Cheddar & Salsa
Picante Cheese Flavored Snacks

Natural White Cheddar Puffs Cheese
Flavored Snacks
Puffs Cheese Flavored Snacks
Twisted Cheese Flavored Snacks
EatSmart Naturals ✓
Multigrain Cheese Puffs
Fresh & Easy ⟨⟩
Cheese Puffs & Curls
Great Value (Wal-Mart)
Cheddar Cheese Crunch
Cheddar Cheese Puffs
Cheddar Flavor Cheese Sensations
Herr's
Cheese Curls
Crunchy Cheese Sticks
Honey Cheese Curls
Hot Cheese Curls
Meijer
Cheese Pops
Cheese Puffs
Cheezy Treats
White Cheddar Puffs
Michael Season's
Baked Cheddar Cheese Curls
Baked Cheddar Cheese Puff
Baked Hot Chili Pepper Curl
Baked Jalapeno Puff
Baked White Cheddar Pops
Ultimate Cheddar Cheese Curls
Ultimate Cheddar Cheese Puffs
Ultimate White Cheddar Cheese Puffs
Pirate's Booty ☕ ✓
Pirate's Booty (All)
Publix ⟨⟩
Crunchy Cheese Curls
Crunchy Cheese Puffs
Snikiddy ✓
Cheddar Cheese Fries
Grilled Cheese Puffs
Ketchup Fries
Mac 'n Cheese Puffs
Nacho Cheese Puffs
Original Fries
Parmesan Garlic Fries
Pizza Puffs
Utz ⓘ
Baked Cheese Curls and Balls

Crunchy Cheese Curls
Puff 'N Corn - Cheese
White Cheddar Cheese Curls

Valu Time (Marsh)
Snack Cheese Baked Puffs

CHIPS & CRISPS, OTHER

Bashas'
Corn Chips
Corn Chips Shovels
Corn Crisp & Sweet
Snack Big Dipper Corn Chip

Brothers All Natural 🏅
Fruit Crisps

Bubbies 🏅
Bread & Butter Chips

Cheetos ⓘ
Fantastix Chili Cheese Flavored Baked
   Corn/Potato Snacks
Fantastix Flamin' Hot Flavored Baked
   Corn/Potato Snacks

Chester's ⓘ
Chili Cheese Flavored Fries
Flamin' Hot Flavored Puffcorn Snacks
Flamin' Hot Flavored Fries

Chifles
Chifles (All)

Corn Nuts ⌇
Barbecue Crunchy Corn Snacks
Chile Picante Con Limon Crunchy Corn
   Snacks
Chile Picante Crunchy Corn Snack
Chorizo Chipotle Crunchy Corn Snacks
Limon Crunchy Corn Snacks
Nacho Cheese Crunchy Corn Snacks
Original Crunchy Corn Snacks
Ranch Crunchy Corn Snacks
Salsa Jalisco Crunchy Corn Snacks

EatSmart Naturals ✓
Corn and Rice Puffs

Eden Foods ⓘ ✓
Brown Rice Chips

Fresh & Easy ()
Soy Crisps - Sweet BBQ Flavored
Soy Crisps - White Cheddar Flavored

Tomato Basil Veggie Crisps
Veggie Chips & Crisps

Fritos ⓘ
Flavor Twists Honey BBQ Flavored
   Corn Chips
Lightly Salted Corn Chips
Original Corn Chips
Scoops! Corn Chips
Spicy Jalapeño Flavored Corn Chips

Funyuns ⓘ
Flamin' Hot Onion Flavored Rings
Onion Flavored Rings

Great Value (Wal-Mart)
Bigger Corn Chips
Corn Chips

Herr's
Veggie Crisps

Kitchen Table Bakers ✓
Kitchen Table Bakers (All)

Lundberg Family Farms 🏅 ✓
Rice Chips - Fiesta Lime
Rice Chips - Honey Dijon
Rice Chips - Nacho Cheese
Rice Chips - Pico De Gallo
Rice Chips - Santa Fe Barbecue
Rice Chips - Sea Salt
Rice Chips - Sesame & Seaweed
Rice Chips - Wasabi

Michael Season's
Cheddar Baked Multigrain Chips
Honey Chipotle Baked Multigrain Chips
Original Baked Multigrain Chips

Mr. Krispers 🏅
Baked Rice Snack Products (All)

Mrs. May's Naturals ✓
Mrs. May's Naturals (All)

New York Style
Parmesan and Roasted Garlic Risotto
   Chips
Sea Salt Risotto Chips
Spicy Marinara Risotto Chips

Newman's Own Organics () ⓘ
Barbeque Soy Crisps
Cinnamon Sugar Soy Crisps
Lightly Salted Soy Crisps
White Cheddar Soy Crisps

Orgran ✓
  Crispibites
  Toasted Corn Dippers
Pirate's Booty ♨ ✓
  Pirate's Booty (All)
Publix ()
  Corn Chips - King Size
Sabritas ⓘ
  Rancheritos Flavored Corn Chips
  Turbos Flamas Flavored Corn Chips
Utz ⓘ
  Corn Chips - Barbeque
  Corn Chips - Plain

CHIPS & CRISPS, POTATO

Baked! Lay's ⓘ
  Cheddar & Sour Cream Flavored Potato
    Crisps
  Original Potato Crisps
  Parmesan and Tuscan Herb Flavored
    Potato Crisps
  Sour Cream & Onion Artificially
    Flavored Potato Crisps
  Southwestern Ranch Flavored Potato
    Crisps
Baked! Ruffles ⓘ
  Cheddar & Sour Cream Flavored Potato
    Crisps
  Original Potato Crisps
Bashas'
  Potato Chips - Barbecue
  Potato Chips - Classic
  Potato Chips - Kettle Cooked - BBQ
  Potato Chips - Kettle Cooked - Original
  Potato Chips - Regular
  Potato Chips - Ripple
  Potato Chips - Sour Cream & Onion
Brothers All Natural ♨
  Potato Crisps
Cape Cod ⓘ
  Cape Cod Products (All)
Food Club (Marsh)
  Potato Sticks
  Snack Potato Chips - Regular
  Snack Potato Chips Kettle - Bbq
  Snack Potato Chips Kettle - Original

Fresh & Easy ()
  Kettle Chips - BBQ
  Kettle Chips - Cheddar Jalapeno
  Kettle Chips - Limon
  Kettle Chips - Salt & Pepper
  Kettle Chips - Salted
Good Health Natural Products ♨
  Avocado Oil Potato Chips (All)
  Glories Sweet Potato Chips
  Olive Oil Potato Chips (All)
Herr's
  Cheddar & Sour Cream Potato Chips
  Crisp N' Tasty Potato Chips
  Honey BBQ Potato Chips
  Jalapeno Kettle Potato Chips
  Ketchup Potato Chips
  Lightly Salted Potato Chips
  Mesquite BBQ Kettle Potato Chips
  No Salt Potato Chips
  Old Bay Potato Chips
  Old Fashioned Potato Chips
  Original Kettle Potato Chips
  Potato Sticks
  Red Hot Potato Chips
  Ripple Potato Chips
  Russet Kettle Potato Chips
  Salt & Pepper Potato Chips
  Salt & Vinegar Potato Chips
Kettle Brand ♨
  Potato Chips (All)
Kroger ⓘ
  Plain Potato Chips
Lay's ⓘ
  Balsamic Sweet Onion Flavored Potato
    Chips
  Cajun Herb & Spice Flavored Potato
    Chips
  Cheddar & Sour Cream Artificially
    Flavored Potato Chips
  Chile Limon Potato Chips
  Classic Potato Chips
  Deli Style Original Potato Chips
  Dill Pickle Flavored Potato Chips
  Garden Tomato & Basil Flavored Potato
    Chips
  Honey BBQ Flavored Potato Chips

Hot & Spicy Barbecue Flavored Potato Chips

Kettle Cooked Crinkle Cut BBQ Potato Chips

Kettle Cooked Crinkle Cut Original Potato Chips

Kettle Cooked Jalapeno Flavored Extra Crunchy Potato Chips

Kettle Cooked Original Potato Chips

Kettle Cooked Reduced Fat Original Flavored Potato Chips

Kettle Cooked Sea Salt & Cracked Pepper Flavored Potato Chips

Kettle Cooked Sea Salt & Vinegar Flavored Potato Chips

Kettle Cooked Sharp Cheddar Flavored Potato Chips

Kettle Cooked Sweet Chili & Sour Cream Flavored Potato Chips

Light Original Potato Chips

Lightly Salted Potato Chips

Limon Tangy Lime Flavored Potato Chips

Natural Sea Salt Thick Cut Potato Chips

Pepper Relish Flavored Potato Chips

Salt & Vinegar Artificially Flavored Potato Chips

Sour Cream & Onion Artificially Flavored Potato Chips

Southwest Cheese & Chiles Flavored Potato Chips

Sweet & Spicy Buffalo Wing Flavored Potato Chips

Sweet Southern Heat BBQ Flavored Potato Chips

Tangy Carolina BBQ Flavored Potato Chips

Wavy Au Gratin Flavored Potato Chips

Wavy Hickory BBQ Flavored Potato Chips

Wavy Ranch Flavored Potato Chips

Wavy Regular Potato Chips

Lay's Stax ⚕

Cheddar Flavored Potato Crisps

Jalapeno Cheddar Flavored Potato Crisps

Mesquite Barbecue Flavored Potato Crisps

Original Flavored Potato Crisps

Ranch Flavored Potato Crisps

Salt & Vinegar Flavored Potato Crisps

Sour Cream & Onion Flavored Potato Crisps

Manischewitz

Potato Chips (All Varieties)

Maui Style ⓘ

Regular Potato Chips

Salt & Vinegar Flavored Potato Chips

Meijer

Potato Sticks

Michael Season's

Baked Thin Potato Crisps - Cheddar & Sour Cream

Baked Thin Potato Crisps - Original

Baked Thin Potato Crisps - Sweet Barbeque

Thin & Crispy Potato Chips - Honey Barbeque

Thin & Crispy Potato Chips - Lightly Salted

Thin & Crispy Potato Chips - Mediterranean

Thin & Crispy Potato Chips - Ripple

Thin & Crispy Potato Chips - Salt & Pepper

Thin & Crispy Potato Chips - Unsalted

Miss Vickie's ⓘ

Hand Picked Jalapeno Kettle Cooked Flavored Potato Chips

Sea Salt & Cracked Pepper Flavored Potato Chips

Sea Salt & Vinegar Kettle Cooked Flavored Potato Chips

Simply Sea Salt Kettle Cooked Potato Chips

Smokehouse BBQ Kettle Cooked Flavored Potato Chips

Munchos ⓘ

Regular Potato Crisps

Old Dutch Foods ()

Original Dutch Crunch Potato Chips (NOT Flavored)

Original Regular Potato Chips (NOT Flavored)

Original Rip-L Potato Chips (NOT Flavored)

Original Ripples Potato Chips (NOT Flavored)

Pik-Nik ⚕

50% Reduced Salt Shoestrings (Original Flavor Only)

Fabulous Fries (Original Flavor Only)

Regular Shoestrings (Original Flavor Only)

Pirate's Booty ⚕ ✓

Pirate's Booty (All)

Popchips ()

Popchips (All)

Pringles ⓘ

Fat Free Original

Fat Free Sour Cream & Onion

Publix ()

Potato Chips - Dip Style

Potato Chips - Original Thins

Potato Chips - Salt & Vinegar

Ruffles ⓘ

Authentic Barbecue Flavored Potato Chips

Cheddar & Sour Cream Flavored Potato Chips

Light Original Potato Chips

Lightly Salted Potato Chips

Natural Reduced Fat Sea Salted Potato Chips

Original Potato Chips

Queso Flavored Potato Chips

Reduced Fat Original Potato Chips

Sour Cream & Onion Flavored Potato Chips

Sabritas ⓘ

Adobadas Flavored Potato Chips

Chile Piquin Flavored Potato Chips

Habanero Limon Flavored Potato Chips

Utz ⓘ

All Natural Kettle Cooked Potato Chips - Dark Russet

All Natural Kettle Cooked Potato Chips - Gourmet Medley

All Natural Kettle Cooked Potato Chips - Lightly Salted

All Natural Kettle Cooked Potato Chips - Sea Salt & Vinegar

Barbeque Potato Chips

Carolina BBQ Potato Chips

Cheddar & Sour Cream Potato Chips

Crab Potato Chips

Grandma Utz Kettle Cooked Potato Chips - Barbeque

Grandma Utz Kettle Cooked Potato Chips - Plain

Homestyle Kettle Cooked Potato Chips - Plain

Honey BBQ Potato Chips

Kettle Classics Potato Chips - Dark Russet

Kettle Classics Potato Chips - Jalapeno

Kettle Classics Potato Chips - Plain

Kettle Classics Potato Chips - Smokin' Sweet BBQ

Kettle Classics Potato Chips - Sour Cream & Chive

Kettle Classics Potato Chips - Sweet Potato

Mystic Kettle Cooked Potato Chips - Dark Russet

Mystic Kettle Cooked Potato Chips - Plain

Mystic Kettle Cooked Potato Chips - Sea Salt & Vinegar

No Salt BBQ Potato Chips

No Salt Potato Chips

Red Hot Potato Chips

Reduced Fat Potato Chips

Ripple Potato Chips - Regular, Plain

Salt & Pepper Potato Chips

Salt & Vinegar Potato Chips

Sour Cream & Onion Potato Chips

Wavy Cut Potato Chips - Regular, Plain

Valu Time (Marsh)

Snack Potato Chips Bbq

Snack Potato Chips Sour Cream & Onion

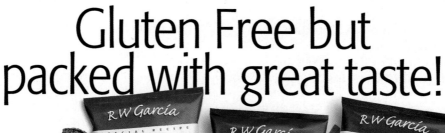

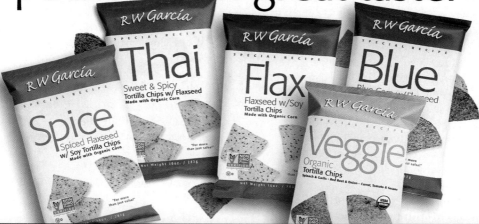

Available at fine retailers near you or online at RWGarcia.com

Chips, Tortilla

Baked! Doritos ⓘ
Nacho Cheese Flavored Tortilla Chips

Baked! Tostitos ⓘ
Scoops! Tortilla Chips

Bashas'
Tortilla Chips Bite Size 100% White Corn
Tortilla Chips Crispy Rounds 100% White Corn
Tortilla Chips Crispy Rounds 100% Yellow Corn
Tortilla Chips Restaurant Style

Casa Fiesta
Nach-Ole Tortilla Chips

Chi-Chi's ⓘ
Chips (All Varieties)

Doritos ⓘ
1st Degree Burn Blazin' Jalapeno Flavored Tortilla Chips
2nd Degree Burn Fiery Buffalo Flavored Tortilla Chips

Black Pepper Jack Cheese Flavored Tortilla Chips
Blazin' Buffalo & Ranch Flavored Tortilla Chips
Collisions Cheesy Enchilada & Sour Cream Flavored Tortilla Chips
Collisions Hot Wings and Blue Cheese Flavored Tortilla Chips
Collisions Pizza Cravers and Ranch Flavored Tortilla Chips
Cool Ranch Flavored Tortilla Chips
Diablo Flavored Tortilla Chips
Last Call Jalapeño Pepper Flavored Tortilla Chips
Late Night All Nighter Cheeseburger Flavored Tortilla Chips
Reduced Fat Cool Ranch Flavored Tortilla Chips
Salsa Verde Flavored Tortilla Chips
Smokin' Cheddar BBQ Flavored Tortilla Chips
Spicy Nacho Flavored Tortilla Chips
Tacos at Midnight Flavored Tortilla Chips

Toasted Corn Tortilla Chips

EatSmart Naturals ✓
Multigrain Tortilla Chips

Food Club (Marsh)
Snack Tortilla Chips - Yellow, Round

Food Should Taste Good 🏅
Chips (All)

Fresh & Easy ()
Blue Corn Tortilla Chips
Jalapeno Flavored Tortilla Chips
Lime Flavored Tortilla Chips
Monterey Jack & Chili Tortilla Chips
Organic Fiesta Mix Tortilla Chips
Organic Unsalted Yellow Corn Tortilla
Chips
Organic White Corn Tortilla Chips
Organic Yellow Corn Tortilla Chips
Restaurant Style White Corn Tortilla
Chips
Spinach & Artichoke Tortilla Chips

Green Mountain Gringo ⓘ
Tortilla Strips - Organic Blue Corn
Tortilla Strips - Organic White Corn
Tortilla Strips - Original

Guiltless Gourmet
Baked Tortilla Chips (All) ⓘ

HealthMarket (Hy-Vee)
Organic Blue Corn Tortilla Chips
Organic White Corn Tortilla Chips
Organic Yellow Corn Tortilla Chips

Herr's
Corn (NOT Multigrain) Tortilla Chips
(All)

Kroger ⓘ
Plain Tortilla Chips
Tortilla Strips Salad Toppers

Mission Foods 🏅
Corn Tortilla Chips (All)

Nash Brothers
Premium Tortilla Chips

Old Dutch Foods ()
Restaurante Bite Size Tortilla Chips
(NOT Flavored)
Restaurante Style Tortilla Chips (NOT
Flavored)

Restaurante Tostados Tortilla Chips
(NOT Flavored)
Restaurante White Corn Tostados
Tortilla Chips (NOT Flavored)

Ortega
Round Tortilla Chips

Publix ()
GreenWise Market Blue Tortilla Chips
GreenWise Market Yellow Tortilla Chips
White Corn Tortilla Chips - Restaurant
Style
Yellow Corn Tortilla Chips - Round
Style

R.W. Garcia
Blue Corn Tortilla Chips
Classic Tortilla Chips
Flaxseed
MixtBag
Stone Ground Yellow Corn Tortilla
Chips
Veggie

Ricos ✓
Chips (All)

Santitas ⓘ
White Corn Restaurant Style Tortilla
Chips
Yellow Corn Tortilla Chips

Tostitos ⓘ
100% White Corn Restaurant Style
Tortilla Chips
Bite Size Rounds Tortilla Chips
Blue Corn Restaurant Style Tortilla
Chips
Crispy Rounds Tortilla Chips
Dipping Strips Tortilla Chips
Natural Blue Corn Restaurant Style
Tortilla Chips
Natural Yellow Corn Restaurant Style
Tortilla Chips
Restaurant Style with A Hint of Lime
Flavor Tortilla Chips
Salsa Verde Tortilla Chips
Scoops! Hint of Jalapeno Tortilla Chips
Scoops! Tortilla Chips

Utz ⓘ
Baked Tortilla Chips
Cheesier Nacho Tortilla Chips

Restaurant Style Tortilla Chips
White Corn Tortilla Chips

Valu Time (Marsh)
Snack Tortillas Chips Round Yellow

COOKIES

Andean Dream
Quinoa Cookies - Chocolate Chip
Quinoa Cookies - Cocoa-Orange
Quinoa Cookies - Coconut
Quinoa Cookies - Orange Essence
Quinoa Cookies - Raisins & Spice

Annie's Homegrown
Gluten Free Bunny Cookies

Biscottea
Gluten-Free Blueberry with White Tea
Gluten-Free Chai
Gluten-Free Earl Grey with Darjeeling
   Tea

Cookies... for Me?
Cookies… For Me? (All)

Ener-G
Biscotti Cranberry Cookies
Biscotti Raisin Cookies
Chocolate Chip Biscotti Cookies
Chocolate Chip Potato Cookies
Chocolate Cookies
Cinnamon Cookies
Ginger Cookies
Sunflower Cookies
Vanilla Cookies
White Chocolate Chip Cookies

Enjoy Life Foods
Chewy Chocolate Chip Cookie Pack
Chewy Chocolate Chip Cookies
Double Chocolate Brownie Cookies
Gingerbread Spice Cookies
Happy Apple Cookies
Lively Lemon Cookies
No-Oats "Oatmeal" Cookies
Snickerdoodle Cookie Pack
Snickerdoodle Cookies

EnviroKidz
Vanilla Animal Cookies

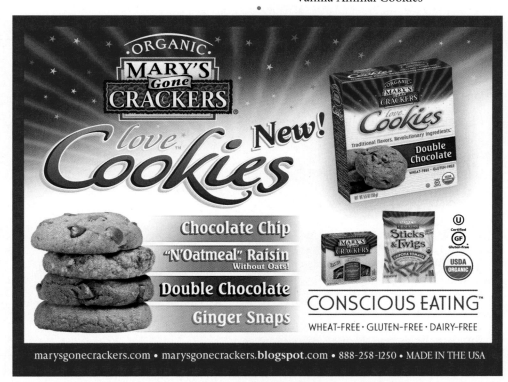

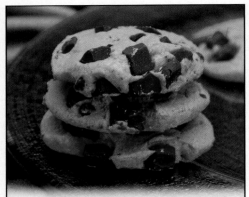

French Meadow Bakery
Gluten-Free Chocolate Chip Cookie

Gillian's Foods ⅊
Gillian's Foods (All)

Gluten Free & FABULOUS ✓
Butterscotch Cookie Bites
Chocolate Chip Cookie Bites
Shortbread Cookie Bites

Glutino
Chocolate Vanilla Cream Sandwich
Cookies
Chocolate Wafers - Chocolate Coated
Lemon Wafers
Strawberry Wafers
Vanilla Cream Sandwich Cookies
Vanilla Wafers - Chocolate Coated

Grainless Baker, The ⅊
The Grainless Baker (All)

Ian's Natural Foods
Wheat and Gluten-Free Animal Cookies
Wheat and Gluten-Free Chocolate Chip
Cookie Buttons

Wheat and Gluten-Free Chocolate
Wafer Bites
Wheat and Gluten-Free Crunchy
Cinnamon Cookie Buttons

Joan's GF Great Bakes ⅊
Joan's GF Great Bakes (All)

Jo-Sef ⅊
Jo-Sef (All)

Katz Gluten Free ⅊
Katz Gluten Free (All)

Kinnikinnick Foods ⅊
Kinnikinnick Foods (All)

Manischewitz
Tender Coconut Patties

Mary's Gone Crackers ⅊
Chocolate Chip Cookies
Double Chocolate Chip Cookies
Ginger Snap Cookies
N'Oatmeal Raisin Cookies

Mi-Del
Gluten-Free Arrowroot Cookies
Gluten-Free Chocolate Chip Cookies
Gluten-Free Chocolate Sandwich
Cookies
Gluten-Free Cinnamon Snaps
Gluten-Free Ginger Snaps
Gluten-Free Pecan Cookies
Gluten-Free Royal Vanilla Sandwich
Cookies

Miss Meringue ⓘ
Meringue Cookies (All)

Nana's
No Gluten Cookie - Chocolate
No Gluten Cookie - Chocolate Crunch
No Gluten Cookie - Ginger
No Gluten Cookie - Lemon
No Gluten Cookie Bars - Berry Vanilla
No Gluten Cookie Bars - Chocolate
Munch
No Gluten Cookie Bars - Nana Banana
No Gluten Cookie Bites - Fudge
No Gluten Cookie Bites - Ginger Spice
No Gluten Cookie Bites - Lemon
Dreams

Orgran ✓
Biscotti Range (All)
Classic Choc Cookie

Dinosaur Wholefruit Cookies -
Wildberry Flavour
Itsy Bitsy Bears
Mini Outback Animals Cookies
Multipack (All)
Outback Animals Cookies Range (All)
Premium Shortbread Hearts
Wild Raspberry Biscuits

Outside the Breadbox 🍺 ✓
Outside the Breadbox (All)

Pamela's Products ✓
Biscotti - Almond Anise
Biscotti - Chocolate Walnut
Biscotti - Lemon Almond
Organic Cookies - Chocolate Chunk
Pecan Shortbread
Organic Cookies - Dark Chocolate,
Chocolate Chunk
Organic Cookies - Espresso Chocolate
Chunk
Organic Cookies - Old Fashioned Raisin
Walnut
Organic Cookies - Peanut Butter
Chocolate Chip
Organic Cookies - Spicy Ginger with
Crystallized Ginger
Simplebites Mini Cookies - Chocolate
Chip Mini Cookies
Simplebites Mini Cookies - Extreme
Chocolate Mini Cookies
Simplebites Mini Cookies - Ginger Mini
Snapz
Traditional Cookies - Butter Shortbread
Traditional Cookies - Chocolate Chip
Walnut
Traditional Cookies - Chunky Chocolate
Chip
Traditional Cookies - Ginger with Sliced
Almonds
Traditional Cookies - Lemon Shortbread
Traditional Cookies - Peanut Butter
Traditional Cookies - Pecan Shortbread
Traditional Cookies - Shortbread Swirl

Schar 🍺 ✓
Chocolate O's
Chocolate Sandwich Cremes
Chocolate-Dipped Cookies

Cocoa Wafers
Hazelnut Wafers
Ladyfingers
Shortbread Cookies
Vanilla Sandwich Cremes
Vanilla Wafers

Shabtai Gourmet Gluten-Free Bakery
🍺 ✓
Gluten Free Chocolate Chip Biscotti
Gluten Free Chocolate Chip Cookie
Gluten Free Florentine Lace Cookie
Gluten Free Lady Fingers
Gluten Free Meltaway Crumb Cookie
Gluten Free Mini Black & White
Cookies
Gluten Free Rainbow Cookie Squares

Smart Treat 🍺
Smart Treat (All)

CRACKERS

Blue Diamond Growers ✓
Almond Nut Thins

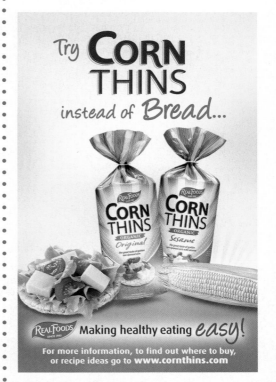

Barbeque Nut Thins
Cheddar Cheese Nut Thins
Country Ranch Nut Thins
Hazelnut Nut Thins
Hint of Sea Salt Nut Thins (Low Sodium)
Pecan Nut Thins
Smokehouse Nut Thins

Brown Rice Snaps ✓
Black Sesame (with organic brown rice)
Cheddar (with organic brown rice)
Onion Garlic
Salsa (with organic brown rice)
Tamari Seaweed
Tamari Sesame
Toasted Onion (with organic brown rice)
Unsalted Plain (with organic brown rice)
Unsalted Sesame
Vegetable (with organic brown rice)

Corn Thins ☷
Cracked Pepper & Lemon Corn Thins

Flax & Soy Corn Thins
Multigrain Corn Thins
Original Corn Thins
Sesame Corn Thins

Crunchmaster
Crunchmaster (All)

Eden Foods ⓘ ✓
Brown Rice Crackers
Nori Maki Rice Crackers

Ener-G ☷ ✓
Cinnamon Crackers
Ener-G Gourmet Crackers
Seattle Crackers

Exotic Rice Toast ✓
Jasmine Rice & Spring Onion
Purple Rice & Black Sesame
Thai Red Rice & Flaxseeds

Gluten Free & FABULOUS ✓
Sweet Savory Bites

Glutino
Breadsticks Pizza
Breadsticks Sesame

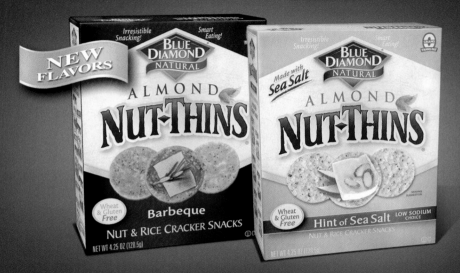
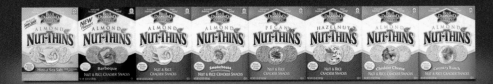

Crackers - Cheddar
Crackers - Multigrain
Crackers - Original
Crackers - Vegetable
Table Crackers

Grainless Baker, The ⚕
The Grainless Baker (All)

Hol-Grain
Brown Rice Crackers - Lightly Salted
Brown Rice Crackers - No Salt
Brown Rice Crackers - Onion & Garlic Flavor
Brown Rice Crackers - Sesame Lightly Salted

Kinnikinnick Foods ⚕
Kinnikinnick Foods (All)

Lydia's Organics ⚕
Lydia's Organics (All)

Mariposa Baking Company ⚕ ✓
Crostini

Mary's Gone Crackers ⚕
Black Pepper Crackers
Caraway Crackers
Herb Crackers
Onion Crackers
Original Seed Crackers

Mr. Krispers ⚕
Baked Rice Snack Products (All)

Orgran ✓
Deli Crackers - Multigrain with Poppyseed
Essential Fibre Crispibread
Essential Fibre Rotondo Biscuits

Outside the Breadbox ⚕
Outside the Breadbox (All)

R.W. Garcia
5 Seed Crackers

Rice Snax ✓
Bar-B-Que
Lightly Salted
Onion Garlic
Salt & Vinegar

Rice Thins ⚕
Wholegrain Rice Thins

San-J ⓘ ✓
Gluten Free Black Sesame Rice Crackers

Gluten Free Brown Rice Crackers
Gluten Free Sesame Rice Crackers

Schar ⚕ ✓
Cheese Bites
Crispbread
Snack Crackers
Table Crackers

SESMARK ⓘ
Rice Thins - Brown
Rice Thins - Cheddar
Rice Thins - Sesame
Rice Thins - Teriyaki

Skinny Crisps ⚕
Skinny Crisps (All)

DRIED FRUIT

Bashas'
Dried Plums - Prunes
Raisins
Raisins Seedless

Craisins
Original Sweetened Dried Cranberries

Eden Foods ⓘ ✓
Dried Cranberries - Organic
Dried Wild Blueberries - Organic
Montmorency Dried Tart Cherries
Wild Berry Mix - Organic

Equal Exchange
Cranberries ⚕

Food Club (Marsh)
Raisins Canister
Raisins Seedless Carton
Raisins Thompson Seedless Canister

Fresh & Easy ⟨⟩
Freeze-Dried Bananas & Strawberries

Great Value (Wal-Mart)
California Pitted Prunes
California Sun-Dried Raisins

Haggen
Raisins - Seedless
Raisins (Canister)

Hy-Vee
California Sun Dried Raisins

Just Tomatoes
Just Tomatoes (All)

Made in Nature ☃
  Organic Dried Fruit Products (All)
Mariani
  Mariani (All)
Meijer
  Prunes - Pitted
  Raisins
  Raisins - Seedless
Newman's Own Organics () ⓘ
  Berry Blend
  Dried Apples
  Dried Apricots
  Dried Cranberries
  Dried Pitted Prunes
  Raisins
Publix ()
  Dinosaurs Dry Fruit
  Raisins
  Rescue Heroes Dry Fruit
  Sharks Dry Fruit
  Snoopy Dry Fruit
St. Dalfour ⓘ
  Dried Fruits (All)
Sunsweet ☃
  Sunsweet (All BUT Chocolate Covered
    PlumSweets)
Welch's
  Welch's (All)
Winn-Dixie ()
  Raisins

FRUIT CUPS

Del Monte ⓘ
  Fruit Snack Cups (Metal or Plastic)
Fruit Roll-Ups ✓
  Flavor Wave
Hy-Vee
  Diced Peaches Fruit Cups
  Mandarin Oranges in Light Syrup Fruit
    Cups
  Mandarin Oranges in Orange Gel Fruit
    Cups
  Mixed Fruit in Light Syrup Fruit Cups
  Peaches in Strawberry Gel Fruit Cups
  Pineapple in Lime Gel Fruit Cups

  Pineapple Tidbit Fruit Cups
  Tropical Fruit Cups
Kroger ⓘ
  Fruit - Cups

FRUIT SNACKS

Annie's Homegrown ⓘ ✓
  Organic Berry Patch Fruit Snacks
  Organic Tropical Treat Bunny Fruit
    Snacks
  Summer Strawberry Fruit Snacks
  Sunny Citrus Fruit Snacks
Food Club (Marsh)
  Fruit Snacks - Build-A-Bear Workshop
  Fruit Snacks - Curious George
  Fruit Snacks - Dinosaurs
  Fruit Snacks - Sharks
  Fruit Snacks - Variety Pack
  Fruit Snacks - Veggie Tales
Fruit by the Foot ✓
  Berry Blast
  Berry Tie-Dye
  Berry Tie-Dye/Color by the Foot Value
    Pack
  Boo Berry
  Color By the Foot
  Franken Berry
  Minis - Berry Wave
  Minis - Wicked Webs Halloween
  Razzle Blue Blitz
  Strawberry
  Tropical Twist
  Variety Pack (14 ct, 28 ct, and 42 ct)
  Variety Pack (Monsters)
  Variety Pack (Strawberry, Color by the
    Foot, Berry Tie-Dye)
  Watermelon
Fruit Gushers ✓
  Blue Raspberry
  Flavor Shock
  Halloween Tropical Mix
  Mouth Mixers Punch Berry
  Strawberry
  Strawberry/Tropical
  Triple Berry Shock
  Tropical

Tropical Flavors
Value Pack (Strawberry, Tropical)
Variety Pack (Strawberry, Watermelon,
Tropical)
Watermelon Blast

Fruit Roll-Ups ✓

Around the World
Blastin' Berry Hot Colors
Bonus Value Pack
Minis - Strawberry Craze
Minis - Wildberry Punch
Scoops Fruity Ice Cream Flavors
Simply…Fruit Variety Pack (Wildberry/
Strawberry)
Stickerz Berry Cool Punch
Stickerz Mixed Berry
Stickerz Tropical Berry Flavor
Stickerz Value Pack (Mixed Berry/
Tropical Berry)
Stickerz Variety Pack
Strawberry
Strawberry Sensation
Tropical Tie-Dye
Value Pack (Strawberry/Berry Cool
Punch)
Variety Pack (Strawberry/Tie-Dye/
Wildfire)

Fruit Shapes ✓

Care Bears
Comics
Create-A-Bug
Dora the Explorer
Easter Fruit Flavored Snacks
Halloween
My Little Pony
Nickelodeon
Scooby-Doo
Shark Bites
Spiderman
Sponge Bob
Sunkist Mixed Fruit
Transformers
Valentine Hearts
Value Pack Sunkist
Variety Pack Scooby-Doo/Looney Tunes

FruitaBu

Fruitabu (All)

Golden Valley Natural

All Natural Fruit Stix (All)

Hy-Vee

Dinosaurs Fruit Snacks
Fruit Snacks (Variety Pack)
Sharks Fruit Snacks
Snoopy Fruit Snacks
Veggie Tales Fruit Snacks

Kellogg's ()

Fruit Flavored Snacks

Kroger ⓘ

Fruit Snacks

Meijer

Fruit Roll - Justice League Berry
Fruit Roll - Rescue Heroes
Fruit Roll - Strawberry
Fruit Roll - Wildberry Rush
Fruit Snack - Dinosaurs
Fruit Snack - Sharks
Fruit Snack - Veggie Tales
Fruit Snacks - African Safari
Fruit Snacks - Curious George
Fruit Snacks - Jungle Adventure
Fruit Snacks - Justice League
Fruit Snacks - Peanuts
Fruit Snacks - Underwater
Fruit Snacks Variety Pack

Publix ()

Veggie Tales Dry Fruit

Sharkies

Sharkies (All)

Stretch Island

Stretch Island (All)

Yogos ()

Yogos

GELATIN SNACKS & MIXES

Bashas'

Gelatin Dessert Cherry
Gelatin Dessert Cherry Sugar Free
Gelatin Dessert Lemon
Gelatin Dessert Lime
Gelatin Dessert Lime Sugar Free
Gelatin Dessert Orange
Gelatin Dessert Orange Sugar Free
Gelatin Dessert Raspberry

Gelatin Dessert Raspberry Sugar Free
Gelatin Dessert Strawberry
Gelatin Dessert Strawberry Sugar Free
Gelatin Dessert Strawberry/Banana
Gelatin Dessert Unflavored

Food Club (Marsh)

Gelatin Dessert - Cherry
Gelatin Dessert - Lemon
Gelatin Dessert - Lime
Gelatin Dessert - Orange
Gelatin Dessert - Orange Sugar Free
Gelatin Dessert - Raspberry
Gelatin Dessert - Raspberry Sugar Free
Gelatin Dessert - Strawberry
Gelatin Dessert - Strawberry Sugar Free
Gelatin Dessert - Unflavored

Fresh & Easy ()

Berry Gelatin
Cherry Gelatin
Mango Gelatin
Pear Gelatin

Great Value (Wal-Mart)

Cherry Gelatin Dessert
Lemon Gelatin Dessert
Lime Gelatin Dessert
Orange Gelatin Dessert
Peach Gelatin Dessert
Strawberry Banana Gelatin Dessert
Strawberry Gelatin Dessert
Sugar Free Cherry Gelatin Dessert
Sugar Free Lime Gelatin Dessert
Sugar Free Orange Gelatin Dessert
Sugar Free Peach Gelatin Dessert
Sugar Free Raspberry Gelatin Dessert
Sugar Free Strawberry Banana Gelatin
   Dessert
Sugar Free Strawberry Gelatin Dessert

Hy-Vee

Cherry Gelatin
Cranberry Gelatin
Lemon Gelatin
Lime Gelatin
Orange Gelatin
Raspberry Gelatin
Strawberry Gelatin
Sugar Free Cherry Gelatin
Sugar Free Cranberry Gelatin

Sugar Free Lime Gelatin
Sugar Free Orange Gelatin
Sugar Free Raspberry Gelatin
Sugar Free Strawberry Gelatin

Jell-O ✍

Apricot Artificial Flavor Gelatin Dessert
Berry Blue Gelatin Dessert
Black Cherry Gelatin Dessert
Blackberry Fusion Gelatin Dessert
Cherry & Black Cherry Sugar Free
   Gelatin Snacks
Cherry Gelatin Dessert
Cranberry Gelatin Dessert
Island Pineapple Gelatin Dessert
Lemon Gelatin Dessert
Lime & Orange Variety Pack Sugar Free
   Gelatin Snacks
Lime Gelatin Dessert
Low Calorie Sugar Free Raspberry &
   Orange Gelatin Snacks
Margarita Limited Edition Gelatin
   Dessert
Melon Fusion Gelatin Dessert
Mixed Berry Smoothie Snacks
Orange Gelatin Dessert
Peach Artificial Flavor Gelatin Dessert
Peach Gelatin Dessert
Pear Chunks In Cherry Pomegranate
   Gelatin Snacks
Raspberry Gelatin Dessert
Real Chunks Of Pineapple In Tropical
   Fusion Sugar Free Gelatin Snacks
Strawberry & Orange Gelatin Snacks
Strawberry & Orange Variety Pack
   Sugar Free Gelatin Snacks
Strawberry & Raspberry Gelatin Snacks
Strawberry Banana Gelatin Dessert
Strawberry Banana Smoothie Snacks
Strawberry Gelatin Dessert
Strawberry Gelatin Snacks
Strawberry Kiwi Gelatin Dessert
Strawberry Sugar Free Gelatin Snacks
Strawberry-Kiwi & Tropical Berry Sugar
   Free Gelatin Snacks
Sugar Free Black Cherry Low Calorie
   Gelatin Dessert

Sugar Free Cherry Low Calorie Gelatin Dessert
Sugar Free Cranberry Low Calorie Gelatin Dessert
Sugar Free Lemon Low Calorie Gelatin Dessert
Sugar Free Lime Low Calorie Gelatin Dessert
Sugar Free Orange Low Calorie Gelatin Dessert
Sugar Free Peach Low Calorie Gelatin Dessert
Sugar Free Raspberry Low Calorie Gelatin Dessert
Sugar Free Strawberry Banana Low Calorie Gelatin Dessert
Sugar Free Strawberry Low Calorie Gelatin Dessert
Sugar Free Variety Pack Low Calorie Gel Cups
Tropical Fusion Gelatin Dessert
Watermelon Gelatin Dessert
X-Treme Cherry & Blue Raspberry Gel Cups
X-Treme Watermelon & Green Apple Gel Cups

Kool-Aid Gels 〰
Cherry Tropical Punch Gel Snacks
Groovalicious Grape Gel Snacks
Ice Blue Raspberry Gel Snacks
Oh Yeah Orange Gel Snacks
Soarin' Strawberry Gel Snacks

Kroger ⓘ
Gelatin - Flavored
Gelatin - Plain
Gelatin - Snack Cups

Meijer
Gelatin Dessert - Berry Blue
Gelatin Dessert - Cherry
Gelatin Dessert - Cherry Sugar Free
Gelatin Dessert - Cranberry
Gelatin Dessert - Cranberry Sugar Free
Gelatin Dessert - Grape
Gelatin Dessert - Lime
Gelatin Dessert - Lime Sugar Free
Gelatin Dessert - Orange
Gelatin Dessert - Orange Sugar Free

Gelatin Dessert - Raspberry
Gelatin Dessert - Raspberry Sugar Free
Gelatin Dessert - Strawberry
Gelatin Dessert - Strawberry Sugar Free
Gelatin Dessert - Strawberry Wild
Gelatin Dessert - Unflavored

Publix ⟨⟩
Mandarin Oranges in Gel
Sugar Free Black Cherry & Cherry Gelatin
Sugar Free Raspberry & Orange Gelatin
Sugar Free Strawberry Gelatin

V & V Supremo
Gelatins (All)

GUM

5
5

Bazooka Bubble Gum ✓
Bazooka Bubble Gum (All)

Big Red
Big Red Gum (All)

Bubblicious
Bubblicious

Dentyne
Dentyne

Doublemint
Doublemint Gum (All)

Dubble Bubble
Dubble Bubble (All)

Eclipse
Eclipse Gum (All)

Extra
Extra Gum (All)

Freedent
Freedent Gum (All)

Glee Gum ⓘ
Glee Gum (All Flavors)

Juicy Fruit
Juicy Fruit Gum (All)

Orbit
Orbit Gum (All)
Orbit White Gum (All)

Publix ⟨⟩
Super Bubble Bubble Gum

Stride
Stride Gum

Trident
Trident

Winterfresh
Winterfresh Gum (All)

Wrigley's Spearmint
Wrigley's Spearmint Gum (All)

Nuts, Seeds & Mixes

Almond Accents
Almond Accents (All BUT Roasted Garlic Caesar)

Arrowhead Mills ✓
Mechanically Hulled Sesame Seeds

B. Lloyd's
B. Lloyd's (All)

Bashas'
Cashews - Halves & Pieces
Cashews - Whole
Mixed Nuts
Nuts - Deluxe Mixed, No Peanuts
Peanuts - Honey Roasted
Peanuts - Party
Peanuts - Unsalted, Dry

Carrington
Organic Flax Seed Products (All)

Central Market Classics (Price Chopper)
Almond Cashew Macadamia Nut Mix
Honey Roasted Almonds
Jumbo Honey Roasted Cashews
Roasted Salted Almonds
Roasted Salted Macadamia Nuts
Slow Roasted Pecans
Smoked Almonds

Eden Foods ⓘ ✓
All Mixed Up
All Mixed Up Too
Pistachios, Shelled and Dry Roasted, Organic
Pumpkin Seeds, Dry Roasted & Salted, Organic
Spicy Pumpkin Seeds, Dry Roasted w/ Tamari, Organic

Tamari Almonds - Dry Roasted - Organic
Tamari Roasted Almonds, Organic

Equal Exchange
Almonds ⚇
Pecans ⚇

Fannie May
Assorted Nuts
Cashews

Fire Dancer
Fire Dancer (All)

Fisher Nuts ()
Almonds
Butter Toffee Peanuts
Cashews
Chef's Naturals (All)
Culinary Touch Almond/Cranberry Blend
Culinary Touch Pecan/Cranberry/Orange Blend
Culinary Touch Slivered Almonds
Culinary Touch Toasted Cashews
Culinary Touch Toasted Pine Nuts
Culinary Touch Walnut/Apple/Blueberry Blend
Dry Roasted Sunflower Kernels
Fusions Energy Blend Snack Mix
Fusions Ice Cream Sundae Snack Mix
Fusions Tropical Twist Snack Mix
Honey Roasted Peanuts (Oil Roasted, Can)
In-Shell Peanuts (All Types)
Macadamia Nuts
Mixed Nuts
Nature's Nut Mix
Party Peanuts
Pecans
Pine Nuts (Pignolas)
Pistachios
Salted In-Shell Sunflower Seeds
Spanish Peanuts
Sunflower Nuts/Seeds
Unsalted Golden Roast Peanuts
Walnuts

Frito Lay ⓘ
Cashews
Deluxe Mixed Nuts

Honey Roasted Peanuts
Hot Peanuts
Praline Pecans
Ranch Sunflower Seeds
Salted Peanuts
Smoked Almonds
Sunflower Seed Kernels
Sunflower Seeds

Hy-Vee
Black Walnuts
English Walnut Pieces
English Walnuts
Natural Almonds
Natural Sliced Almonds
Pecan Halves
Pecan Pieces
Raw Spanish Peanuts
Salted Blanched Peanuts
Salted Spanish Peanuts
Slivered Almonds

I.M. Healthy ♀
Roasted Sweet Corn - Chili Lime
Roasted Sweet Corn - Regular

Manitoba Harvest ♀ ✓
Manitoba Harvest Hemp Foods & Oils
(All)

Meijer
Almonds - Blanched Sliced
Almonds - Blanched Slivered
Almonds - Natural Sliced
Almonds - Slivered
Almonds - Whole
Blanched Peanuts Slightly Salted
Cashew Halves with Pieces
Cashew Halves with Pieces Lightly
Salted
Cashews Whole
Nut Topping
Nuts - Blanched Peanuts
Nuts - Deluxe Mixed
Nuts - Mixed
Nuts - Mixed Lightly Salted
Peanuts - Dry Roasted
Peanuts - Dry Roasted Lightly Salted
Peanuts - Dry Roasted Unsalted
Peanuts - Honey Roasted
Peanuts - Hot and Spicy

Peanuts - Spanish
Pecan Chips
Pecan Halves
Pine Nuts
Sunflower Seeds
Sunflower Seeds Salted Shell
Walnut Chips
Walnuts Black
Walnuts Halves and Pieces

Mrs. May's Naturals ✓
Mrs. May's Naturals (All)

Nut Harvest ⓘ
Natural Lightly Roasted Almonds
Natural Sea Salted Peanuts
Natural Sea Salted Whole Cashews

Pastene
Pignoli Nuts (Pine Nuts)

Paula Deen ()
Peanuts (All)

Planters ∿
Almonds - Recipe Ready
Almonds - Sliced
Almonds - Slivered
Almonds - Smoked Almonds
Cashew Sesame Mix - Salt & Pepper Nut
Mix Peanuts/Almonds/Cashews
Cashew Sesame Mix Made with Pure
Sea Salt
Cashews - Chocolate Covered 3.5 Oz
Cashews - Chocolate Lovers Milk
Chocolate
Cashews - Deluxe Jumbo with Sea Salt
Cashews - Deluxe Whole Honey
Roasted
Cashews - Deluxe Whole with Sea Salt
Cashews - Dry Roasted
Cashews - Halves & Pieces
Cashews - Halves & Pieces Lightly
Salted
Cashews - Halves & Pieces Made with
Pure Sea Salt
Cashews - Honey Roasted
Cashews - Jumbo All Natural
Cashews - Salted
Cashews - Select Cashews Almonds &
Pecans with Sea Salt
Cashews - Whole

Cashews - Whole Lightly Salted
Cocktail Peanuts
Cocktail Peanuts - Lightly Salted
Cocktail Peanuts - Lightly Salted Made
  with Pure Sea Salt
Cocktail Peanuts - Party Pack
Cocktail Peanuts - Party Size
Cocktail Peanuts - Raging Buffalo Wing
Cocktail Peanuts - Smoky Bacon
Cocktail Peanuts - Unsalted
Cocktail Peanuts - White Hot Wasabi
Cocktail Peanuts - with Sea Salt
Go-Nuts Lightly Salted Heart-Healthy
  Mix 1.5 Oz
Hazelnuts - Chopped
Holiday Collection - Honey Roasted
  Sweet'n Crunchy Peanuts & Cocktail
Macadamia Cashew & Almonds Select
Macadamias
Macadamias - Chopped
Mixed Nuts
Mixed Nuts - Almonds Cashews &
  Mixed Nuts In Milk Chocolate
Mixed Nuts - Deluxe Cashews,
  Almonds, Brazils, Hazelnuts & Pecans
Mixed Nuts - Deluxe Lightly Salted
Mixed Nuts - Deluxe with Sea Salt
Mixed Nuts - Honey Roasted
Mixed Nuts - Lightly Salted
Mixed Nuts - Unsalted
Nut-Rition Heart Healthy Mix
Nut-Rition Lightly Salted Mix
Nut-Rition Mix - South Beach Diet
  Recommended Cashews Almonds &
  Macadamias
Nut-Rition Smoked Almonds Lightly
  Salted
Peanuts - Cocktail Party Pack
Peanuts - Dry Roasted
Peanuts - Dry Roasted Honey Roasted
Peanuts - Dry Roasted Lightly Salted
Peanuts - Dry Roasted Lightly Salted
  with Sea Salt
Peanuts - Dry Roasted Party Size
Peanuts - Dry Roasted Unsalted
Peanuts - Dry Roasted with Sea Salt
Peanuts - Heat
Peanuts - Honey & Dry Roasted

Peanuts - Honey Roasted
Peanuts - Honey Roasted Big Bag
Peanuts - Honey Roasted Go-Paks 1.75
  0Z
Peanuts - Honey Roasted Party Size
Peanuts - Rich Roasted Whole In Milk
  Chocolate
Peanuts - Roasted In-Shell Salted
Peanuts - Salted
Peanuts - Salted Big Bag
Peanuts - Sweet N' Crunchy
Peanuts - Wicked Hot Chipotle
Pecan Chips - Recipe Ready
Pecan Halves
Pecan Halves - Recipe Ready
Pecan Lovers with Cashews & Pistachios
Pecan Pieces
Pecan Pieces - Recipe Ready
Pine Nuts
Pistachios - Dry Roasted
Redskin Spanish Peanuts
Roasted Salted Pepitas
Sunflower Kernels
Sunflower Kernels - Big Bag
Sunflower Kernels - Dry Roasted
Sunflower Seeds - Roasted & Salted
Sweet Roasts - Honey Roasted
Trail Mix - Nuts Seeds & Raisins
Walnuts
Walnuts - Recipe Ready
Walnuts Black - Recipe Ready
Wicked Hot Chipotle Pepitas

Price Chopper
Chopped Pecans
Pecan Halves
Slivered Almonds
Walnut Chips
Walnut Halves
Whole Almonds

Publix ()
Almonds - Natural Whole
Almonds - Salted
Almonds - Sliced
Cashews - Dry Roasted
Cashews - Halves & Pieces
Cashews - Halves & Pieces, Lightly
  Salted

Cashews - Whole
Mixed Nuts
Mixed Nuts - Deluxe
Mixed Nuts - Dry Roasted
Mixed Nuts - Lightly Salted
Peanuts - Dry Roasted, Lightly Salted
Peanuts - Dry Roasted, Salted
Peanuts - Dry Roasted, Unsalted
Peanuts - Oil Roasted, Honey Roasted
Peanuts - Salted Party
Pecans
Pistachios
Sunflower Seeds
Sunflower Seeds - Raw-Shelled, All
   Natural
Walnuts

Sabritas ⓘ
Picante Peanuts
Salt & Lime Peanuts

Seapoint Farms
Dry Roasted Edamame (All)

South Beach Living 〰
Dark Chocolate Covered Soynuts 7 Pk
   Snack Pack Delights

Spitz ⓘ
Chili Lime Sunflower Seeds
Cracked Pepper Sunflower Seeds
Dill Pickle Sunflower Seeds
Salted Sunflower Seeds
Seasoned Pumpkin Seeds
Seasoned Sunflower Seeds
Smoky BBQ Sunflower Seeds
Spicy Sunflower Seeds

True North ⓘ
Almond Clusters
Almond Cranberry Vanilla Clusters
Almond Cranberry Vanilla Clusters in
   White Chocolate
Almond Pecan Cashew Clusters
Almonds Pistachios Walnuts Pecans
Citrus Burst Nut Clusters
Pecan Almond Peanut Clusters

Wine Nuts
Chardonnay
Choco~Late
Lemoncella
Margarita Mix

Merlot

POPCORN

Bashas'
Popcorn - Microwave Butter
Popcorn - Microwave Extra Butter
Popcorn - Microwave Kettle Corn
Popcorn - Microwave Lite Butter Crazy
Popcorn - Yellow

Cape Cod ⓘ
Cape Cod Products (All)

Chester's ⓘ
Butter Flavored Puffcorn Snacks
Cheddar Cheese Flavored Popcorn
Cheese Flavored Puffcorn Snacks

Cracker Jack ⓘ
Original Caramel Coated Popcorn &
   Peanuts

Eden Foods ⓘ ✓
Popcorn - Yellow - Organic

Food Club (Marsh)
Popcorn Microwave Butter
Popcorn Microwave Butter Crazy
Popcorn Microwave Butter Lite
Popcorn Microwave Natural

Fresh & Easy ◊
Organic Lightly Salted Popcorn

Haggen
Popcorn - Microwave Butter
Popcorn - Microwave Butter Crazy
Popcorn - Microwave Butter Lite
Popcorn - Microwave Kettle Corn
Popcorn - Microwave Natural
Popcorn - Yellow

Herr's
Light Popcorn
Original Popcorn
White Cheddar Popcorn

Hy-Vee
94% Fat Free Butter Microwave Popcorn
Butter Microwave Popcorn
Extra Butter Lite Microwave Popcorn
Extra Butter Microwave Popcorn
Kettle Microwave Popcorn
Light Butter Microwave Popcorn
Natural Flavor Microwave Popcorn

White Popcorn
Yellow Popcorn

Jolly Time 🏅
American's Best 94% Fat Free Butter
  Flavor
Better Butter
Blast O Butter
Blast O Butter Light
Butter-Licious
Butter-Licious Light
Crispy'n White
Crispy'n White Light
Healthy Pop 94% Fat Free Butter Flavor
Healthy Pop 94% Fat Free Butter Flavor
  Low Sodium
Healthy Pop 94% Fat Free Caramel
  Apple
Healthy Pop 94% Fat Free Crispy White
  Naturally Flavored
Healthy Pop 94% Fat Free Kettle Corn
Kernel Corn - American's Best White
Kernel Corn - American's Best Yellow
Kernel Corn - Jolly Time Select Yellow
Kernel Corn - White Pop Corn
Kernel Corn - Yellow Pop Corn
KettleMania
Mallow Magic
Sassy Salsa
Sea Salt & Cracked Pepper
The Big Cheez
White & Buttery

Kroger ⓘ
Plain Popcorn Kernels

Meijer
Caramel Corn
Cheese Popcorn
Chicago Style Popcorn
Popcorn
Popcorn - Micro Kettle Sweet & Salty
Popcorn - Microwave 94% Fat Free
Popcorn - Microwave Butter
Popcorn - Microwave Butter 75% Fat
  Free
Popcorn - Microwave Extra Butter
Popcorn - Microwave Extra Butter Lite
Popcorn - Microwave Hot n' Spicy
Popcorn - Microwave Natural Lite

Popcorn - White
Popcorn - Yellow
Purple Cow Butter Popcorn
White Cheddar Popcorn

Newman's Own ⓘ
Microwave Popcorn - 94% Fat Free
Microwave Popcorn - Butter
Microwave Popcorn - Butter Boom
Microwave Popcorn - Light Butter
Microwave Popcorn - Natural
Microwave Popcorn - Natural 100
  Calorie Mini Bags
Microwave Popcorn - Tender White
  Kernel
Microwave Popcorn - White Cheddar
  Cheese
Regular Pop (Jar)

Newman's Own Organics ⟨⟩ ⓘ
Pop's Corn - Butter Flavored
Pop's Corn - Light Butter
Pop's Corn - No Butter/No Salt

Old Dutch Foods ⟨⟩
White Popcorn (NOT Flavored)

Oogie's
Oogie's (All)

Pirate's Booty 🏅 ✓
Pirate's Booty (All)

Ricos ✓
Popcorn (All)

Smartfood ⓘ
Cranberry Almond Flavored Popcorn
  Clusters
Peanut Butter Apple Flavored Popcorn
  Clusters
Reduced Fat White Cheddar Cheese
  Flavored Popcorn
White Cheddar Cheese Flavored
  Popcorn

Utz ⓘ
Butter Popcorn
Cheese Popcorn
Puff 'N Corn - Caramel
Puff 'N Corn - Plain
White Cheddar Popcorn

Valu Time (Marsh)
Snack Popcorn Cheese

PORK SKINS & RINDS

Baken-Ets ⓘ
BBQ Flavored Fried Pork Skins
Fried Pork Skins
Hot 'N Spicy Flavored Pork Skins
Hot 'n Spicy Flavored Fried Pork
  Cracklins
Hot Sauce Flavored Fried Pork Cracklins

Herr's
BBQ Flavored Pork Rinds
Original Pork Rinds

PRETZELS

Ener-G ⚕ ✓
Crisp Pretzels
Sesame Pretzel Rings
Wylde Pretzels
Wylde Sesame Pretzels

Glutino
Chocolate Covered Pretzels
Pretzel Twists

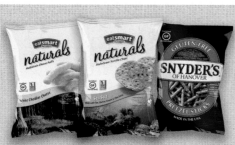

Certified Delicious!

Celebrate your freedom to enjoy snacks again! Snyder's of Hanover and EatSmart Naturals offer many unique taste experiences that meet the needs of a gluten-free diet. So go ahead, pack a snack. Add crunch to your lunch. Today, some of the best things in life are gluten-free!

eatsmartnaturals.com

Certified
GF
Gluten-Free ®
These products are certified gluten-free by the Gluten-Free Certification Organization. For more information, visit GFCO.org.

©2010
SNYDER'S
OF HANOVER

Pretzels
Unsalted Pretzel Twists
Yogurt Covered Pretzels

Mary's Gone Crackers ⚕
Sticks & Twigs - Chipotle Tomato
Sticks & Twigs - Curry
Sticks & Twigs - Sea Salt

Snyder's of Hanover ✓
Gluten-Free Pretzel Sticks

PUDDING & PUDDING MIXES

Bar Harbor ⓘ
Indian Pudding

Bashas'
Pudding Instant - Banana Cream
Pudding Instant - Butterscotch
Pudding Instant - Chocolate
Pudding Instant - Chocolate Sugar Free
Pudding Instant - Coconut Cream
Pudding Instant - French Vanilla
Pudding Instant - Lemon
Pudding Instant - Pistachio
Pudding Instant - Vanilla
Pudding Instant - Vanilla Sugar Free
Pudding Ref. Chocolate
Pudding Ref. Chocolate/Vanilla Swirl
Pudding Ref. Vanilla
Pudding Snack Butterscotch
Pudding Snack Chocolate
Pudding Snack Tapioca
Pudding Snack Vanilla

Ensure
Ensure Pudding (All)

Food Club (Marsh)
Pudding - Chocolate 6 Pack
  (Refrigerated)
Pudding - Chocolate/Vanilla Swirl 6
  Pack (Refrigerated)
Pudding Cook & Serve - Butterscotch
Pudding Cook & Serve - Chocolate
Pudding Cook & Serve - Vanilla
Pudding Instant - Banana Cream
Pudding Instant - Butterscotch
Pudding Instant - Chocolate
Pudding Instant - Chocolate Sugar Free
Pudding Instant - Lemon

Pudding Instant - Vanilla
Pudding Instant - Vanilla Sugar & Fat
  Free
Pudding Snack - Banana
Pudding Snack - Butterscotch
Pudding Snack - Chocolate
Pudding Snack - Chocolate Lite Fat Free
Pudding Snack - Tapioca
Pudding Snack - Vanilla

Fresh & Easy ()

Dark Chocolate Pudding
Flan
French Vanilla Pudding
Rice Pudding
Tapioca Pudding

Great Value (Wal-Mart)

Banana Cream Instant Pudding & Pie
  Filling
Banana Cream Instant Pudding
Chocolate Family Size Instant Pudding
Chocolate Instant Pudding
French Vanilla Instant Pudding & Pie
  Filling
French Vanilla Instant Pudding
Pistachio Instant Pudding & Pie Filling
Pistachio Instant Pudding
Sugar Free Chocolate Instant Pudding
Sugar Free French Vanilla Instant
  Pudding
Vanilla Family Size Instant Pudding
Vanilla Instant Pudding & Pie Filling
Vanilla Instant Pudding

Handi-Snacks Pudding ⌒

Banana Pudding
Baskin Robbins Banana Split Pudding
  Doubles
Baskin Robbins Chocolate Chip Cookie
  Pudding Doubles
Baskin Robbins Chocolate Vanilla
  Sundae Pudding Doubles
Baskin Robbins Fudge Rocky Road
  Pudding Doubles
Butterscotch Pudding
Chocolate Pudding
Rice Pudding
Sugar Free Chocolate Reduced Calorie
  Pudding

Sugar Free Creamy Caramel Reduced
  Calorie Pudding
Sugar Free Vanilla Reduced Calorie
  Pudding
Vanilla Pudding

Hy-Vee

Chocolate Fudge Pudding Cups
Chocolate Pudding Cups
Cooked Chocolate Pudding
Cooked Vanilla Pudding
Fat Free Chocolate Pudding Cups
Instant Butterscotch Pudding
Instant Chocolate Pudding
Instant Fat Free/Sugar Free Chocolate
  Pudding
Instant Fat Free/Sugar Free Vanilla
  Pudding
Instant Lemon Pudding
Instant Pistachio Pudding
Instant Vanilla Pudding
Tapioca Pudding Cups
Vanilla Pudding Cups

Jell-O ⌒

Americana Fat Free Rice Pudding
Caramel Creme Sugar Free Mousse
  Temptations
Chocolate Fudge Sundaes Pudding
  Snacks
Chocolate Indulgence Sugar Free
  Mousse Temptations
Chocolate Sugar Free Pudding Snacks
Cook & Serve Banana Cream Pudding
  & Pie Filling
Cook & Serve Butterscotch Pudding &
  Pie Filling
Cook & Serve Chocolate Fudge Pudding
  & Pie Filling
Cook & Serve Chocolate Pudding & Pie
  Filling
Cook & Serve Chocolate Sugar Free
  Pudding & Pie Filling
Cook & Serve Coconut Cream Pudding
  & Pie Filling
Cook & Serve Lemon Pudding & Pie
  Filling
Cook & Serve Vanilla Pudding & Pie
  Filling

Cook & Serve Vanilla Sugar Free Pudding & Pie Filling
Creamy Caramel Sugar Free Pudding Snacks
Dark Chocolate Decadence Sugar Free Mousse Temptations
Devil's Food & Chocolate Fat Free Pudding Snacks
Double Chocolate Sugar Free Pudding Snacks
Fat Free Chocolate Pudding Snacks
Fat Free Chocolate Vanilla Swirls Pudding Snacks
Fat Free Tapioca Pudding Snacks
Grape Gelatin Dessert
Instant Banana Cream Pudding & Pie Filling
Instant Banana Cream Sugar Free & Fat Free Pudding & Pie Filling
Instant Butterscotch Pudding & Pie Filling
Instant Butterscotch Sugar Free & Fat Free Pudding & Pie Filling
Instant Cheesecake Pudding & Pie Filling
Instant Cheesecake Sugar Free & Fat Free Pudding & Pie Filling
Instant Chocolate Fudge Pudding & Pie Filling
Instant Chocolate Fudge Sugar Free & Fat Free Pudding & Pie Filling
Instant Chocolate Pudding & Pie Filling
Instant Chocolate Sugar Free & Fat Free Pudding & Pie Filling
Instant Coconut Cream Pudding & Pie Filling
Instant Devil's Food Fat Free Pudding & Pie Filling
Instant French Vanilla Pudding & Pie Filling
Instant Lemon Pudding & Pie Filling
Instant Lemon Sugar Free & Fat Free Pudding & Pie Filling
Instant Pistachio Pudding & Pie Filling
Instant Pistachio Sugar Free & Fat Free Pudding & Pie Filling
Instant Vanilla Pudding & Pie Filling

Instant Vanilla Sugar Free & Fat Free Pudding & Pie Filling
Instant White Chocolate Fat Free Pudding & Pie Filling
Instant White Chocolate Sugar Free & Fat Free Pudding & Pie Filling
Original Chocolate Pudding Snacks
Original Chocolate Vanilla Swirls Pudding Snacks
Original Strawberry Cheesecake Snacks
Original Tapioca Pudding Snacks
Original Vanilla Pudding Snacks
Original with The Taste Of Oreo Cookies Pudding Snacks
Peach & Watermelon Sugar Free Gelatin Snacks
Reduced Calorie Sugar Free Chocolate Vanilla Swirls Pudding Snacks
Strawberries & Creme Swirled Pudding Snacks Creme Savers
Vanilla & Chocolate 100 Calorie Packs Fat Free Pudding Snacks

Kroger ⓘ
Pudding - Boxed
Pudding - Snack Cups

Kunzler
Pan Pudding

Meijer
Pudding - Cook & Serve Butterscotch
Pudding - Cook and Serve Chocolate
Pudding - Cook and Serve Vanilla
Pudding and Pie Filling Instant - Chocolate
Pudding and Pie Filling Instant - Coconut Cream
Pudding and Pie Filling Instant - French Vanilla
Pudding and Pie Filling Instant - Pistachio
Pudding and Pie Filling Instant - Vanilla
Pudding Instant - Banana Cream
Pudding Instant - Butterscotch Fat Free & Sugar Free
Pudding Instant - Vanilla Fat Free and Sugar Free
Pudding Premium - Chocolate Peanut Butter
Pudding Premium - French Vanilla
Pudding Premium - Orange Dream
Pudding Snack - Banana
Pudding Snack - Butterscotch

Pudding Snack - Chocolate
Pudding Snack - Chocolate Fat Free
Pudding Snack - Chocolate Fudge
Pudding Snack - Multi-Pack Chocolate
and Vanilla
Pudding Snack - Vanilla
Publix ()
Chocolate Pudding
Fat Free Chocolate Pudding
Fat Free Chocolate-Vanilla Swirl
Pudding
Rice Pudding
Sugar Free Chocolate-Vanilla Swirl
Pudding
Tapioca Pudding

Rice Cakes

Lundberg Family Farms 🏅 ✓
Apple Cinnamon Rice Cakes
Brown Rice Cakes (Salt Free)
Brown Rice Cakes (Salted)
Buttery Caramel Rice Cakes
Honey Nut Rice Cakes
Mochi Sweet Rice Cake
Organic Brown Rice Cakes (Salt Free)
Organic Brown Rice Cakes (Salted)
Organic Caramel Corn Rice Cakes
Organic Cinnamon Toast Rice Cakes
Organic Flax with Tamari Rice Cake
Organic Green Tea with Lemon Rice
Cake
Organic Koku Seaweed Rice Cakes
Organic Mochi Sweet Rice Cakes
Organic Popcorn Rice Cakes
Organic Sesame Tamari Rice Cakes
Organic Wild Rice Rice Cakes
Sesame Tamari Rice Cakes
Toasted Sesame Rice Cakes
Wild Rice Rice Cake
Publix ()
Lightly Salted Rice Cakes
Mini Caramel Rice
Mini Cheddar Rice
Mini Ranch Rice
Unsalted Rice Cakes
White Cheddar Rice Cakes

Quaker ()
Gluten-Free Apple Cinnamon Large
Rice Cakes
Gluten-Free Butter Popped Corn Large
Rice Cakes
Gluten-Free Caramel Corn Large Rice
Cakes
Gluten-Free Chocolate Crunch Large
Rice Cakes
Gluten-Free Lightly Salted Large Rice
Cakes
Gluten-Free Salt Free Large Rice Cakes
Gluten-Free White Cheddar Large Rice
Cakes

Trail Mix

Enjoy Life Foods 🏅 ✓
Not Nuts! Beach Bash Nut-Free Mix
Not Nuts! Mountain Mambo Nut-Free
Mix
Fisher Nuts ()
Fusions Trail Blazer Snack Mix
Fresh & Easy ()
Dried Fruits & Nuts (Assorted Varieties)
Frito Lay ⓘ
Nut & Chocolate Trail Mix
Nut & Fruit Trail Mix
Original Trail Mix
Lydia's Organics 🏅
Lydia's Organics (All)
Nut Harvest ⓘ
Natural Nut & Fruit Mix
Planters 〰
Trail Mix - Fruit & Nut
Trail Mix - Mixed Nuts & Raisins
Publix ()
Party Time Mix

Miscellaneous

Cerrone Cone
Ice Cream Cone
Let's Do… ✓
Gluten-Free Ice Cream Cones
Gluten-Free Sugar Cones

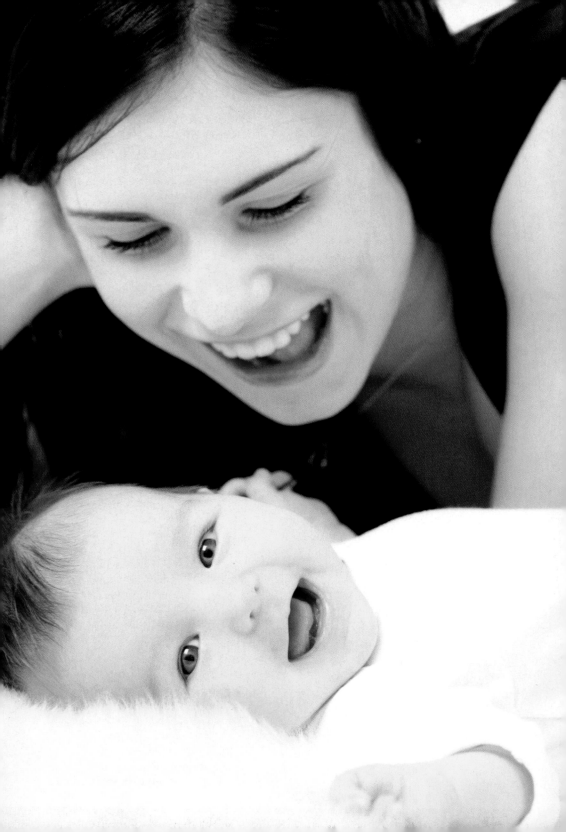

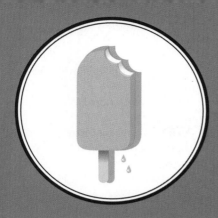

FROZEN FOODS

Beans

Bashas'
Frozen Blackeye Peas
Frozen Lima Beans - Baby

Food Club (Marsh)
Frozen Baby Lima Beans

Great Value (Wal-Mart)
Microwavable Cut Green Beans

Hanover Foods ⓘ
Baby Lima Beans
Fordhook Lima Beans

Hy-Vee
Baby Lima Beans

Meijer
Frozen Beans - Baby Lima
Frozen Beans - Lima Fordhook

Publix ◖◗
Green Beans - Cut
Green Beans - French Cut
Peas - Blackeye
Special Butter Beans

Thrifty Maid (Winn-Dixie) ◖◗
Green Beans, Cut
Peas, Sweet Green

Winn-Dixie ◖◗
Butter Beans
Lima Beans, Baby
Lima Beans, Fordhook
Lima Beans, Petite
Lima Beans, Speckled

Cookie Dough

French Meadow Bakery
Gluten-Free Chocolate Chip Cookie
Dough

Glutenfreeda ♉
Cookie Dough (All)

Dough

Chebe ♉ ✓
Bread Sticks
Frozen Rolls
Sandwich Buns
Tomato-Basil Breadsticks

Frozen Yogurt

Dreyer's
Fat Free Vanilla Yogurt
Frozen Yogurt Mini Cups - Cappuccino
Chip
Frozen Yogurt Mini Cups - Caramel
Praline Crunch
Frozen Yogurt Mini Cups - Peach
Slow Churned Yogurt Blends Black
Cherry Vanilla Swirl
Slow Churned Yogurt Blends
Cappuccino Chip
Slow Churned Yogurt Blends Caramel
Praline Crunch
Slow Churned Yogurt Blends Chocolate
Vanilla Swirl
Slow Churned Yogurt Blends Peach
Slow Churned Yogurt Blends Strawberry

Slow Churned Yogurt Blends Tart
  Mango
Slow Churned Yogurt Blends Vanilla

Edy's
also see Dreyer's

Gifford's Ice Cream
Black Raspberry w/Chocolate Chips
Cappuccino
Chocolate Peanut Butter Cup
Low Fat / No Sugar Added Butter Pecan
Mint Chocolate Chip
Moose Tracks
No Fat / No Sugar Added Black
  Raspberry
No Fat / No Sugar Added Vanilla w/
  Raspberry Swirl

Häagen-Dazs
Coffee
Dulce de Leche
Peach
Snack Size Mini Cups - Vanilla Yogurt
Tart Natural
Vanilla
Vanilla Raspberry Swirl
Wildberry

Hood
Frozen Tangy Yogurt (All)
Frozen Yogurt - Chocolate Fat Free
Frozen Yogurt - Maine Blueberry &
  Sweet Cream Fat Free
Frozen Yogurt - Mocha Fudge Fat Free
Frozen Yogurt - Strawberry Fat Free
Frozen Yogurt - Strawberry-Banana Fat
  Free
Frozen Yogurt - Vanilla Fat Free

Oberweis Dairy
Chocolate Yogurt
French Vanilla Yogurt

Prairie Farms
Chocolate Frozen Yogurt
Strawberry Frozen Yogurt
Vanilla Frozen Yogurt

Publix ()
Black Cherry Premium Low Fat Frozen
  Yogurt
Butter Pecan Premium Low Fat Frozen
  Yogurt

Chocolate Premium Low Fat Frozen
  Yogurt
Neapolitan Premium Low Fat Frozen
  Yogurt
Peach Premium Low Fat Frozen Yogurt
Peanut Butter Cup Premium Low Fat
  Frozen Yogurt
Strawberry Premium Low Fat Frozen
  Yogurt
Vanilla Orange Premium Low Fat
  Frozen Yogurt
Vanilla Premium Low Fat Frozen Yogurt

Turkey Hill
Frozen Yogurt - Banana Split
Frozen Yogurt - Chocolate Cherry
  Cordial
Frozen Yogurt - Chocolate
  Marshmallow
Frozen Yogurt - Fudge Ripple
Frozen Yogurt - Limited Edition
  Caramel Caribou
Frozen Yogurt - Neapolitan
Frozen Yogurt - Orange Cream Swirl
Frozen Yogurt - Peach Mango Smoothie
Frozen Yogurt - Vanilla Bean
Limited Edition - Nutty Caramel
  Caribou (Frozen Yogurt)

FRUIT

Bashas'
Frozen Berry Medley
Frozen Blackberries
Frozen Blueberries
Frozen Mixed Fruit - Individually Quick
  Frozen
Frozen Peaches - Sliced - Individually
  Quick Frozen
Frozen Pitted Dark Sweet Cherries
Frozen Raspberries Red - Individually
  Quick Frozen
Frozen Strawberries - Sliced
Frozen Strawberries - Sliced in Sugar
Frozen Strawberries - Whole -
  Individually Quick Frozen

Food Club (Marsh)
Frozen Berry Medley

Frozen Blackberries Individually Quick Frozen
Frozen Blueberries
Frozen Blueberries Individually Quick Frozen
Frozen Cherries - Dark Sweet
Frozen Peach Slices - Individually Quick Frozen
Frozen Raspberries - Red, Individually Quick Frozen
Frozen Strawberries - Whole, Individually Quick Frozen
Frozen Strawberries Whole

Fresh & Easy ()
Fruits (Assorted Variety)

Great Value (Wal-Mart)
Berry Medley
Sliced Strawberries

Haggen
Berry Medley
Blackberries - Individually Quick Frozen
Blueberries - Individually Quick Frozen
Mixed Fruit
Peaches Sliced - Individually Quick Frozen
Raspberries - Individually Quick Frozen
Raspberries Red w/Heavy Syrup (Tub)
Strawberry Whole - Individually Quick Frozen

Hy-Vee
Blueberries
Cherry Berry Blend
Red Raspberries
Sliced Strawberries
Whole Strawberries

Kroger ⓘ
Plain Frozen Fruit

Meijer
Frozen Berry Medley
Frozen Blackberries
Frozen Blueberries
Frozen Dark Sweet Cherries
Frozen Mango Chunks
Frozen Mango Sliced
Frozen Mixed Fruit

Frozen Mixed Fruit Individually Quick Frozen
Frozen Organic Blueberries
Frozen Organic Peaches
Frozen Organic Raspberries
Frozen Organic Strawberries
Frozen Pineapple Chunks
Frozen Raspberries
Frozen Raspberries - Individually Quick Frozen
Frozen Sliced Peaches
Frozen Strawberries - Individually Quick Frozen
Frozen Strawberries - Sliced
Frozen Tart Cherries
Frozen Triple Berry Blend
Frozen Tropical Fruit Blend

Nash Brothers
Organic Frozen Fruit

Publix ()
Blackberries
Blueberries
Cherries - Dark Sweet
Cranberries
Mixed Berries
Mixed Fruit
Peaches - Sliced
Raspberries
Strawberries - Sliced, Sweetened
Strawberries - Whole

Raley's
Berry Medley
Blackberries
Dark Sweet Cherries
Mixed Fruit
Strawberries

Stahlbush Island Farms ⓘ ✓
Stahlbush Island Farms (All)

Winn-Dixie ()
Berry Medley
Blackberries
Blueberries
Dark Sweet Cherries
Mango Chunks
Mixed Fruit
Red Raspberries
Sliced Peaches

Strawberries - No Sugar Added
Strawberries - Sugar Added
Whole Strawberries

Wyman's
Wyman's (All)

ICE CREAM

Ciao Bella ⓘ
Gelato Pints (All BUT Malted Milk Ball, Key Lime Graham, and Maple Ginger Snap)

Dreyer's
Banana Split (Limited Edition)
Eggnog (Limited Edition)
Fat Free No Sugar Added Vanilla Chocolate
Fun Flavors - Butter Pecan
Fun Flavors - Cherry Chocolate Chip
Fun Flavors - Chocolate Peanut Butter Cup
Fun Flavors - Dulce de Leche
Fun Flavors - Mango
Fun Flavors - Mocha Almond Fudge
Fun Flavors - Nestle Butterfinger
Fun Flavors - Rocky Road
Fun Flavors - Spumoni
Grand Ice Cream - Butter Pecan (Pint)
Grand Ice Cream - Chocolate
Grand Ice Cream - Chocolate Chip
Grand Ice Cream - Coffee
Grand Ice Cream - Double Vanilla
Grand Ice Cream - French Vanilla
Grand Ice Cream - Mint Chocolate Chip
Grand Ice Cream - Neapolitan
Grand Ice Cream - Real Strawberry
Grand Ice Cream - Rocky Road
Grand Ice Cream - Vanilla
Grand Ice Cream - Vanilla Bean
Grand Ice Cream - Vanilla Chocolate
Maxx Cherry Chocolate Bomb
Maxx Chocolate Peanut Butter Chunk
Maxx Java MashUp
Maxx Nestle Butterfinger
Peppermint (Limited Edition)
Pumpkin (Limited Edition)
Root Beer Float (Limited Edition)

Slow Churned Eggnog (Limited Edition)
Slow Churned Hot Cocoa (Limited Edition)
Slow Churned Light Butter Pecan
Slow Churned Light Caramel Delight
Slow Churned Light Chocolate
Slow Churned Light Chocolate Chip
Slow Churned Light Chocolate Fudge Chunk
Slow Churned Light Coffee
Slow Churned Light French Vanilla
Slow Churned Light Fudge Tracks
Slow Churned Light Mint Chocolate Chip
Slow Churned Light Neapolitan
Slow Churned Light Peanut Butter Cup
Slow Churned Light Rocky Road
Slow Churned Light Strawberry
Slow Churned Light Take the Cake
Slow Churned Light Vanilla
Slow Churned Light Vanilla Bean
Slow Churned No Sugar Added Butter Pecan
Slow Churned No Sugar Added French Vanilla
Slow Churned No Sugar Added Fudge Tracks
Slow Churned No Sugar Added Mint Chocolate Chip
Slow Churned No Sugar Added Neapolitan
Slow Churned No Sugar Added Triple Chocolate
Slow Churned No Sugar Added Vanilla
Slow Churned No Sugar Added Vanilla Bean
Slow Churned Peppermint (Limited Edition)
Slow Churned Pumpkin (Limited Edition)

Edy's
also see Dreyer's
Fun Flavors - Espresso Chip

Fresh & Easy ⟨⟩
Butter Pecan Ice Cream
Chocolate Chip Ice Cream
Chocolate Ice Cream

Coffee Ice Cream
Dulce De Leche Ice Cream
Espresso Fudge Ice Cream
Gelato - Cappucino
Gelato - Chocolate Hazelnut
Gelato - Dark Chocolate
Gelato - Pistachio
Gelato - Roasted Banana
Mint Chocolate Chip Ice Cream
Mocha Java Ice Cream
Neapolitan Ice Cream
Rocky Road Ice Cream
Strawberry Ice Cream
Vanilla Ice Cream

Gifford's Ice Cream
Black Raspberry
Butter Almond
Butter Pecan
Caramel Caribou
Cherry Amaretto Chocolate
Cherry Vanilla
Chocolate
Chocolate Chip
Chocolate Moose Tracks
Chocolate Rainforest Crunch
Coffee
French Vanilla
Joyful Coconut Almond
M&M
Maine Black Bear
Maine Deer Tracks
Maine Maple Walnut
Maine Wild Blueberry
Mint Chocolate Chip
Moose Tracks
Old Fashioned Vanilla
Peanut Butter Cup
Pink Peppermint Stick
Pistachio Nut
Pumpkin
Rocky Road
Rum Raisin
Smurf (Cotton Candy)
Strawberry
White Chocolate Caramel Cashew

Häagen-Dazs
Amaretto Almond Crunch (Limited Edition)
Banana Split
Bananas Foster (Limited Edition)
Butter Pecan
Cherry Vanilla
Chocolate
Chocolate Chocolate Chip
Chocolate Peanut Butter
Coffee
Crème Brulee
Dark Chocolate
Dark Chocolate Mint (Limited Edition)
Dulce de Leche
Five Caramel
Five Coffee
Five Ginger
Five Lemon
Five Milk Chocolate
Five Mint
Five Passion Fruit
Five Strawberry
Five Vanilla Bean
Green Tea
Java Chip
Mango
Mint Chip
Peanut Butter Brittle (Limited Edition)
Peppermint Bark (Limited Edition)
Pineapple Coconut
Pistachio
Rocky Road
Rum Raisin
Snack Size Mini Cups - Chocolate
Snack Size Mini Cups - Chocolate Chocolate Chip
Snack Size Mini Cups - Chocolate Peanut Butter
Snack Size Mini Cups - Coffee
Snack Size Mini Cups - Dulce de Leche
Snack Size Mini Cups - Strawberry
Snack Size Mini Cups - Vanilla
Strawberry
Vanilla
Vanilla Bean
Vanilla Chocolate Chip
Vanilla Honey Bee

Vanilla Swiss Almond
White Chocolate Raspberry Truffle

Haggen
Ice Cream - Black Cherry
Ice Cream - Caramel Vanilla
Ice Cream - French Vanilla
Ice Cream - Mint Chocolate Chip
Ice Cream - Mocha Almond Fudge
Ice Cream - Neapolitan
Ice Cream - Orange Vanilla
Ice Cream - Rocky Road
Ice Cream - Strawberry
Ice Cream - Tin Roof Sundae

Hood
Chocolate
Chocolate Chip
Classic Trio
Creamy Coffee
Fudge Twister
Golden Vanilla
Maple Walnut
Natural Vanilla Bean
New England Creamery - Bear Creek
   Caramel
New England Creamery - Boston
   Vanilla Bean
New England Creamery - Cape Cod
   Fudge Shop
New England Creamery - Light Butter
   Pecan
New England Creamery - Light
   Chocolate Chip
New England Creamery - Light Coffee
New England Creamery - Light Martha's
   Vineyard Black Raspberry
New England Creamery - Light Under
   The Stars
New England Creamery - Light Vanilla
New England Creamery - Maine
   Blueberry & Sweet Cream
New England Creamery - Martha's
   Vineyard Black Raspberry
New England Creamery - Moosehead
   Lake Fudge
New England Creamery - Mystic
   Lighthouse Mint

New England Creamery - New England
   Homemade Vanilla
New England Creamery - Rhode Island
   Lighthouse Coffee
New England Creamery - Vermont
   Maple Nut
Patchwork
Red Sox Ice Cream (All Flavors)
Strawberry

Horizon Organic ⓘ
Horizon Organic (All BUT Ice Cream
   Sandwiches)

Hy-Vee
Butter Crunch Ice Cream
Cherry Nut Ice Cream
Chocolate Chip Ice Cream
Chocolate Chip Light Ice Cream
Chocolate Ice Cream
Chocolate Marshmallow Ice Cream
Chocolate/Vanilla Flavored Ice Cream
Dutch Chocolate Light Ice Cream
Fudge Marble Ice Cream
Mint Chip Ice Cream
Neapolitan Ice Cream
Neapolitan Light Ice Cream
New York Vanilla Ice Cream
Peppermint Stick Ice Cream
Strawberry Ice Cream
Vanilla Flavored Ice Cream
Vanilla Light Ice Cream

It's Soy Delicious
Almond Pecan
Awesome Chocolate
Black Leopard
Carob Peppermint
Chocolate Almond
Chocolate Peanut Butter
Espresso
Green Tea
Mango Raspberry
Pistachio Almond
Raspberry
Tiger Chai
Vanilla
Vanilla Fudge

Kroger ⓘ
Private Selection Gelato

Lactaid
Butter Pecan Ice Cream
Chocolate Ice Cream
Vanilla Ice Cream

Lindy's Homemade
Lindy's (All)

Living Harvest ⓘ ✓
Tempt Frozen Dessert

Luna & Larry's Coconut Bliss ⓘ
Coconut Bliss (All)

Meijer
Awesome Strawberry Ice Cream
Bordeaux Cherry Chocolate Ice Cream
Butter Pecan Ice Cream
Candy Bar Swirl Ice Cream
Carb Conquest Chocolate Ice Cream
Carb Conquest Vanilla Ice Cream
Chocolate Chip Ice Cream
Chocolate Ice Cream
Chocolate Peanut Butter Fudge Ice
    Cream
Chocolate Thunder Ice Cream
Combo Cream
Cotton Candy Ice Cream
Dulce De Leche Ice Cream
Fat Free No Sugar Added Caramel
Fat Free No Sugar Added Vanilla with
    Splenda
Fudge Swirl Ice Cream
Gold Caramel Toffee Swirl Ice Cream
Gold Double Nut Chocolate Ice Cream
Gold Georgian Bay Butter Pecan Ice
    Cream
Gold Peanut Butter Fudge Swirl Ice
    Cream
Gold Peanut Butter Fudge Tracks Ice
    Cream
Gold Thunder Bay Cherry Ice Cream
Gold Victorian Vanilla
Heavenly Hash Ice Cream
Lite Neapolitan Ice Cream
Lite No Sugar Added Butter Pecan Ice
    Cream with Splenda
Lite No Sugar Added Vanilla with
    Splenda
Mackinac Fudge Ice Cream
Mint Chocolate Ice Cream

Neapolitan Ice Cream
Peppermint Ice Cream
Praline Pecan Ice Cream
Scooperman Ice Cream
Tin Roof Ice Cream
Vanilla Ice Cream

Midwest Country Fare (Hy-Vee)
Chocolate Chip Ice Cream
Chocolate Ice Cream
Light Vanilla Ice Cream
Neapolitan Ice Cream
Vanilla Ice Cream

Oberweis Dairy
Apple Strudel
Birthday Cake
Black Cherry
Black Walnut
Brandy
Butter Brickle
Butter Pecan
Chocolate
Chocolate Almond
Chocolate Chip
Chocolate Chocolate Chip
Chocolate Marshmallow
Chocolate Peanut Butter
Cinnamon
Coffee
Cotton Candy
Dark Chocolate
Dulce de Leche
Egg Nog
Lowfat Chocolate
Lowfat Chocolate Marshmallow
Lowfat Strawberry
Lowfat Vanilla
Mango Pomegranate
Mint Chocolate Chip
No Sugar Added Chocolate
No Sugar Added Vanilla
Peach
Peppermint
Pistachio
Pumpkin
Rocky Road
Rum Raisin
Strawberry

Udderly Truffles
Vanilla
Vanilla Soft Serve

Prairie Farms
Belgian Chocolate Ice Cream
Chocolate Chip Ice Cream
Chocolate Ice Cream
French Vanilla Ice Cream
Mint Chip Ice Cream
Neapolitan Ice Cream
Vanilla Bean Ice Cream
Vanilla Ice Cream
Vanilla/Orange Ice Cream

Prestige (Winn-Dixie) ()
Chocolate Almond Ice Cream
Chocolate Ice Cream
Vanilla Ice Cream

Private Selection Brand (Kroger) ⓘ
Gelato

Publix ()
Banana Split Premium Ice Cream
Bear Claw Premium Ice Cream
Black Jack Cherry Premium Ice Cream
Buckeye's & Fudge Premium Limited
   Edition Ice Cream
Butter Pecan Premium Homemade Ice
   Cream
Butter Pecan Premium Ice Cream
Butter Pecan Premium Light Ice Cream
Caramel Mountain Tracks Premium
   Limited Edition Ice Cream
Cherry Nut Premium Ice Cream
Chocolate Almond Premium Ice Cream
Chocolate Cherish Passion Premium Ice
   Cream
Chocolate Chip Premium Homemade
   Ice Cream
Chocolate Chip Premium Ice Cream
Chocolate Ice Cream
Chocolate Low Fat Ice Cream
Chocolate Marshmallow Swirl Ice
   Cream
Chocolate Peanut Butter Swirl Ice
   Cream
Chocolate Premium Ice Cream
Chocolate Premium Light Ice Cream

Coffee Almond Fudge Premium Light
   Ice Cream
Coffee Premium Ice Cream
Double Chocolate Chunk Premium
   Homemade Ice Cream
Dulce de Leche Premium Ice Cream
Egg Nog Premium Limited Edition Ice
   Cream
French Silk Duo Premium Limited
   Edition Ice Cream
French Vanilla Premium Ice Cream
Fudge Royal Ice Cream
Fudge Royal Low Fat Ice Cream
Heavenly Hash Premium Ice Cream
Maple Walnut Premium Limited Edition
   Ice Cream
Mint Chocolate Chip Premium Ice
   Cream
Monkey Business Premium Limited
   Edition Ice Cream
Neapolitan Ice Cream
Neapolitan Low Fat Ice Cream
Neapolitan Premium Ice Cream
Neapolitan Premium Light Ice Cream
Otter Paws Premium Ice Cream
Peanut Butter Goo Goo Premium Ice
   Cream
Peppermint Stick Premium Limited
   Edition Ice Cream
Rum Raisin Premium Limited Edition
   Ice Cream
Santa's White Christmas Premium Ice
   Cream
Strawberry Premium Homemade Ice
   Cream
Strawberry Premium Ice Cream
Strawberry Premium Light Ice Cream
Vanilla Ice Cream
Vanilla Low Fat Ice Cream
Vanilla Premium Homemade Ice Cream
Vanilla Premium Ice Cream
Vanilla Premium Light Ice Cream
Vanilla Strawberry Ice Cream

Purely Decadent Dairy Free
Cherry Nirvana
Chocolate Obsession
Coconut Craze

Cookie Dough (Gluten-Free)
Mint Chocolate Chip
Mocha Almond Fudge
Peanut Butter Zig Zag
Pomegranate Chip
Praline Pecan
Purely Vanilla
Rocky Road
So Very Strawberry
Swinging Anna Banana
Turtle Tracks
Vanila Swiss Almond

Rice Dream ✓

Cocoa Marble Fudge
Neapolitan
Vanilla

So Delicious Dairy Free

Organic - Butter Pecan
Organic - Chocolate Peanut Butter
Organic - Chocolate Velvet
Organic - Creamy Lemon
Organic - Creamy Orange
Organic - Creamy Raspberry
Organic - Creamy Vanilla
Organic - Dulce De Leche
Organic - Mint Marble Fudge
Organic - Mocha Fudge
Organic - Neapolitan
Organic - Strawberry

Soy Dream ✓

Butter Pecan Frozen Dessert
French Vanilla Frozen Dessert
Green Tea Frozen Dessert
Mocha Fudge Frozen Dessert
Vanilla Frozen Dessert
Vanilla Fudge Frozen Dessert

Talenti

Talenti (All BUT Caramel Cookie
Crunch Gelato)

Turkey Hill

All Natural Recipe - Cherry Vanilla
All Natural Recipe - Chocolate
All Natural Recipe - Coffee
All Natural Recipe - Mint Chocolate
Chip
All Natural Recipe - Neapolitan
All Natural Recipe - Nutty Neapolitan

All Natural Recipe - Vanilla Bean
Duetto Gelati - Cherry
Duetto Gelati - Lemon
Duetto Gelati - Limited Edition Bananas
Foster
Duetto Gelati - Limited Edition Caramel
Apple
Duetto Gelati - Mango
Duetto Gelati - Pomegranate Blueberry
Duetto Gelati - Raspberry
Duetto Gelati - Root Beer
Duetto Gelati - Strawberry Banana
Dynamic Duos - Movie Night
Dynamic Duos - PB Explosion
Frozen Yogurt - Limited Edition
PomBlueberry Chocolate Chunk
Light Recipe - Banana Split
Light Recipe - Bavarian Espresso
Light Recipe - Chocolate Moose Nutty
Tracks
Light Recipe - Coconut Almond Fudge
Light Recipe - Dulce de Chocolate
Light Recipe - Moose Tracks
Light Recipe - Raspberry Chocolate
Chunk
Light Recipe - Vanilla Bean
Limited Edition - Box of Chocolates
Limited Edition - Caramel Caribou
Limited Edition - Chunky Peanut Butter
Limited Edition - Eagles Touchdown
Sundae
Limited Edition - Junior Mint
Limited Edition - Peaches 'n Cream
Limited Edition - Peppermint Pattie
Limited Edition - Peppermint Stick
Limited Edition - Vanilla Swiss Almond
No Sugar Added Recipe - Cherry Fudge
Ripple
No Sugar Added Recipe - Dutch
Chocolate
No Sugar Added Recipe - Moosetracks
(Light)
No Sugar Added Recipe - Peanut Brittle
(Light)
No Sugar Added Recipe - Vanilla Bean
Premium Ice Cream - Banana Split
Premium Ice Cream - Black Cherry
Premium Ice Cream - Black Raspberry

Premium Ice Cream - Butter Pecan
Premium Ice Cream - Choco Mint Chip
Premium Ice Cream - Chocolate
  Marshmallow
Premium Ice Cream - Chocolate Peanut
  Butter Cup
Premium Ice Cream - Colombian Coffee
Premium Ice Cream - Dutch Chocolate
Premium Ice Cream - Egg Nog
  (Seasonal)
Premium Ice Cream - French Vanilla
Premium Ice Cream - Fudge Ripple
Premium Ice Cream - Neapolitan
Premium Ice Cream - Orange Cream
  Swirl
Premium Ice Cream - Original Vanilla
Premium Ice Cream - Peanut Butter
  Ripple
Premium Ice Cream - Rocky Road
Premium Ice Cream - Rum Raisin
Premium Ice Cream - Strawberries & Cream
Premium Ice Cream - Vanilla & Chocolate
Premium Ice Cream - Vanilla Bean
Stuff'd - Chocolate Mint Moose Tracks
Stuff'd - Chocolate Nutty Moose Tracks
Stuff'd - Moose Tracks
Stuff'd - Praline Pecan Paradise

Valu Time (Marsh)
Ice Cream Chocolate
Ice Cream Chocolate Chip
Ice Cream Fudge Swirl
Ice Cream Neapolitan
Ice Cream Rainbow Sherbet
Ice Cream Strawberry Swirl
Ice Cream Vanilla

Winn-Dixie ()
Classic Chocolate Ice Cream
Classic Neapolitan Ice Cream
Classic Strawberry Ice Cream
Classic Vanilla Ice Cream

JUICE & JUICE DRINKS

Bashas'
Frozen Apple Juice Concentrate
Frozen Grapefruit Juice Concentrate
Frozen Lemonade Concentrate

Frozen Orange Juice Concentrate
Frozen Orange Juice Concentrate with
  Calcium
Frozen Pink Lemonade Concentrate

Food Club (Marsh)
Frozen Juice - Apple Concentrate
Frozen Juice - Orange Concentrate
Frozen Juice - Orange Concentrate, No Pulp
Frozen Juice - Orange with Calcium
Frozen Lemonade
Frozen Pink Lemonade

Fresh & Easy ()
Frozen Juice Concentrate - Apple
Frozen Juice Concentrate - Cran
Frozen Juice Concentrate - Orange

Great Value (Wal-Mart)
Frozen Concentrate Pulp Free Orange Juice
Frozen Concentrated 100% Grape Juice
Frozen Concentrated Apple Juice
Frozen Concentrated Country Style
  Orange Juice
Frozen Concentrated Florida Grapefruit
  Juice
Frozen Concentrated Fruit Punch
Frozen Concentrated Grape Juice Drink
Frozen Concentrated Lemonade
Frozen Concentrated Limeade
Frozen Concentrated Orange Juice
Frozen Concentrated Orange Juice w/
  Calcium
Frozen Concentrated Pink Lemonade

Hy-Vee
Apple Juice Concentrate
Fruit Punch Concentrate
Grape Juice Cocktail Concentrate
Lemonade Concentrate
Limeade Concentrate
Orange Juice Frozen Concentrate
Orange Juice with Added Calcium
  Frozen Concentrate
Pineapple Juice From Concentrate
Pink Lemonade Frozen Concentrate

Kroger ⓘ
Frozen Lemonade

Meijer
Frozen Apple Juice Concentrate
Frozen Fruit Punch Concentrate

Frozen Grape Juice Concentrate
Frozen Grapefruit Juice Concentrate
Frozen Lemonade Concentrate
Frozen Limeade Concentrate
Frozen Orange Juice Concentrate
Frozen Orange Juice Concentrate High Pulp
Frozen Pink Lemonade Concentrate

Midwest Country Fare (Hy-Vee)
100% Concentrated Orange Juice

Publix ()
Frozen Concentrated Orange Juice

Meat & Sausage

Bashas'
Shrimp - Cooked
Bubba Burger ⍩
Bubba Burgers (All)
Byron's ()
Pork BBQ
Empire Kosher
Frozen Chicken
Frozen Ground Turkey
Frozen Whole Turkey & Turkey Breasts
Individually Quick Frozen Chicken
Parts
Holten Meat
Holten Meat (All)
Jennie-O Turkey Store ⓘ
Frozen Ground Seasoned Turkey
Frozen Ground Turkey
Frozen Turkey Burgers
Jones Dairy Farm
All Natural Golden Brown Fully Cooked
Beef Sausage Links
All Natural Golden Brown Fully Cooked
Light Pork & Rice Sausage Links
All Natural Golden Brown Fully Cooked
Maple Pork Sausage Links
All Natural Golden Brown Fully Cooked
Maple Sausage Patties
All Natural Golden Brown Fully Cooked
Mild Pork Sausage Links
All Natural Golden Brown Fully Cooked
Mild Sausage Patties
All Natural Golden Brown Fully Cooked
Pork & Uncured Bacon Sausage Links

All Natural Golden Brown Fully Cooked
Spicy Pork Sausage Links
All Natural Golden Brown Fully Cooked
Turkey Sausage Links
All Natural Hearty Pork Sausage Links
All Natural Light Pork Sausage & Rice
Links Sausage
All Natural Little Maple Pork Sausage
Links
All Natural Little Pork Sausage Links
All Natural Little Turkey Sausage Links
All Natural Original Pork Sausage Roll
All Natural Pork Sausage Patties
Kroger ⓘ
Frozen Plain Chicken Breast
Frozen Plain Chicken Thighs
Frozen Plain Chicken Wings
Frozen Plain Turkey Breast
Frozen Plain Turkey Thighs
Meijer
Frozen Duckling
Frozen Turkey Breast
Frozen Turkey Breast Young
Organic Prairie
Beef Hot Dogs
Beef Liver Steak
Boneless Skinless Chicken Breasts
Bratwurst
Breakfast Sausage
Brown-n-Serve Breakfast Links
Chicken Hot Dogs
Chicken Italian Sausage
Ground Beef
Ground Beef Patties
Ground Chicken
Ground Turkey
Hardwood Smoked Bacon
Hardwood Smoked Boneless Half Ham
Hardwood Smoked Turkey Bacon
Italian Sausage
New York Strip Steak
Pork Chops
Ribeye Steak
Whole Young Chicken
Whole Young Turkey
Perdue
Individually Frozen - Chicken Breasts

FAN GLUTENFREE TASTIC

Why are we calling attention to the fact that Jones All Natural Sausage contains no gluten and none of the ingredients hidden in other brands? Because we thought you'd like to know. It's just pork, salt and spices—has been for over 120 years. Plus our sausage is frozen so it's always fresh. Always fantastic. Visit **jonesdairyfarm.com/glutenfree** for great recipes and special savings.

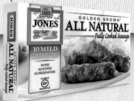

No nitrites

No MSG

No artificial flavors

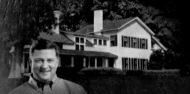

– *Philip Jones*
President, Jones Dairy Farm

PURE FLAVOR SIMPLE PLEASURE

ALL NATURAL SAUSAGE • HAM • BACON • CANADIAN BACON • BRAUNSCHWEIG

Individually Frozen - Chicken Tenderloins

Individually Frozen - Chicken Wings

Philly-Gourmet ⓘ
100% Pure Beef Patties

All Beef Sandwich Steaks

Pilgrim's Pride
Marinated Individually Quick Frozen - Boneless/Skinless Breasts

Marinated Individually Quick Frozen - Boneless/Skinless Thighs

Marinated Individually Quick Frozen - Drum

Marinated Individually Quick Frozen - Drummettes

Marinated Individually Quick Frozen - Split Breast

Marinated Individually Quick Frozen - Tenderloins

Marinated Individually Quick Frozen - Thigh

Marinated Individually Quick Frozen - Wing Sections

Publix ⟨⟩
Frozen Boneless Skinless Chicken Breasts

Frozen Boneless Skinless Chicken Cutlets

Frozen Chicken Breast Tenderloins

Frozen Chicken Wingettes

Quaker Maid Meats ⓘ
100% Pure All Beef Sandwich Steaks (All)

Shelton's
Chicken Franks

Smoked Chicken Franks

Smoked Turkey Franks

Turkey Breakfast Sausage

Turkey Breakfast Strips

Turkey Burgers

Turkey Franks

Turkey Italian Sausage

Turkey Sausage Patties

Uncured Turkey Bologna

Steak-umm
Burgers - Original

Burgers - Sweet Onion

Sliced Steaks

NOVELTIES

Bashas'
Chocolate Sundae Ice Cream Cups

Ice Cream Bars

Orange Cream Bars

Strawberry Sundae Ice Cream Cups

Cool Fruits
Freezer Pops (All)

Del Monte ⓘ
Fruit Chillers (Cups or Freeze & Eat Tubes)

Diana's Banana Babies
Diana's Banana Babies (All)

Dibs
Chocolate

Mint

Vanilla

Dreyer's
Acai Blueberry Fruit Bar

Black Cherry/Strawberry Kiwi/Mixed Berry No Sugar Added Fruit Bar Pack

Cherry/Grape/Tropical Mini Snack Size Fruit Bars

Creamy Coconut Fruit Bar

Grape Fruit Bar

Lemonade Fruit Bar

Lime Fruit Bar

Orange & Cream Fruit Bar

Orange & Cream/Raps Cream/Lime Cream Mini Snack Size Fruit Bars

Pineapple Fruit Bar

Pomegranate Fruit Bar

Raspberry/Strawberry/Tangerine No Sugar Added Fruit Bar Variety Pack

Strawberry Fruit Bar

Tangerine Fruit Bar

Edy's
also see Dreyer's

Eskimo Pie
Vanilla with Dark Chocolate

Vanilla with Dark Chocolate Club

Vanilla with Dark Chocolate No Sugar Added

Fat Boy Ice Cream ()
  Nut Sundaes
  Vanilla Sundaes

Food Club (Marsh)
  Frozen Novelties - Fudge Bars
  Frozen Novelties - Ice Cream Bars

Fresh & Easy ()
  Fudge Bar
  Pomegranate Cherry Fruit Bar

Gaga's SherBetter
  SherBetter (All)

Häagen-Dazs
  Chocolate Dark Chocolate Ice Cream
    Bar
  Coffee Almond Crunch Mini Bars
  Vanilla Dark Chocolate Ice Cream Bar
  Vanilla Milk Chocolate Almond Ice
    Cream Bar
  Vanilla Milk Chocolate Almond Mini
    Bars
  Vanilla Milk Chocolate Ice Cream Bar

Haggen
  Frozen Novelties Fudge Bars
  Ice Cream Bars
  Merry-Go-Round Bars
  Orange Cream Bars Bag

Hood
  Fudge Stix
  Hoodsie Cups
  Hoodsie Pops - 6 Flavor Assortment
    Twin Pops
  Hoodsie Sundae Cups
  Ice Cream Bar
  Kids Karnival Stix
  Orange Cream Bar

Hy-Vee
  Assorted Twin Pops
  Chocolate & Strawberry Sundae Cups
  Fat Free No Sugar Added Fudge Bars
  Fudge Bars
  Galaxy Bars
  No Sugar Added Low Fat Ice Cream
    Bars
  Orange Galaxy Bars
  Pops - Cherry, Orange, Grape
  Reduced Fat Galaxy Bars

Single Serve Chocolate Chip Ice Cream
    Cups
  Vanilla Ice Cream Cups

Julie's Organic (i) ✓
  Gluten-Free Lemon Yogurt Ice Cream
    Sandwich with Vanilla Cookies
  Gluten-Free Vanilla Ice Cream
    Sandwich with Chocolate Cookies

Luigi's Real Italian Ice
  Luigi's Real Italian Ice (All)

Meijer
  Brr Bar
  Dream Bars
  Frozen Novelties - Gold Bar
  Frozen Novelties - Toffee Bar
  Fudge Bars
  Ice Cream Bars
  Juice Stix
  No Sugar Added Fudge Bars
  No Sugar Added Party Pops (Assorted)
  Orange Glider
  Party Pops Orange/Cherry/Grape
  Red White and Blue Pops
  Toffee Bars
  Twin Pops

Minute Maid
  Juice Bars - Cherry
  Juice Bars - Grape
  Juice Bars - Orange

Nestlé Ice Cream
  (ICED) ENrG Bar
  Butterfinger Bar
  Frozen Lemonade Cup
  Frozen Strawberry Lemonade Cup
  Fruit Mania Push-Up
  Fudge Bar
  Itzakadoozie Ice Pop
  Laffy Taffy Push Up
  Nesquik Push-Up
  Orange Push-Up
  Rainbow Push-Up
  Rainbow Twisters Push-Up
  Vanilla Bar with Chocolatey Coating

North Star
  Fudge Bars

Prairie Farms
- Chocolate Coated Vanilla Flavored Ice Cream Bars
- Chocolate Ice Cream Cups
- Old Recipe Bars
- Reduced Fat Ice Cream Bars
- Strawberry Ice Cream Cups
- Vanilla Ice Cream Cups

Publix ()
- Banana Pops
- Cream Pops
- Fudge Bar
- Fudge Sundae Cups
- Ice Cream Bar
- Ice Cream Squares
- No Sugar Added Fudge Pops
- No Sugar Added Ice Cream Bars
- No Sugar Added Ice Pop
- Orange, Cherry and Grape Junior Ice Pops
- Red White and Blue Junior Ice Pops
- Toffee Bar
- Twin Pops
- Vanilla Cups

Purely Decadent Dairy Free
- Purely Vanilla Bar
- Vanilla Almond Bar

Skinny Cow, The
- Caramel Skinny Truffle Bars
- Chocolate Skinny Truffle Bars
- Dulce De Leche Skinny Cups
- French Vanilla Skinny Truffle Bars
- Low Fat Fudge Bars
- Skinny Mini Fudge Bars
- White Mint Skinny Truffle Bars

So Delicious Dairy Free
- Creamy Orange Bar
- Creamy Raspberry Bar
- Kidz - Assorted Fruit Pops
- Kidz - Fudge Pops
- Organic - Creamy Fudge Bar
- Organic - Creamy Vanilla Bar
- Organic - Vanilla & Almonds Bar
- Sugar Free - Fudge Bar
- Sugar Free - Vanilla Bar

Sweet Nothings
- Fudge Bar

- Mango Raspberry Bar

Turkey Hill
- Fudge Bars
- Ice Cream Bars

Whole Fruit
- Fruit Bars

Winn-Dixie ()
- Banana Pops
- Fudge Bars

PIZZA & CRUSTS

Against the Grain ⚇
- Against the Grain (All)

Amy's Kitchen ⓘ ✓
- Rice Crust Cheese Pizza
- Rice Crust Spinach Pizza

Chebe ⚇ ✓
- Pizza Crusts

Foods by George ⚇
- Pizza
- Pizza Crusts

Gluten Free & FABULOUS ✓
- Cheese Pizza
- Pepperoni Pizza
- Pesto Margherita Pizza
- Spinach Feta Pizza
- Vegetable Margherita Pizza

Glutino
- 3 Cheese Brown Rice Crust Pizza
- BBQ Chicken Pizza
- Pepperoni Brown Rice Crust Pizza
- Spinach & Feta Pizza
- Spinach Soy Cheese Brown Rice Crust Pizza

Udi's Gluten Free Foods ⚇
- Pizza Crusts

POTATOES

Alexia Foods ⓘ ⚇
- Potato Products (All)

Bashas'
- Frozen French Fried Potatoes
- Frozen French Fried Potatoes - Steak Cut

Frozen French Fries - Crinkle Cut
Frozen Hashbrowns Shredded
Frozen Hashbrowns, Southern Style
Frozen Hashbrowns Western Style
Frozen Tater Treats

Diner's Choice
Diner's Choice (All)

Dr. Praeger's ✓
Potato Littles
Sweet Potato Littles
Sweet Potato Pancakes

Food Club (Marsh)
Frozen Potato French Fries
Frozen Potato French Fries - Crinkle
  Cut
Frozen Potato Hash Brown Patties
Frozen Potato Hashbrowns - Southern
  Style
Frozen Potato Steak Fry
Frozen Potato Tater Treats
Frozen Potatoes O'Brien
Frozen Shredded Potato Hash Browns

Fresh & Easy ()
French Fries (Assorted Varieties)
Hashbrowns (Assorted Varieties)

Hy-Vee
Country Style Hash Brown Potatoes
Crinkle Cut Fries
Criss Cut Potatoes
Hash Browns Real Russet Potatoes
Steak Fries

McCain Foods ⓘ
5 Minute Fries
Classic Cut Fries
Crinkle Cut Fries
HomeStyle BabyCakes
Mash-Bites Potatoes
Popcorn Potatoes
Premium Gold Crisp Crinkle Cut Fry
Premium Golden Crisp Fast Food Fries
  Shoestring Cut
Premium Golden Crisp Straight Cut
  French Fry
Roasters - All American
Roasters - Grilled Garlic & Onion
Smiles Fun Shaped Potatoes
Steak Fries

Tasti Taters Shaped Potatoes

Meijer
Frozen French Fries
Frozen French Fries Crinkle Cut
Frozen French Fries Quickie Crinkles
Frozen French Fries Shoestring
Frozen French Fries Steak Cut
Frozen Hashbrowns
Frozen Hashbrowns - Shredded
Frozen Hashbrowns - Southern Style
Frozen Hashbrowns - Western Style
Frozen Potatoes - French Fried Crinkle
  Cut
Frozen Potatoes - Tater Treats

Ore-Ida ⓘ
ABC Tater Tots
Cottage Fries
Country Fries
Country Style Hashbrowns
Country Style Steak Fries
Crispers
Extra Crispy Crinkle Cut
Extra Crispy Fast Food Fries
Extra Crispy Seasoned Crinkle Cut
Fast Food Fries
French Fries
Golden Crinkles
Golden Fries
Golden Patties
Golden Twirls
Pixie Crinkles
Potatoes O'Brien
Shoestrings
Southern Style Hash Browns
Steak Fries
Steam n' Mash Cut Russets
Steam n' Mash Cut Sweet Potatoes
Steam n' Mash Garlic Seasoned Potatoes
Sweet Potato Fries
Tater Tots (All Varieties)
Waffle Fries
Zesties
Zesty Twirls

Publix ()
Crinkle Cut Fries
Golden Fries
Shoestring Fries

Southern Style Hash Browns
Steak Fries
Tater Bites
Tater Puffs

Smart Ones ⓘ
Broccoli & Cheddar Potatoes

Valu Time (Marsh)
Frozen Potato French Fry Regular

Winn-Dixie ()
Instant Potato Flakes

PREPARED MEALS & SIDES

Amy's Kitchen ⓘ ✓
Asian Noodle Stir-Fry
Baked Ziti Bowl
Black Bean & Vegetable Enchilada
Black Bean & Vegetable Enchilada -
  Light in Sodium
Black Bean Enchilada Whole Meal
Brown Rice & Vegetable Bowl
Brown Rice & Vegetables Bowl - Light
  in Sodium

Brown Rice with Black-Eyed Peas &
  Veggies Bowl
Cheese Enchilada
Cheese Enchilada Whole Meal
Garden Vegetable Lasagna
Indian Mattar Paneer
Indian Mattar Paneer - Light in Sodium
Indian Mattar Tofu
Indian Palak Paneer
Indian Paneer Tikka
Indian Vegetable Korma
Mexican Casserole Bowl
Mexican Casserole Bowl - Light in
  Sodium
Mexican Tamale Pie
Rice Macaroni & Cheese
Santa Fe Enchilada Bowl
Shepard's Pie
Teriyaki Bowl
Thai Stir-Fry
Tofu Rancheros
Tofu Scramble

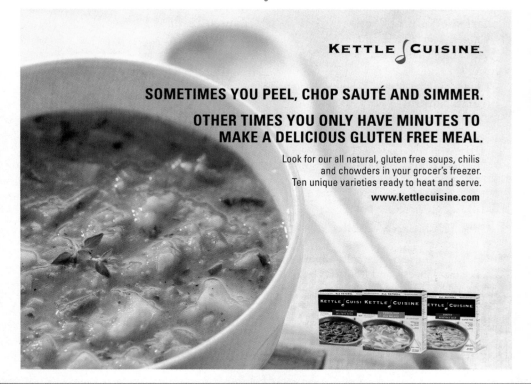

Applegate Farms
Natural Gluten-Free Chicken Nuggets

Bashas'
Frozen Vegetable Stew Mix

Bell & Evans ⓘ ✓
Chicken Wings - Buffalo
Chicken Wings - Honey BBQ
Gluten-Free Breaded Chicken Breasts
Gluten-Free Breaded Chicken Nuggets
Gluten-Free Breaded Chicken Patties
Gluten-Free Breaded Chicken Tenders
Gluten-Free Breaded Italian Chicken
    Patties
Gluten-Free Garlic Parmesan Breaded
    Chicken Breast
Grilled Chicken Breasts - Buffalo
Grilled Chicken Breasts - Honey BBQ
Grilled Chicken Breasts - Plain

Blue Horizon
Albacore Tuna Bites
Fish & Chip Bites
Gluten-Free Crab Cakes
Gluten-Free Fish Sticks
Salmon Cake Bites

CedarLane Natural Foods
Garden Vegetable Enchiladas
Three Layer Enchilada Pie

Chung's
Chung's For 2 - Sweet 'N Sour Chicken

Coleman Natural ⓘ
Gluten Free Chicken Breast Nuggets
Gourmet Chicken Meatballs - Buffalo
    Style ✓
Gourmet Chicken Meatballs - Chipotle
    Cheddar ✓
Gourmet Chicken Meatballs - Italian
    Parmesan ✓
Gourmet Chicken Meatballs - Pesto
    Parmesan ✓
Gourmet Chicken Meatballs - Spinach,
    Fontina Cheese, and Roasted Garlic ✓
Gourmet Chicken Meatballs - Sun-
    Dried Tomato Basil Provolone ✓

Coleman Organic ⓘ
Chicken Wings - Buffalo Style

Delimex ⓘ
3-Cheese Taquitos

Beef Grande Taquitos
Beef Tamales
Beef Taquitos
Chicken & Cheese Tamales
Chicken Grande Taquitos
Chicken Taquitos

Dr. Praeger's ✓
Broccoli Littles
Potato Crusted Fillet Fish Sticks
Potato Crusted Fish Fillets
Potato Crusted Fishies
Spinach Littles

Empire Kosher
Fully Cooked Barbecue Chicken -
    Frozen
Fully Cooked Barbecue Turkey - Frozen

Fast Fixin' ⓘ
Ham and Cheese Omelet On-the-Go
Southwest Style Omelet On-the-Go

Gluten Free Café ✓
Asian Noodles
Fettuccini Alfredo
Lemon Basil Chicken
Pasta Primavera

Glutenfreeda ⚇
Burritos (All)

Glutino
Chicken Penne Alfredo
Chicken Ranchero
Duo Cheese Pizza
Macaroni & Cheese
Pad Thai w/Chicken
Penne Alfredo
Pomodoro Chicken

Hans All Natural ⓘ
Gourmet Chicken Meatballs - Buffalo
    Style ✓
Gourmet Chicken Meatballs - Sweet
    Basil Parmesan ✓

Ian's Natural Foods
Wheat and Gluten-Free Recipe
    Alphatots
Wheat and Gluten-Free Recipe Chicken
    Finger Kids Meal
Wheat and Gluten-Free Recipe Chicken
    Nuggets

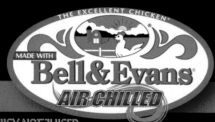
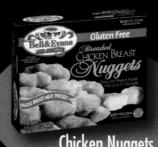
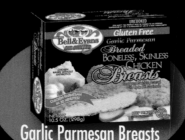
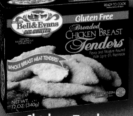
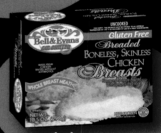
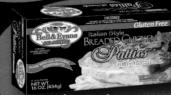
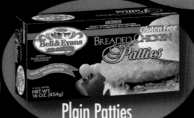

Wheat and Gluten-Free Recipe Chicken Patties

Wheat and Gluten-Free Recipe Chicken Tenders

Wheat and Gluten-Free Recipe Egg & Maple Cheddar Wafflewich

Wheat and Gluten-Free Recipe Fish Sticks

Wheat and Gluten-Free Recipe Lightly Battered Fish

Wheat and Gluten-Free Recipe Mac & Meat Sauce

Wheat and Gluten-Free Recipe Mac & NO Cheese

Wheat and Gluten-Free Recipe Maple Sausage and Egg Wafflewich

Wheat and Gluten-Free Recipe Popcorn Turkey Corn Dogs

John Soules Foods ⓘ

Fully Cooked Products (All)

Kettle Cuisine ✓

Angus Beef Steak Chili with Beans

Chicken Chili with White Beans

Chicken Soup with Rice Noodles

New England Clam Chowder

Organic Mushroom and Potato Soup

Roasted Vegetable Soup

Southwestern Chicken and Corn Chowder

Thai Curry Chicken Soup

Three Bean Chili

Tomato Soup with Garden Vegetables

Mama Lucia ⓘ

Fully Cooked Sausage Meatballs Made with Beef

Rosina ()

Rosina Sausage Meatballs

SeaPak

Shrimp Scampi

Smart Ones ⓘ

Chicken Santa Fe

Cranberry Turkey Medallions

Fiesta Chicken

Honey Dijon Chicken

Lemon Herb Chicken Piccata

Santa Fe Rice & Beans

Starfish ⚇ ✓

Gluten Free Battered Cod

Gluten Free Battered Haddock

Gluten Free Battered Halibut

Tabatchnick Fine Foods

Balsamic Tomato & Rice Soup

Black Bean Soup

Cabbage Soup

Corn Chowder

Cream of Broccoli Soup

Cream of Spinach Soup

Creamed Spinach

Lentil Soup

New England Potato Soup

No Salt Spilt Pea Soup

Old Fashioned Potato Soup

Southwest Bean Soup

Split Pea Soup

Vegetarian Chili

Wilderness Wild Rice Soup

Yankee Bean Soup

SHERBET & SORBET

Dreyer's

Berry Rainbow Sherbet

Orange Cream Sherbet

Tropical Rainbow Sherbet

Edy's

also see Dreyer's

Food Club (Marsh)

Sherbet Cherry Lemon

Sherbet Lime

Sherbet Orange

Sherbet Pineapple

Sherbet Rainbow

Sherbet Raspberry

Fresh & Easy ()

Blackberry Rum Sorbet

Lemon Sorbet

Mango Sorbet

Pine Orange Sorbet

Pome & Blueberry Sorbet

Gaga's SherBetter

SherBetter (All)

Gifford's Ice Cream

Orange

Rainbow

Red Raspberry

Häagen-Dazs

Chocolate Sorbet

Cranberry Blueberry Sorbet

Mango Sorbet

Orchard Peach Sorbet

Raspberry Sorbet

Snack Size Mini Cups - Mango Sorbet

Snack Size Mini Cups - Raspberry
Sorbet

Strawberry Sorbet

Zesty Lemon Sorbet

Haggen

Sherbet - Orange

Sherbet - Rainbow

Sherbet - Red Raspberry

Hood

New England Creamery - Black
Raspberry Sherbet

New England Creamery - Orange
Sherbet

New England Creamery - Rainbow
Sherbet

New England Creamery - Wildberry
Sherbet

Sherbet (All)

Hy-Vee

Lime Sherbet

Orange Sherbet

Pineapple Sherbet

Rainbow Sherbet

Raspberry Sherbet

Kroger ⓘ

Private Selection Sorbet

Private Selection Sorbetto

Lindy's Homemade ♜

Lindy's (All)

Meijer

Cherry Sherbert

Lime Sherbert

Orange Sherbert

Pineapple Sherbert

Rainbow Sherbert

Raspberry Sherbert

Oberweis Dairy

Lemon Sorbet

Mango Pomegranate Sorbet

Orange Sherbet

Raspberry Sherbet

Prairie Farms

Sherbet (All Flavors)

Private Selection Brand (Kroger) ⓘ

Sorbet

Sorbetto

Publix ()

Cool Lime Sherbet

Exotic Fruit Medley Sherbet

No Sugar Added Sunny Orange Sherbet

Peach Mango Passion Sherbet

Rainbow Dream Sherbet

Raspberry Blush Sherbet

Sunny Orange Sherbet

Tropic Pineapple Sherbet

Tropical Swirl Sherbet

Sambazon

Sambazon (All)

Talenti

Talenti (All BUT Caramel Cookie
Crunch Gelato)

Turkey Hill

Sherbet - Cherry Orchard

Sherbet - Fruit Rainbow

Sherbet - Orange Grove

Venice Ice - Lemon & Cherry

Venice Ice - Mango

Venice Ice - Peach Green Tea

Venice Ice - Pomegranate Blueberry &
Cream with Acai

Venice Ice - Pomegranate Lemonade

Venice Ice - Raspberry

Whole Fruit

Sorbet

VEGETABLES

Bashas'

Frozen Broccoli - Cut

Frozen Brussels Sprouts

Frozen Carrots - Crinkle Cut

Frozen Cauliflower Florets

Frozen Corn Cob

Frozen Corn Cob - Mini Ear

Frozen Corn Gold

Frozen Green Beans - Cut
Frozen Mixed Vegetables
Frozen Okra - Cut
Frozen Peas
Frozen Spinach - Chopped
Frozen Squash - Cooked

Central Market Classics (Price Chopper)

Butternut Squash
White Asparagus

Food Club (Marsh)

Frozen Broccoli Baby Florets
Frozen Broccoli Cuts
Frozen Brussel Sprouts
Frozen Carrots - Crinkle Cut
Frozen Carrots - Whole Baby
Frozen Cauliflower Florets
Frozen Chopped Broccoli
Frozen Corn - White, Super Sweet
Frozen Corn - Whole Kernel
Frozen Corn On Cob
Frozen Cut Green Beans
Frozen French Cut Green Beans
Frozen Green Peas
Frozen Green Peas - Petite
Frozen Mixed Vegetables
Frozen Onions - Diced
Frozen Peas & Carrots
Frozen Spinach - Chopped
Frozen Spinach - Cut Leaf
Frozen Steamin' Easy - Broccoli Cuts
Frozen Steamin' Easy - California Style
Frozen Steamin' Easy - Cut Green Beans
Frozen Steamin' Easy - Florentine
Frozen Steamin' Easy - French Cut Green Beans
Frozen Steamin' Easy - Peas & Carrots
Frozen Steamin'Easy - Green Peas
Frozen Steamin'Easy - Mixed Vegetables
Frozen Steamin'Easy - Whole Kernel Corn
Frozen Sugar Snap Peas
Frozen Vegetable Stir Fry
Frozen Vegetables - California Style
Frozen Vegetables - Florentine
Frozen Vegetables - Italian
Frozen Whole Green Beans

Fresh & Easy ()

Vegetables (Assorted Variety)

Grand Selections (Hy-Vee)

Caribbean Blend Vegetables
Normandy Blend Vegetables
Petite Green Peas
Petite Whole Carrots
Riviera Blend Vegetables
Sugar Snap Peas
Super Sweet Cut Corn
White Shoepeg Corn
Whole Green Beans

Great Value (Wal-Mart)

"Golden" Whole Kernel Corn Microwavable
Broccoli & Cauliflower
Broccoli Cuts
Broccoli Florets
Broccoli, Cauliflower, & Carrots
California Style Vegetable Mix
Cauliflower
Corn On The Cob
Cut Broccoli
Cut Corn On The Cob
Cut Green Beans
Cut Leaf Spinach
Extra Long, All Green Asparagus Spears
Golden Sweet Whole Kernel Corn No Salt Added Corn
Microwavable Diced Carrots
Microwaveable Sweet Peas
Mixed Vegetables
Seasoned Mixed Garden Medley
Vegetable Medley

Green Giant ✓

Valley Fresh Steamers - Broccoli Cuts
Valley Fresh Steamers - Chopped Broccoli
Valley Fresh Steamers - Cut Green Beans
Valley Fresh Steamers - Extra Sweet Niblets Corn
Valley Fresh Steamers - Mixed Vegetables
Valley Fresh Steamers - Niblets Corn
Valley Fresh Steamers - Select Baby Sweet Peas

Valley Fresh Steamers - Select Broccoli
Florets

Valley Fresh Steamers - Select Sugar
Snap Peas

Valley Fresh Steamers - Select White
Shoepeg Corn

Valley Fresh Steamers - Select Whole
Green Beans

Valley Fresh Steamers - Sweet Peas

Haggen

Broccoli Cuts
Broccoli Florets
Brussel Sprouts
Corn Petite White
Corn Whole Kernel
Country Trio Vegetables
Cut Green Beans
French Style Green Beans
Mixed Vegetables
Peas - Green Petite
Petite Peas & Carrots
Petite Whole Green Beans
Spinach - Chopped
Vegetable - California Style
Vegetable - Stir Fry
Vegetables - Fiesta Style
Vegetables Winter Mix

Hanover Foods ⓘ

Asparagus Spears
Blue Lake Cut Green Beans
Blue Lake French Green Beans
Blue Lake Whole Green Beans
Broccoli & Cauliflower Blend
Broccoli Cuts
Broccoli Florets
Broccoli Florets Petite
Broccoli, Water Chestnuts, Red Peppers,
Yellow Peppers
Brussel Sprouts Petite
California Blend
Carrots Sliced
Carrots Whole Baby
Cauliflower Clusters
Green Beans Cut
Green Beans Italian Cut
Green Beans Petite
Green Beans Whole

Green Peppers Diced
Oriental Blend
Peas - Petite
Peas - Snow
Peas - Sugar Snap
Peas - Sweet
Spinach Cut Leaf
White Sweet Corn
Whole Golden Beans

Hy-Vee

Baby Lima Beans
Broccoli Florets
Brussels Sprouts
California Mix
Cauliflower Florets
Chopped Broccoli
Chopped Spinach
Cream Style Golden Corn
Crinkle Cut Carrots
Cut Golden Corn
Cut Green Beans
Fiesta Blend
French Cut Green Beans
Italian Blend
Leaf Spinach
Mini Corn on the Cob
Mixed Vegetables
Oriental Vegetables
Sweet Peas
Winter Mix

Kroger ⓘ

Plain Frozen Vegetables

Meijer

Frozen Beans - Green Cut
Frozen Beans - Green French Cut
Frozen Beans - Green Italian Cut
Frozen Broccoli Chopped
Frozen Broccoli Cuts
Frozen Broccoli Spears
Frozen Brussels Sprouts
Frozen Carrots Crinkle Cut
Frozen Carrots Whole Baby
Frozen Cauliflower Florets
Frozen Chinese Pea Pods
Frozen Collards Chopped
Frozen Corn - Whole Kernel
Frozen Corn - Whole Kernel Golden

Frozen Corn Cob Mini Ear
Frozen Corn on Cob
Frozen Edamame (Soybeans)
Frozen Mixed Vegetables
Frozen Okra - Chopped
Frozen Okra - Whole
Frozen Onions - Chopped
Frozen Organic Green Peas
Frozen Organic Mixed Vegetables
Frozen Peas - Green
Frozen Peas - Green Petite
Frozen Peas & Carrots
Frozen Peppers - Green, Chopped
Frozen Spinach - Chopped
Frozen Spinach - Leaf
Frozen Squash - Cooked
Frozen Vegetables - California Style
Frozen Vegetables - Fiesta
Frozen Vegetables - Florentine
Frozen Vegetables - Italian
Frozen Vegetables - Mexican
Frozen Vegetables - Oriental
Frozen Vegetables - Parisian Style
Frozen Vegetables - Stew Mix
Frozen Vegetables - Stir Fry

Midwest Country Fare (Hy-Vee)
Broccoli Cuts
Brussels Sprouts
California Blend
Cauliflower
Chopped Broccoli
Cut Corn
Green Peas
Mixed Vegetables

Publix ()
Alpine Blend
Broccoli - Chopped
Broccoli - Cuts
Broccoli - Spears
Brussels Sprouts
California Blend
Carrots - Crinkle Cut
Carrots - Whole Baby
Cauliflower
Collard Greens, Chopped
Corn - Cut
Corn On The Cob

Del Oro Blend
Field Peas with Snap
Green Peppers - Diced
Gumbo Mix
Italian Blend
Japanese Blend
Mixed Vegetables
Okra - Cut
Okra - Whole Baby
Onions - Diced
Oriental Blend
Peas
Peas - Butter
Peas - Crowder
Peas - Green
Peas - Petite
Peas - Purple Hull
Peas and Carrots
Rhubarb
Roma Blend
Soup Mix with Tomatoes
Spinach - Chopped
Spinach - Cut Leaf
Spinach - Leaf
Squash - Cooked
Squash - Yellow Sliced
Succotash
Turnip Greens - Chopped
Turnip Greens with Diced Turnips

Seapoint Farms
Frozen Edamame (All)
Frozen Edamame Veggie Blends (All)

Stahlbush Island Farms ⓘ ✔
Stahlbush Island Farms (All)

Thrifty Maid (Winn-Dixie) ()
Mixed Vegetables

Valu Time (Marsh)
Frozen Beans Green Cut
Frozen Corn Whole Kernel
Frozen Juice Orange Concentrate
Frozen Mixed Vegetables
Frozen Peas Green

Winn-Dixie ()
Broccoli Cuts
Broccoli Florets
Broccoli Spears
Broccoli, Chopped

Brussels Sprouts
Carrots, Crinkle Cut
Carrots, Whole Baby
Cauliflower
Collard Greens, Chopped
Corn on the Cob, Mini
Corn on the Cob, Regular
Corn, White, Cut
Corn, Yellow, Cut
Green Beans, Cut
Green Beans, French Style Sliced
Green Beans, Italian
Green Beans, Whole
Green Peppers, Diced
Mixed Vegetables
Mustard Greens
Okra, Cut
Okra, Whole
Onions, Diced
Organic Corn, Yellow, Cut
Organic Green Beans, Cut
Organic Mixed Vegetables
Organic Peas, Green
Pearl Onions
Peas & Carrots
Peas, Butter
Peas, Crowder
Peas, Field with Snaps
Peas, Green
Peas, Petite Green
Spinach, Chopped
Spinach, Cut Leaf
Squash, Yellow
Steamable Broccoli, Cut
Steamable Corn, Yellow, Cut
Steamable Green Beans, Cut
Steamable Mixed Vegetables
Steamable Peas, Sweet Green
Succotash
Turnip Greens, Chopped
Turnip Greens, with Turnips

Vegetarian Meat

Quorn ()
Recipe Tenders
Turkey-Style Roast

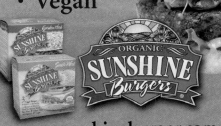
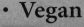
Veggie Burgers

Dr. Praeger's ✓
Gluten-Free California Veggie Burger
Sunshine Burger ♡ ✓
Barbecue Organic Sunshine Burger
Breakfast Organic Sunshine Burger
Falafel Organic Sunshine Burger
Garden Herb Organic Sunshine Burger
Original Natural Sunshine Burger
South West Organic Sunshine Burger

Waffles & French Toast

Ian's Natural Foods
Wheat and Gluten-Free Recipe French
Toast Sticks
Nature's Path ⓘ ✓
Buckwheat Wildberry Waffles
Homestyle Waffles
Mesa Sunrise Waffles

Van's Natural Foods

Wheat-Gluten Free Apple Cinnamon
Waffles
Wheat-Gluten Free Blueberry Waffles
Wheat-Gluten Free Buckwheat Waffles
Wheat-Gluten Free Flax Waffles
Wheat-Gluten Free Minis Totally
Natural Waffles
Wheat-Gluten Free Totally Natural
Waffles

WHIPPED TOPPINGS

Bashas'

Frozen Whipped Topping
Frozen Whipped Topping - Extra
Creamy
Frozen Whipped Topping - Fat Free
Frozen Whipped Topping - Lite

Cool Whip ↩

Free Whipped Topping
Regular Extra Creamy Whipped
Topping
Regular Original Twin Pack 16 Oz
Plastic Tubs Whipped Topping
Regular Original Whipped Topping
Sugar Free Whipped Topping
Whipped Topping Lite

Food Club (Marsh)

Frozen Whipped Topping
Frozen Whipped Topping - Extra
Creamy
Frozen Whipped Topping - Fat Free
Frozen Whipped Topping - Lite

Great Value (Wal-Mart)

Fat Free Whipped Topping
Light Whipped Topping
Whipped Topping

Hy-Vee

Extra Creamy Whipped Topping
Fat Free Whipped Topping
Lite Whipped Topping
Whipped Topping

Meijer

Frozen Whipped Topping
Frozen Whipped Topping Fat Free
Frozen Whipped Topping Lite

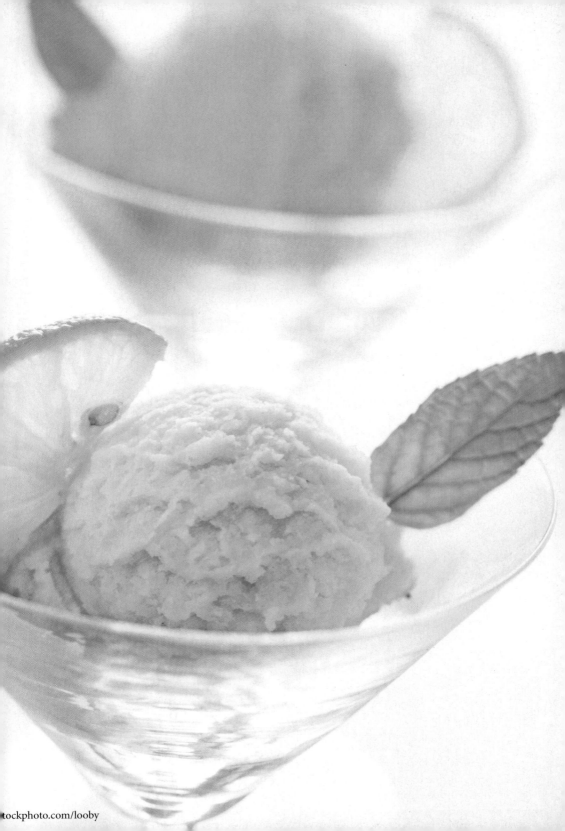

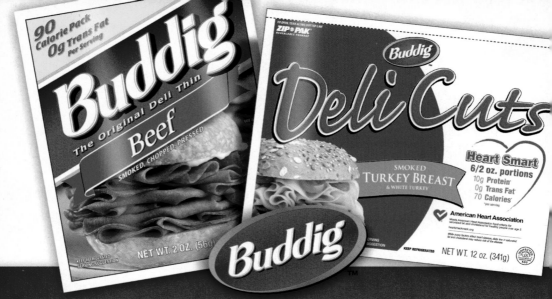

Free of Gluten. Full of Flavor

Go gluten free with Buddig and Old Wisconsin® Buddig Original and Deli Cuts are great-tasting, naturally high in protein and low in fat. Deli Cuts have recently been certified by the American Heart Association® to display their heart-check mark, making them an even better way to help you control your diet. Old Wisconsin products offer a wide range of hardwood-smoked beef and turkey meat snacks to fit your lifestyle. Enjoy naturally gluten free lunchmeat and snacks with the Buddig and Old Wisconsin family of products.

Visit *buddig.com* and *oldwisconsin.com* to learn more or visit your local grocery retailer.

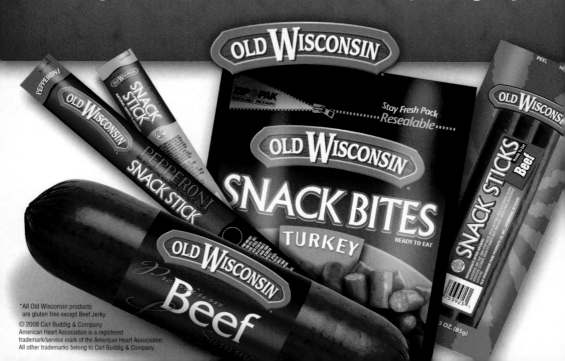

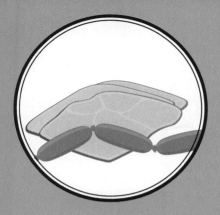

MEAT

BACON

Bashas'
  Bacon - Center Cut Sliced
  Bacon - Sliced
  Bacon - Thick Sliced
Beeler's ⚇
  Beeler's (All)
Boar's Head
  Meats (All)
Coleman Natural ⓘ
  Uncured Hickory Smoked Bacon
Farmer John ⓘ
  Bacon - Center Cut
  Bacon - Dry Salt Pork
  Bacon - Ends and Pieces
  Bacon - Maple Ends & Pieces
  Bacon - Old Fashioned Maple Table
    Brand
  Bacon - Premium Applewood
  Bacon - Premium Cracked Peppercorn
  Bacon - Premium Low Sodium
  Bacon - Premium Old Fashioned Maple
  Bacon - Premium Regular Smoked
  Bacon - Premium Thick Sliced
  Bacon - Quick Serve Fully Cooked
  Bacon - Table Brand
  Bacon - Thick Smoked
Great Value (Wal-Mart)
  Hickory Fully Cooked Bacon
  Hickory Smoked Bacon
  Lower Sodium Bacon
  Peppered Bacon
Haggen
  L Board Regular Bacon

Thick L Board Bacon
Hormel ⓘ
  Black Label - Bacon
  Canadian Style Bacon
  Fully Cooked Bacon
  Microwave Bacon
  Natural Choice - Canadian Bacon
  Natural Choice - Uncured Bacon
Hy-Vee
  Fully Cooked Turkey Bacon
  Hickory Smoked Fully Cooked Bacon
  Turkey Bacon
Jennie-O Turkey Store ⓘ
  Extra Lean Turkey Bacon
  Regular Turkey Bacon
Jones Dairy Farm
  Slab Bacon
  Sliced Bacon, Regular
  Sliced Bacon, Thick
Kroger ⓘ
  Bacon - Plain
Kunzler
  Kunzler & Authentic Select Brand
    Bacon (All Types)
Meijer
  Bacon
  Bacon Lower Sodium
Organic Prairie
  Hardwood Smoked Bacon
  Hardwood Smoked Turkey Bacon
  Sliced Canadian Bacon
Oscar Mayer ✍
  Bacon
  Center Cut Bacon
  Center Cut Naturally Smoked Bacon

Center Cut Smokehouse Thick Sliced
Bacon
Lower Sodium Bacon
Natural Smoked Uncured Bacon
Ready To Serve Canadian Bacon Fully
Cooked Bacon
Ready To Serve Hearty Thick Cut Bacon
Real Bacon Bits
Smoked Cured 55% Less Fat Turkey
Bacon

Plumrose
Plumrose (All)

Publix ()
Bacon (All Varieties)

Range Brand (i)
Bacon

Smith's
Smith's (All)

Sugardale (i)
Low Salt Bacon
Peppered Bacon
Peppered Ready Bacon
Ready Bacon
Regular Sliced Bacon
Thick Sliced Bacon
Thin Sliced Bacon

Superior's (i)
Low Salt Bacon
Regular Sliced Bacon
Thick Sliced Bacon
Thin Sliced Bacon

Thumann's ✓
Meat (All BUT Deep Fry Hot Dogs)

Valu Time (Marsh)
Tux Bacon

Winn-Dixie ()
Hickory Sweet Lower Sodium Bacon
Hickory Sweet Sliced Bacon
Hickory Sweet Thick Sliced Bacon
Hickory Sweet Thin Sliced Bacon

BEEF

Always Tender (i)
Flavored Fresh Beef Peppercorn
Non-Flavored Fresh Beef

Beeler's 😋
Beeler's (All)

Boar's Head
Meats (All)

Buddig 😋
Buddig Original - Beef
Buddig Original - Corned Beef
Buddig Original - Pastrami
Deli Cuts - Pastrami
Deli Cuts - Roast Beef

Columbus Salame
Deli Meats (All)

Extra Value
Extra Value (All)

Fast Classics (i)
Bacon Cheeseburger
Beef Burger
Black Angus Burger
Cheese Burger
Vidalia Onion Burger

Food Club (Marsh)
Corned Beef Hash

Fresh & Easy ()
Luncheon Meat Tub - Roast Beef

Great Value (Wal-Mart)
100% Pure Beef Patties (75/25)
100% Pure Beef Patties (80/20)
100% Pure Beef Patties (85/15)
Beef Philly Steak
Thinly Sliced Seasoned Roast Beef

Hebrew National ()
Hebrew National (All BUT Hebrew
National Beef Franks in a Blanket)

Hormel (i)
Beef Tamales
Natural Choice - Roast Beef

Hy-Vee
Deli Thin Sliced Roast Beef
Quarter Pounders
Thin Sliced Beef
Thin Sliced Corned Beef
Thin Sliced Pastrami

Kunzler
Roast Beef Presliced
Roast Beef Whole

Land O'Frost
Lunchmeats (All BUT Taste Escapes Lemon Pepper Chicken)

Meijer
Corned Beef Sliced Chipped
Ground Beef Chuck Fine
Ground Beef Fine
Pastrami Sliced Chipped Meat

Old Neighborhood
Old Neighborhood (All)

Organic Prairie
Sliced Roast Beef

Oscar Mayer ᕗ
Deli Fresh Meats - Roast Beef Slow Roasted Shaved
Deli Fresh Meats - Shaved French Dip 7 Oz. Tray
Slow Roasted 96% Fat Free Roast Beef

Plumrose
Plumrose (All)

Publix ()
Beef Bottom Round Roast (Pre-Packed Sliced Deli Lunch Meats)
Corned Beef (Pre-Packed Sliced Deli Lunch Meats)
GreenWise Market Beef Back Ribs
GreenWise Market Beef Cubed Steak
GreenWise Market Beef for Stew
GreenWise Market Bottom Round
GreenWise Market Bottom Round Steak
GreenWise Market Brisket Flat
GreenWise Market Chuck Eye Steak
GreenWise Market Chuck Roast, Boneless
GreenWise Market Chuck Short Ribs
GreenWise Market Chuck Short Ribs, Boneless
GreenWise Market Chuck Steak, Boneless
GreenWise Market Eye Round
GreenWise Market Eye Round Steak
GreenWise Market Flank Steak
GreenWise Market Flap Meat
GreenWise Market Flat Iron Steak
GreenWise Market Ground Chuck
GreenWise Market Ground Chuck for Chili

GreenWise Market Ground Chuck Patties
GreenWise Market Ground Round
GreenWise Market Ground Round Patties
GreenWise Market Inside Skirt Steak
GreenWise Market Outside Skirt Steak
GreenWise Market Porterhouse Steak
GreenWise Market Rib Eye Roast, Boneless
GreenWise Market Rib Eye Steak, Bone-In
GreenWise Market Rib Eye Steak, Boneless
GreenWise Market Rib Roast
GreenWise Market Round Cubes
GreenWise Market Rump Roast
GreenWise Market Shoulder Roast, Boneless
GreenWise Market Shoulder Steak
GreenWise Market Sirloin Flap Meat
GreenWise Market Sirloin for Kabobs
GreenWise Market Sirloin for Stir Fry
GreenWise Market Sirloin Tip Roast
GreenWise Market Sirloin Tip Side Steak
GreenWise Market Sirloin Tip Steak
GreenWise Market Strip Steak Boneless
GreenWise Market T-Bone Steak
GreenWise Market Tenderloin Roast
GreenWise Market Tenderloin Steak
GreenWise Market Top Blade Roast, Boneless
GreenWise Market Top Blade Steak
GreenWise Market Top Round
GreenWise Market Top Round for Stir Fry
GreenWise Market Top Round London Broil
GreenWise Market Top Round Steak
GreenWise Market Top Round Steak, Thin Sliced
GreenWise Market Top Sirloin Filet Steak
GreenWise Market Top Sirloin Steak, Boneless
GreenWise Market Tri Tip Roast
GreenWise Market Tri Tip Steaks

Peppered Beef (Pre-Packed Sliced Deli Lunch Meats)

Premium Certified Beef

Redi-Serve ⓘ ✓

Beef Burgers

Rib Quik

Saag's

Saag's (All BUT British Bangers)

Sabrett

Hamburgers

Sausages by Amylu

Burgers by Amylu (All BUT Chicken Chorizo Sausage and Chicken Wieners)

Meatballs by Amylu (All BUT Chicken Chorizo Sausage and Chicken Wieners)

Shady Brook Farms

Shady Brook Farms (All BUT Beer Smoked Turkey Bratwurst Fully Cooked, Italian Style Meatballs, Appetizer Sized Meatballs, Cajun Fried Turkey, and Teriyaki Turkey Breast Tenderloins)

Smith's

Smith's (All)

Thin 'n Trim

Thin 'n Trim (All)

Thumann's ✓

Meat (All BUT Deep Fry Hot Dogs)

Bologna

Boar's Head

Meats (All)

Empire Kosher

Chicken Bologna - Slices

Turkey Bologna - Slices

Turkey Bologna Roll

Farmer John ⓘ

Lunch Meats - Bologna

Hebrew National ⟨⟩

Hebrew National (All BUT Hebrew National Beef Franks in a Blanket)

Hy-Vee

Beef Bologna

Bologna

Garlic Bologna

German Brand Bologna

Thick Bologna

Thin Bologna

Turkey Bologna

Johnsonville

Johnsonville (All BUT Cooked Beer Brats and Beer n' Bratwurst)

Kunzler

Bologna - All Beef

Bologna - Regular

Garlic Ring Bologna

German Bologna

Lancaster County Brand Bologna

Non-Garlic Ring Bologna

Old Fashion Bologna

Plain Ring Bologna

Midwest Country Fare (Hy-Vee)

Sliced Bologna

Thick Sliced Bologna

Old Neighborhood

Old Neighborhood (All)

Old Wisconsin ⓘ

Ring Bologna

Oscar Mayer ⌐

98% Fat Free Bologna

Beef Bologna

Beef Light Bologna

Bologna Made with Chicken & Pork

Bologna/Chopped Ham & White Smoked Turkey Variety Pack

Light Bologna

Lower Fat Turkey Bologna

Turkey Lower Fat Bologna

Perdue

Deli Turkey Bologna

Publix ⟨⟩

Beef Bologna (Pre-Packed Sliced Deli Lunch Meats)

German Bologna (Pre-Packed Sliced Deli Lunch Meats)

Saag's

Saag's (All BUT British Bangers)

Smith's

Smith's (All)

Sugardale ⓘ
- Beef Bologna
- Bologna
- Cleveland Bologna
- Emberdale Chunk Bologna
- Garlic Bologna
- Leona Bologna
- Thick Bologna

Superior's ⓘ
- Beef Bologna
- Bologna
- Cleveland Bologna
- Garlic Bologna
- German Bologna
- Leona Bologna
- Thick Sliced Bologna

Thumann's ✓
- Meat (All BUT Deep Fry Hot Dogs)

CHICKEN

Allen Family Foods, Inc.
- Allen Family Foods, Inc. (All)

Bell & Evans ⓘ ✓
- Fresh Chicken (All)

Boar's Head
- Meats (All)

Buddig ⚉
- Buddig Original - Chicken
- Deli Cuts - Rotisserie Chicken
- Fix Quix - Chicken

Coleman Natural ⓘ
- Bone-in Skin-on Chicken Thigh
- Boneless Skinless Chicken Breast
- Boneless Skinless Chicken Thigh
- Drummettes
- Drumsticks
- Fresh for the Freezer Chicken
- Split Breast
- Whole Chicken
- Wings

Coleman Organic ⓘ
- Bone-in Skin-on Chicken Thigh
- Boneless Skinless Chicken Breast
- Boneless Skinless Chicken Thigh
- Chicken Breast Tenders
- Drummettes

- Drumsticks
- Fresh for the Freezer Chicken
- Split Breast
- Whole Chicken
- Wings

Empire Kosher
- Fresh Chill Pack Chicken & Turkey
- Fresh Rotisserie Chicken

Fast Classics ⓘ
- Boneless Wingz
- Buffalo Wings
- Flame Roasted Chicken Breast
- Honey BBQ Chicken Wings

Fast Fixin' ⓘ
- Chicken Breast Mesquite
- Grilled Chicken Breast

FreeBird
- Chicken Products (All)

Great Value (Wal-Mart)
- 100% Natural Boneless Skinless Chicken Breasts
- Boneless Skinless Chicken Breast Fillets
- Chicken Drumsticks
- Chicken Thighs
- Chicken Wing Drumettes
- Chicken Wing Sections

Hormel ⓘ
- Natural Choice - Grilled Chicken Strips
- Natural Choice - Oven Roasted Chicken Strips

Hy-Vee
- 100% Natural Fresh Boneless Skinless Chicken
- 100% Natural Fresh Chicken Breast Tenderloins
- 100% Natural Fresh Chicken Drumsticks
- 100% Natural Fresh Chicken For Roasting with Neck & Giblets
- 100% Natural Fresh Chicken Gizzards
- 100% Natural Fresh Chicken Leg Quarters
- 100% Natural Fresh Chicken Split Breasts with Ribs
- 100% Natural Fresh Chicken Thighs
- 100% Natural Fresh Chicken Wing Drummettes

100% Natural Fresh Chicken Wings

100% Natural Fresh Skinless Chicken
Split Breasts

100% Natural Fresh Whole Cut Up
Chicken with Neck & Giblets

100% Natural Fresh Young Chicken with
Neck & Giblets

100% Natural Pick of the Chick Fresh
Chicken

Boneless Skinless Chicken Thighs
Flavored For Fajitas

Herb Garlic Flavored Chicken Breasts
with Rib Meat

Lemon Butter Flavored Chicken Breasts
with Rib Meat

Thin Sliced Chicken

Jennie-O Turkey Store ⓘ

Deli Chicken Breast - Buffalo Style

Deli Chicken Breast - Mesquite Smoked

Deli Chicken Breast - Oven Roasted

Kroger ⓘ

Fresh Plain Chicken Breast

Fresh Plain Chicken Thighs

Fresh Plain Chicken Wings

Land O' Frost

Lunchmeats (All BUT Taste Escapes
Lemon Pepper Chicken)

Meijer

Chicken Slice Chipped Meat

Organic Prairie

Sliced Roast Chicken Breast

Oscar Mayer ⌇

Chicken White Oven Roasted

Deli Fresh Cold Cuts Rotisserie
Seasoned Shaved 98% Fat Free Family
Size

Deli Fresh Meats - Chicken Breast
Rotisserie Style Shaved

Deli Fresh Meats - Shaved Cajun
Seasoned 8 Oz. Tray

Deli Fresh Shaved/Sliced Barbecue
Seasoned

Deli Fresh Singles Chicken Breast Oven
Roasted Shaved 2 Pack

Homestyle Oven Roasted White
Chicken

Perdue

Buffalo Style Jumbo Chicken Wings

Carving - Chicken Breast, Oven Roasted

Grilled Chicken Breast Strips - All
Natural

Ground Breast of Chicken

Ground Chicken

Ground Chicken Burgers

Honey BBQ Jumbo Chicken Wings

Hot & Spicy Jumbo Chicken Wings

Perfect Portions Boneless Skinless
Chicken Breasts - All Natural

Perfect Portions Boneless Skinless
Chicken Breasts - Herb & Pepper

Perfect Portions Boneless Skinless
Chicken Breasts - Italian Style

Perfect Portions Boneless Skinless
Chicken Breasts - Roasted Garlic with
White Wine

Rotisserie Chicken - Barbecue

Rotisserie Chicken - Chesapeake
Seasoned

Rotisserie Chicken - Italian

Rotisserie Chicken - Lemon Pepper

Rotisserie Chicken - Oven Roasted

Rotisserie Chicken - Smokey
Peppercorn

Rotisserie Chicken - Toasted Garlic

Rotisserie Chicken - Tuscany Herb
Roasted

Rotisserie Oven Stuffer Roaster

Rotisserie Oven Stuffer Roaster Breast

Sauce N Toss Buffalo Style Chicken
Wings

Sauce N Toss Honey BBQ Chicken
Wings

Seasoned Oven Ready Cornish Hens

Seasoned Oven Ready Roaster

Seasoned Oven Ready Roaster Bone-In
Breast

Short Cuts Carved Chicken Breast -
Grilled Southwestern Style

Short Cuts Carved Chicken Breast -
Honey Roasted

Short Cuts Carved Chicken Breast -
Original Roasted

Short Cuts Carved Chicken Breasted
Roasted Garlic with White Wine

Sliced Chicken Breast - Oil Fried Tender & Tasty Products

Pilgrim's Pride
Buffalo Wings - Fully Cooked
Marinated Italian Chicken Breasts - Chill Pack in a Tray
Marinated Lemon-Pepper Chicken Breasts - Chill pack in a Tray

Publix ()
All Natural Fresh Chicken
GreenWise Market Boneless Chicken Breast
GreenWise Market Boneless Chicken Thighs
GreenWise Market Chicken Cutlet
GreenWise Market Chicken Drummettes
GreenWise Market Chicken Drumsticks
GreenWise Market Chicken Fillet
GreenWise Market Chicken Sausage, Herb and Tomato
GreenWise Market Chicken Sausage, Hot Italian
GreenWise Market Chicken Sausage, Mild Italian
GreenWise Market Chicken Tenderloin
GreenWise Market Chicken Thighs
GreenWise Market Chicken Wings
GreenWise Market Ground Chicken
GreenWise Market Skinless Chicken Drumsticks
GreenWise Market Skinless Chicken Thighs
GreenWise Market Split Chicken Breast
GreenWise Market Whole Chicken

Rocky Jr. ⓘ
Bone-In Skin-On Chicken Thigh
Boneless Skinless Chicken Breast
Boneless Skinless Chicken Thigh
Chicken Breast Tenders
Drummettes
Drumsticks
Split Breast
Whole Chicken
Wings

Rocky the Range ⓘ
Whole Chicken

Rosie Organic ⓘ
Bone-In Skin-On Chicken
Boneless Skinless Chicken Breast
Boneless Skinless Chicken Thigh
Chicken Breast Tenders
Drummettes
Drumsticks
Split Breast
Whole Chicken
Wings

Sanderson Farms
Sanderson Farms (All)

Shady Brook Farms
Shady Brook Farms (All BUT Beer Smoked Turkey Bratwurst Fully Cooked, Italian Style Meatballs, Appetizer Sized Meatballs, Cajun Fried Turkey, and Teriyaki Turkey Breast Tenderloins)

Thin 'n Trim
Thin 'n Trim (All)

Thumann's ✓
Meat (All BUT Deep Fry Hot Dogs)

HAM & PROSCIUTTO

Bashas'
Ham Cooked 4X6 95% Fat Free
Honey Ham 96% Fat Free
Luncheon Meat with Ham

Beeler's ⸚
Beeler's (All)

Bilinski Sausage ⸚
Bilinski Sausage (All)

Boar's Head
Meats (All)

Buddig ⸚
Buddig Original - Brown Sugar Ham
Buddig Original - Ham
Buddig Original - Honey Ham
Deli Cuts - Baked Honey Ham
Deli Cuts - Brown Sugar Baked Ham
Deli Cuts - Smoked Ham
Fix Quix - Smoked Ham

Columbus Salame
Deli Meats (All)

Cure 81 ⓘ
Ham

Farmer John ⓘ
Bone-In Ham - Premium Butt and
    Shank Portions
Bone-In Ham - Premium Gold Wrap
Bone-In Ham - Premium Half
Bone-In Ham - Premium Sliced Ham
    Steaks
Bone-In Ham - Premium Spiral Sliced
Bone-In Ham - Premium Spiral Sliced
    Half
Bone-In Ham - Whole
Boneless Ham - Canless Honey Ham
Boneless Ham - Flat Tavern Half
Boneless Ham - Golden Tradition
Boneless Ham - Golden Tradition
    Premium Black Forest
Boneless Ham - Golden Tradition
    Premium Brown Sugar and Honey
Boneless Ham - Golden Tradition
    Premium Original Whole and Half
Boneless Ham - Pee Wee Half
Ham Steaks - Clove
Ham Steaks - Maple
Ham Steaks - Original
Ham Steaks - Pineapple & Mango
Ham Steaks - Smoked
Lunch Meats - Black Forest Ham
Lunch Meats - Brown Sugar & Honey
    Ham
Lunch Meats - Chopped Ham
Lunch Meats - Ham Roll
Lunch Meats - Sliced Cooked Ham

Fresh & Easy ⟨⟩
Luncheon Meat Tub - Ham

Great Value (Wal-Mart)
97% Fat Free Baked Ham
97% Fat Free Cooked Ham
97% Fat Free Honey Ham
Sliced Chopped Ham
Sliced Turkey Ham
Thinly Sliced Smoked Ham
Thinly Sliced Smoked Honey Ham

Hormel ⓘ
Black Label - Chopped Ham
Diced Ham

Ham Patties
Julienne Ham
Natural Choice - Cooked Deli Ham
Natural Choice - Honey Deli Ham
Natural Choice - Smoked Deli Ham

Hy-Vee
96% Fat Free Cubed Cooked Ham
96% Fat Free Diced Cooked Ham
96% Sliced Cooked Ham
Brown Sugar Spiral Sliced Ham
Chopped Ham
Cooked Ham
Deli Thin Sliced Brown Sugar Ham
Deli Thin Slices - Honey Ham
Deli Thin Slices - Smoked Ham
Ham & Cheese Loaf
Honey & Spice Spiral Sliced Ham
Thin Sliced Ham with Natural Juices
Thin Sliced Honey Ham with Natural
    Juices

Jones Dairy Farm
Canadian Bacon Slices
Deli-Style Honey & Brown Sugar Cured
    Ham Slices
Ham Slices
Ham Steaks
Whole Hams

Kunzler
Kunzler Brand Hams (All Types)

Land O'Frost
Lunchmeats (All BUT Taste Escapes
    Lemon Pepper Chicken)

Meijer
Double Smoked Ham
Honey Ham - 97% Fat Free
Honey Roasted Ham
Sliced Cooked Ham - 97% Fat Free

Old Neighborhood
Old Neighborhood (All)

Organic Prairie
Sliced Hardwood Smoked Ham
Spiral Sliced Ham

Oscar Mayer ⌒
Baked Cooked 96% Fat Free Ham
Boiled 96% Fat Free Ham
Chopped Ham

Deli Fresh Meats - Black Forest Shaved 9 Oz. Tray

Deli Fresh Meats - Brown Sugar Thin Sliced

Deli Fresh Meats - Cooked 96% Fat Free

Deli Fresh Meats - Ham Brown Sugar Shaved

Deli Fresh Meats - Ham Honey Shaved

Deli Fresh Meats - Ham Smoked Shaved

Deli Fresh Meats - Ham Virginia Brand Shaved

Deli Fresh Meats - Honey 96% Fat Free

Deli Fresh Meats - Smoked 96% Fat Free

Deli Fresh Singles Ham Home-Style Roasted Shaved 2 Pack

Deli Fresh Singles Ham Honey Smoked Shaved 2 Pack

Fat Free Ham & Turkey Variety Pack

Ham Honey 96% Fat Free Ham

Ham/Turkey Breast/Canadian Style Bacon Variety Pack

Honey 96% Fat Free Ham

Honey Chopped Ham

Honey Thin Sliced Ham

Natural Smoked Ham

Smoked 96% Fat Free Ham

Smoked 98% Fat Free Ham

Turkey Ham

Perdue

Carving - Turkey Ham, Honey Smoked

Deli Pick Ups - Sliced Turkey Ham, Honey Smoked

Deli Turkey Ham - Hickory Smoked

Slicing - Turkey Ham

Plumrose

Plumrose (All)

Publix ()

Cooked Ham (Pre-Packed Sliced Deli Lunch Meats)

Extra Thin Sliced Honey Ham (Pre-Packed Sliced Deli Lunch Meats)

Hickory Smoked Ham, Semi-Boneless, Fully Cooked

Honey Cured Bone-In Ham - Brown Sugar Glazed

Honey Cured Bone-In Ham - with Brown Sugar Glaze Mix Packet

Honey Cured Boneless Ham - with Brown Sugar Glaze

Honey Kut Ham (Pre-Packed Sliced Deli Lunch Meats)

Low Salt Ham (Pre-Packed Sliced Deli Lunch Meats)

Sweet Ham (Pre-Packed Sliced Deli Lunch Meats)

Tavern Ham (Pre-Packed Sliced Deli Lunch Meats)

Virginia Brand Ham (Pre-Packed Sliced Deli Lunch Meats)

Saag's

Saag's (All BUT British Bangers)

Smith's

Smith's (All)

Sugardale ⓘ

Boneless Ham (Whole or Half)

Chopped Ham

Cooked Ham

Cooked Honey Ham

Country Inn Boneless Ham

Country Inn Ham Slices

Half Boneless Petite Spiral Sliced Honey Ham

Prestige Bone-In Ham Steaks

Prestige Portions Ham

Quarter Boneless Spiral Sliced Honey Ham

Semi-Boneless Ham (Whole or Half)

Signature Ham (Whole or Half)

Skinless Shankless Whole Ham

Spiral Sliced Half Ham

Ultra Thin Sliced Deli Meat - Ham

Virginia Classic Ham (Whole or Half)

Superior's ⓘ

Deluxe Semi-Boneless Whole Ham

Easy Carve Boneless Ham (Whole, Half, Quarter, or Sliced)

Prestige Old Fashioned Cooked Ham

Prestige Whole Ham

Semi-Boneless Half Ham

Tavern Boneless Hams (Whole, Half, or Quarter)

Tavern Ham Slices

Village Tavern Ham - Bavarian

Village Tavern Ham - Brown Sugar

Village Tavern Ham - Cajun
Village Tavern Ham - Honey
Village Tavern Honey Half Ham

Thin 'n Trim
Thin 'n Trim (All)

Thumann's ✓
Meat (All BUT Deep Fry Hot Dogs)

HOT DOGS & FRANKS

Beeler's �️
Beeler's (All)

Bilinski Sausage �️
Bilinski Sausage (All)

Boar's Head
Meats (All)

Coleman Natural ⓘ
Beef Hot Dog
Beef-Pork Frank

Empire Kosher
Turkey Franks

Farmer John ⓘ
Franks and Wieners - Dodger Dogs
Franks and Wieners - Premium Beef
  Franks
Franks and Wieners - Premium Jumbo
  Beef Franks
Franks and Wieners - Premium Jumbo
  Meat Wieners
Franks and Wieners - Premium Meat
  Wieners
Franks and Wieners - Premium Quarter
  Pounder Beef Franks

Haggen
Franks - Beef

Hebrew National ()
Hebrew National (All BUT Hebrew
  National Beef Franks in a Blanket)

Honeysuckle White
Honeysuckle White (All BUT Beer
  Smoked Turkey Bratwurst Fully
  Cooked, Italian Style Meatballs, Cajun
  Fried Turkey, and Teriyaki Turkey
  Breast Tenderloins)

Hormel ⓘ
Beef Franks

Jennie-O Turkey Store ⓘ
Turkey Franks

Johnsonville
Johnsonville (All BUT Cooked Beer
  Brats and Beer n' Bratwurst)

Kunzler
Beef Franks
Chicken Franks
Grill Franks
Meat Franks
Turkey Franks

Midwest Country Fare (Hy-Vee)
Bun Length Hot Dogs
Cheezy Jumbo Hot Dogs
Hot Dogs
Jumbo Hot Dogs

Old Neighborhood
Old Neighborhood (All)

Old Wisconsin ⓘ
Natural Casing Wieners

Organic Prairie
Beef Hot Dogs
Chicken Hot Dogs
Classic Hot Dogs
Turkey Hot Dogs

Oscar Mayer ᴼ
30 Ct Wieners
98% Fat Free 8 Ct Made with Turkey
  Wieners
Beef Light 10 Ct Franks
Beef Xxl Premium Hot Dogs
Classic 10 Ct Turkey Hot Dogs
Classic Beef 10 Ct Franks
Classic Bun - Length 8 Ct Beef Franks
Classic Bun - Length 8 Ct Turkey Hot
  Dogs
Classic Bun - Length 8 Ct Wieners
Classic Cheese 10 Ct Turkey Hot Dogs
Classic Light Made with Turkey & Pork
  10 Ct Wieners
Classic Made with Turkey & Chicken/
  Pork 10 Ct Cheese Dogs
Classic Made with Turkey & Chicken/
  Pork 10 Ct Wieners
Premium Beef & Cheddar Franks
Premium Jalapeno & Cheddar Franks
Selects Premium 8 Ct Wieners

Selects Premium Beef 8 Ct Beef Franks
Turkey 30 Ct Hot Dogs

Publix ()
Beef Franks
Beef Hot Dogs
Meat Franks
Meat Hot Dogs

Rocky Dogs ⓘ
Chicken Hot Dogs

Saag's
Saag's (All BUT British Bangers)

Sabrett
All Beef Frankfurters
Pork & Beef Frankfurters

Smith's
Smith's (All)

Sugardale ⓘ
Beef Wieners
Bunfull Coneys
Bunfull Hot Dogs
Coney Longs
Coneys
Hot Dogs
Jumbo Beef Wieners
Jumbo Coneys
New York Brand Beef Wieners

Superior's ⓘ
Beef Frankies
Big As Bunz Hot Dogs
Frankies
Hot Dogs
Jumbo Frankies

Thumann's ✓
Meat (All BUT Deep Fry Hot Dogs)

Meat Alternatives

LightLife ()
Tofu Pups

Pepperoni

Boar's Head
Meats (All)

Haggen
Pillow Pack Pepperoni

Hormel ⓘ
Pepperoni
Turkey Pepperoni

Hy-Vee
Pepperoni

Organic Prairie
Sliced Beef Pepperoni
Sliced Pork Pepperoni

Sugardale ⓘ
Link Pepperoni
Pepperoni
Sandwich Pepperoni
Stick Pepperoni

Thumann's ✓
Meat (All BUT Deep Fry Hot Dogs)

Pork

Always Tender ⓘ
Flavored Fresh Pork - Bourbon Maple
Flavored Fresh Pork - Brown Sugar
  Maple
Flavored Fresh Pork - Citrus
Flavored Fresh Pork - Lemon-Garlic
Flavored Fresh Pork - Mediterranean &
  Olive Oil
Flavored Fresh Pork - Onion-Garlic
Flavored Fresh Pork - Original
Flavored Fresh Pork - Portabella
  Mushroom
Flavored Fresh Pork - Roast Flavor
Flavored Fresh Pork - Sun-Dried
  Tomato
Non-Flavored Fresh Pork

Beeler's ⚇
Beeler's (All)

Coleman Natural ⓘ
Hampshire Pork Baby Back Ribs
Hampshire Pork Chops
Hampshire Pork Loin
Hampshire Pork St. Louis Ribs
Hampshire Pork Tenderloins

Columbus Salame
Deli Meats (All)

Farmer John ⓘ
California Natural - Back Ribs
California Natural - Bone-In Butt Roast

California Natural - Bone-In Pork Loin
California Natural - Bone-In Pork Picnic
California Natural - Boneless Loin
California Natural - Boneless Pork Butt
California Natural - Boneless Pork
  Picnic
California Natural - Boneless Pork
  Shoulder
California Natural - Boneless Pork
  Sirloin
California Natural - Case Ready Pork
  Chops
California Natural - Ground Pork
California Natural - Pork Cushion
California Natural - Spareribs
California Natural - St. Louis Style
  Spareribs
California Natural - Tenderloins
Carefree Cookin' Pork - Boneless Leg
Carefree Cookin' Pork - Boneless Pork
  Loin
Carefree Cookin' Pork - Boneless Sirloin
Carefree Cookin' Pork - Picnics
Carefree Cookin' Pork - Pork Butt
Carefree Cookin' Pork - Pork Cushion
Carefree Cookin' Pork - Riblets
Carefree Cookin' Pork - Ribs
Carefree Cookin' Pork - Spareribs
Carefree Cookin' Pork - St. Louis Style
  Spareribs
Carefree Cookin' Pork - Tenderloins
Lunch Meats - Headcheese
Lunch Meats - Mission Loaf

Fast Fixin' ⓘ
Ribz for Sandwiches

Hormel ⓘ
Pickled Pigs Feet, Hocks & Tidbits

Hy-Vee
Pickle Loaf

Kunzler
BBQ Loaf
Dutch Loaf
Old Fashion Loaf
Olive Loaf
P & P Loaf
Pepper Loaf
Pork BBQ

Midwest Country Fare (Hy-Vee)
Sliced Dutch Brand Loaf
Sliced Pickle Loaf

Publix ()
All Natural Fresh Pork
Cajun Pork Sausage
GreenWise Market Boston Butt Roast
GreenWise Market Boston Butt Roast,
  Boneless
GreenWise Market Butterfly Pork Chop
GreenWise Market Center Cut Pork
  Loin Chop
GreenWise Market Center Cut Pork
  Loin Roast, Boneless
GreenWise Market Center Cut Pork Rib
  Chop
GreenWise Market Center Cut Pork
  Roast
GreenWise Market Cubed Steak
GreenWise Market Ground Pork
GreenWise Market Pork Back Ribs
GreenWise Market Pork Chop, Boneless
GreenWise Market Pork for Stew
GreenWise Market Pork for Stir Fry
GreenWise Market Pork Ham, Rump
  Portion
GreenWise Market Pork Ham, Shank
  Portion
GreenWise Market Pork Ham, Whole
GreenWise Market Pork Kabobs
GreenWise Market Pork Loin, Crown
  Roast
GreenWise Market Pork Picnic
GreenWise Market Pork Sage Sausage
GreenWise Market Pork Shoulder
  Country Ribs
GreenWise Market Pork Spare Ribs
GreenWise Market Pork Steak
GreenWise Market Pork Steak, Boneless
GreenWise Market Romano Pork
  Sausage
GreenWise Market Sirloin Cutlets
GreenWise Market St. Louis Pork Spare
  Ribs
GreenWise Market Whole Pork
  Tenderloin

Olive Loaf (Pre-Packed Sliced Deli Lunch Meats)

Pickle & Pimento Loaf (Pre-Packed Sliced Deli Lunch Meats)

Spanish Style Pork (Pre-Packed Sliced Deli Lunch Meats)

SALAMI

Boar's Head
Meats (All)

Columbus Salame
Salame (All)

Empire Kosher
Turkey Salami - Slices
Turkey Salami Roll

Farmer John ⓘ
Lunch Meats - Cotto Salami

Hebrew National ⟨⟩
Hebrew National (All BUT Hebrew National Beef Franks in a Blanket)

Hormel ⓘ
Hard Salami
Homeland Hard Salami
Natural Choice Hard Salami

Hy-Vee
Cooked Salami

Johnsonville
Johnsonville (All BUT Cooked Beer Brats and Beer n' Bratwurst)

Kunzler
Cooked Salami
Hard Salami

Midwest Country Fare (Hy-Vee)
Sliced Cooked Salami

Oscar Mayer ⌇
Cotto Salami
Cotto Salami/ Bologna/Chopped Ham Variety Pack
Hard Sausage/Salami
Salami Beef Deli Thin
Turkey Cotto Salami 50% Less Fat

Perdue
Deli Turkey Salami

Publix ⟨⟩
Hard Salami - Reduced Fat (Pre-Packed Sliced Deli Lunch Meats)

Saag's
Saag's (All BUT British Bangers)

Smith's
Smith's (All)

Sugardale ⓘ
Cooked Salami
Genoa Salami
Hard Salami
Ultra Thin Sliced Deli Meat - Salami

Superior's ⓘ
Cooked Salami
Paradise Cooked Salami

Thin 'n Trim
Thin 'n Trim (All)

Thumann's ✓
Meat (All BUT Deep Fry Hot Dogs)

SAUSAGE

Al Fresco All Natural ⓘ
Chicken Sausages (All BUT Mango Chipotle Chicken Sausage)

Beeler's ⚇
Beeler's (All)

Bilinski Sausage ⚇
Bilinski Sausage (All)

Boar's Head
Meats (All)

Canino's Sausage Company ⚇
Bratwurst
Breakfast Sausage
German Brand Sausage
Hot Italian Sausage
Hot! Chorizo
Mild Italian Sausage
Polish Sausage
Spicy Cajun Style Sausage
Sweet Italian Sausage

Coleman Natural ⓘ
Bratwurst
Mild Italian Chicken Sausage
Polish Kielbasa
Spicy Andouille Chicken Sausage

Spicy Chipotle Chicken Sausage
Spicy Chorizo Chicken Sausage
Spicy Italian Chicken Sausage
Spinach & Feta Cheese Chicken Sausage
Sun-Dried Tomato and Basil Chicken Sausage
Sweet Apple with Maple Syrup Chicken Sausage

Coleman Organic ⓘ
Mild Italian Chicken Sausage
Spinach & Feta Chicken Sausage
Sun-Dried Tomato & Basil Chicken Sausage
Sweet Apple Chicken Sausage

Farmer John ⓘ
Breakfast Sausage Links & Patties - Firehouse Hot Roll
Breakfast Sausage Links & Patties - Firehouse Hot Skinless Links
Breakfast Sausage Links & Patties - Old Fashioned Maple Skinless
Breakfast Sausage Links & Patties - Original Roll
Breakfast Sausage Links & Patties - Original Skinless
Breakfast Sausage Links & Patties - Premium Original Chorizo
Breakfast Sausage Links & Patties - Premium P C Links Lower Fat
Breakfast Sausage Links & Patties - Premium S C Links
Breakfast Sausage Links & Patties - Premium Sausage Patties Lower Fat
Breakfast Sausage Links & Patties - Premium Spicy Hot Chorizo
Breakfast Sausage Links & Patties - Premium Traditional Chorizo
Breakfast Sausage Links & Patties - Quick Serve Fully Cooked
California Natural - Apple Smoked Chicken Sausage
California Natural - Asiago Smoked Chicken Sausage
California Natural - Brat Smoked Chicken Sausage
California Natural - Cajun Style Smoked Chicken Sausage
California Natural - Lemon Cracked Pepper Smoked Chicken Sausage
California Natural - Mango and Habanero Smoked Chicken Sausage
Dinner Sausage - Hot Louisiana Smoked
Dinner Sausage - Jalapeno Pepper Premium Rope
Dinner Sausage - Jalapeno Pepper Premium Smoked
Dinner Sausage - Premium Beef Rope
Dinner Sausage - Premium Polish
Dinner Sausage - Premium Pork Rope
Dinner Sausage - Red Hots Extra Premium Smoked
Lunch Meats - Original Premium Liverwurst
Lunch Meats - Premium Braunschweiger
Lunch Meats - Premium Liverwurst with Bacon

Great Value (Wal-Mart)
Fully Cooked Beef Breakfast Patties
Fully Cooked Maple Pork Sausage Patties
Fully Cooked Original Pork Sausage Patties
Fully Cooked Sausage Links
Fully Cooked Spicy Pork Sausage Patties
Hot Pork Sausage
Mild Pork Sausage
Sage Pork Sausage

Hans All Natural ⓘ
Organic Breakfast Links Chicken Sausage
Skinless Chicken Breakfast Links
Spinach & Feta Cheese Chicken Sausage
Spinach, Fontina Cheese & Garlic Chicken Sausage
Sun-Dried Tomato Provolone Chicken Sausage

Hebrew National ⟨⟩
Hebrew National (All BUT Hebrew National Beef Franks in a Blanket)

Honeysuckle White
Honeysuckle White (All BUT Beer Smoked Turkey Bratwurst Fully Cooked, Italian Style Meatballs, Cajun Fried Turkey, and Teriyaki Turkey Breast Tenderloins)

Hormel ⓘ
Crumbled Sausage
Smokies

Hy-Vee
Beef Sausage
Little Smokies
Polish Rope Sausage
Polish Sausage
Sausage Links
Sausage Patties
Smoked Bratwurst
Smoked Sausage
Smoked Sausage with Cheddar Cheese

Jennie-O Turkey Store ⓘ
Breakfast Lover's Turkey Sausage
Extra Lean Smoked Kielbasa Turkey Sausage
Extra Lean Smoked Turkey Sausage
Fresh Breakfast Sausage - Maple Links
Fresh Breakfast Sausage - Mild Links
Fresh Breakfast Sausage - Mild Patties
Fresh Dinner Sausage - Hot Italian
Fresh Dinner Sausage - Lean Turkey Bratwurst
Fresh Dinner Sausage - Sweet Italian
Fully Cooked Frozen Sausage Links & Patties

Johnsonville
Johnsonville (All BUT Cooked Beer Brats and Beer n' Bratwurst)

Jones Dairy Farm
Chub Braunschweiger (Liverwurst), Bacon & Onion
Chub Braunschweiger (Liverwurst), Light
Chub Braunschweiger (Liverwurst), Mild & Creamy
Chub Braunschweiger (Liverwurst), Original
Chunk Braunschweiger (Liverwurst), Light
Chunk Braunschweiger (Liverwurst), Original
Slices Braunschweiger (Liverwurst), Original

Kunzler
Braunschweigner (Liverwurst)
Fresh Sausage - Bratwurst
Fresh Sausage - Hot & Sweet Italian
Fresh Sausage - Regular
Smoked Sausages - 5 Pepper & Cheddar
Smoked Sausages - Black Forest Kielbasa
Smoked Sausages - Black Forest Smoked
Smoked Sausages - Jalapeno & Cheddar
Smoked Sausages - Regular Kielbasa
Smoked Sausages - Regular Smoked & Kielbasa
Smoked Sausages - Regular Smoked Hot & Rajin Cajun

Little Sizzlers ⓘ
Original Sausage Links and Patties

Old Neighborhood
Old Neighborhood (All)

Old Wisconsin ⓘ
Festival Bratwurst
Polish Kielbasa
Smoked Sausage with Cheddar

Oscar Mayer ◠
Smoked Turkey Sausage
Turkey Polska Kielbasa

Perdue
Seasoned Fresh Lean Turkey Sausage - Sweet Italian
Turkey Breakfast Sausage

Publix ()
Fresh Bratwurst
Fresh Chorizo
Fresh Italian Sausage, Hot
Fresh Italian Sausage, Mild
Fresh Turkey Italian Sausage, Hot
Fresh Turkey Italian Sausage, Mild

Saag's
Saag's (All BUT British Bangers)

Sabrett
Hot Sausage
Italian Sausage

Sausages by Amylu
Sausages by Amylu (All BUT Chicken
Chorizo and Chicken Wieners)

Smith's
Smith's (All)

Sugardale ⓘ
Kielbassi

Superior's ⓘ
Polish Sausage

Thin 'n Trim
Thin 'n Trim (All)

Thrifty Maid (Winn-Dixie) ()
Mild Pork Sausages

Thumann's ✓
Meat (All BUT Deep Fry Hot Dogs)

V & V Supremo
Chorizo Products (All)

TOFU & TEMPEH

Eden Foods ⓘ ✓
Dried Tofu

Fresh & Easy ()
Tofus

LightLife ()
Garden Veggie Tempeh
Organic Flax Tempeh
Organic Soy Tempeh
Organic Wild Rice Tempeh

Mori-Nu
Organic Silken Tofu
Silken Extra Firm Tofu
Silken Firm Tofu
Silken Lite Firm Tofu
Silken Soft Tofu

Sunergia ()
Sunergia (All)

TURKEY

Bashas'
Turkey Breast Sliced 97% Fat Free

Boar's Head
Meats (All)

Buddig ♈
Buddig Original - Honey Roasted
Turkey
Buddig Original - Mesquite Turkey
Buddig Original - Oven Roasted Turkey
Buddig Original - Turkey
Deli Cuts - Honey Roasted Turkey
Deli Cuts - Oven-Roasted Turkey
Deli Cuts - Smoked Turkey
Fix Quix - Turkey

Columbus Salame
Deli Meats (All)

Empire Kosher
Fresh Ground Turkey
Honey Smoked Turkey Breast-Skinless
Preferred - Signature Edition Smoked
Turkey Breast, Skinless
Preferred - Signature Edition Turkey
Breast Pastrami, Skinless
Preferred - Signature Edition Turkey
Pastrami, Skinless
Premier - Signature Edition All Natural
Turkey Breast Skinless
Premier - Signature Edition All Natural
Turkey Breast with Skin
Signature Edition - Oven Prepared
Turkey Breast
Signature Edition - Smoked Turkey
Breast
Smoked Turkey Breast - Slices
Turkey Breast - Slices
Turkey Pastrami - Slices
White Turkey Roll

Farmer John ⓘ
Lunch Meats - Premium Oven Roasted
Turkey Breast

Fresh & Easy ()
Luncheon Meat Tub - Turkey

Great Value (Wal-Mart)
Fat Free Turkey Breast
Sliced Fat Free Smoked Turkey Breast
Sliced Fat Free Turkey Breast
Sliced Honey Turkey Breast
Thinly Sliced Oven Roasted Turkey
Breast
Thinly Sliced Smoked Turkey Breast

Honeysuckle White

Honeysuckle White (All BUT Beer Smoked Turkey Bratwurst Fully Cooked, Italian Style Meatballs, Cajun Fried Turkey, and Teriyaki Turkey Breast Tenderloins)

Hormel ⓘ

Julienne Turkey
Natural Choice - Honey Deli Turkey
Natural Choice - Oven Roasted Deli Turkey
Natural Choice - Smoked Deli Turkey

Hy-Vee

All Natural Fresh Turkey
All Natural Frozen Turkey
Butter Basted Turkey
Cubed Turkey
Deli Thin Slices - Honey Roasted Turkey Breast
Deli Thin Slices - Oven Roasted Turkey Breast
Moisture Enhanced Fresh Turkey
Moisture Enhanced Frozen Turkey
Organic Turkey
Thin Sliced Honey Turkey
Thin Sliced Turkey

Jennie-O Turkey Store ⓘ

Flavored Tenderloins - Applewood Smoked
Flavored Tenderloins - Balsamic Herb & Olive Oil
Flavored Tenderloins - Garlic & Red Pepper
Flavored Tenderloins - Lemon-Garlic
Flavored Tenderloins - Roast Flavor
Flavored Tenderloins - Smoky SW Style
Flavored Tenderloins - Tequila Lime
Flavored Tenderloins - Tomato Basil
Flavored Tenderloins - Traditional Herb
Fresh Ground Turkey - Extra Lean
Fresh Ground Turkey - Italian
Fresh Ground Turkey - Lean
Fresh Ground Turkey - Taco Seasoned
Fresh Lean Turkey Patties
Fresh Tray - Breast Slices
Fresh Tray - Breast Strips
Fresh Tray - Tenderloins

Grand Champion - Hickory Smoked Turkey Breast (Deli)
Grand Champion - Homestyle Pan Roasted Turkey Breast (Deli)
Grand Champion - Honey Cured Turkey Breast (Deli)
Grand Champion - Mesquite Smoked Turkey Breast (Deli)
Grand Champion - Oven Roasted Turkey Breast (Deli)
Grand Champion - Tender Browned Turkey Breast (Deli)
Hickory Smoked Turkey Breast - Cracked Pepper (Deli)
Hickory Smoked Turkey Breast - Garlic Pesto (Deli)
Hickory Smoked Turkey Breast - Honey Cured (Deli)
Hickory Smoked Turkey Breast - Sun Dried Tomato (Deli)
Natural Choice - Oven Roasted Turkey Breast (Deli)
Natural Choice - Peppered Turkey Breast (Deli)
Natural Choice - Tender Browned Turkey Breast (Deli)
Oven Ready Turkey - Garlic & Herb
Oven Ready Turkey - Homestyle
Oven Roasted Turkey Breast (Deli)
Pan Roasts with Gravy - White
Pan Roasts with Gravy - White/Dark Combo
Refrigerated Honey Cured Turkey Ham
Refrigerated Quarter Turkey Breasts - Cajun-Style
Refrigerated Quarter Turkey Breasts - Cracked Pepper
Refrigerated Quarter Turkey Breasts - Hickory Smoked
Refrigerated Quarter Turkey Breasts - Honey Cured
Refrigerated Quarter Turkey Breasts - Oven Roasted
Refrigerated Quarter Turkey Breasts - Sun-Dried Tomato
Refrigerated Turkey Ham
Smoked Turkey Breast - Hickory (Deli)

Smoked Turkey Breast - Honey Cured (Deli)
Smoked Turkey Breast - Mesquite (Deli)
Smoked Turkey Wings & Drumsticks
So Easy - Slow Roasted Turkey Breast
Turkey Breast - Apple Cinnamon (Deli)
Turkey Breast - Garlic Peppered (Deli)
Turkey Breast - Honey Maple (Deli)
Turkey Breast - Honey Mesquite (Deli)
Turkey Breast - Hot Red Peppered (Deli)
Turkey Breast - Italian Style (Deli)
Turkey Breast - Maple Spiced (Deli)
Turkey Breast - Mesquite Smoked (Deli)
Turkey Breast - Peppered (Deli)
Turkey Breast - Smoked (Deli)
Turkey Breast - Smoked Peppered (Deli)
Turkey Breast - Tender Browned (Deli)
Turkey Breast - Tomato Basil (Deli)

Kroger ⓘ
Fresh Plain Turkey Breast
Fresh Plain Turkey Thighs

Kunzler
Turkey Breast Presliced
Turkey Breast Whole
Turkey Ham - Black Forest
Turkey Ham - Regular

Land O'Frost
Lunchmeats (All BUT Taste Escapes Lemon Pepper Chicken)

Meijer
Fresh Hen Turkey
Fresh Tom Turkey
Gold - Hen Turkey
Gold - Tom Turkey
Hen Turkey
Hickory Smoked Turkey Breast
Honey Roasted Turkey Breast
Tom Turkey
Turkey Basted with Timer
Turkey Breast Fresh
Turkey Breast Zipper 97% Fat Free
Turkey Fresh Natural
Turkey Sliced Chipped Meat

Norwestern ⓘ
Deli Turkey - Hickory Smoked
Deli Turkey - Oven Roasted

Old Neighborhood
Old Neighborhood (All)

Organic Prairie
Sliced Roast Turkey Breast
Sliced Smoked Turkey Breast

Oscar Mayer ⌒
Deli Fresh Meats - Cracked Black Peppered Shaved 8 Oz. Tray
Deli Fresh Meats - Honey Smoked Thin Sliced
Deli Fresh Meats - Mesquite Thin Sliced
Deli Fresh Meats - Oven Roasted & White Turkey 98% Fat Free
Deli Fresh Meats - Oven Roasted 98% Fat Free 20 Oz
Deli Fresh Meats - Oven Roasted Thin Sliced
Deli Fresh Meats - Smoked 98% Fat Free
Deli Fresh Meats - Smoked Thin Sliced
Deli Fresh Meats - Turkey Breast Honey Smoked Shaved
Deli Fresh Meats - Turkey Breast Mesquite Shaved
Deli Fresh Meats - Turkey Breast Oven Roasted Shaved
Deli Fresh Meats - Turkey Breast Smoked Shaved
Deli Fresh Singles Turkey Breast Honey Oven Roasted Shaved 2 Pack
Deli Fresh Singles Turkey Breast Smoked Shaved 2 Pack
Deli Fresh Turkey Breast Oven Roasted Shaved 98% Fat Free
Deli Fresh Turkey Breast Oven Roasted Shaved 98% Fat Free Family Size
Deli Fresh Turkey Breast Smoked Shaved 98% Fat Free Family Size
Deli Fresh Turkey Breast Thick Carved Oven Roasted 98% Fat Free
Lean White Honey Smoked 95% Fat Free Turkey
Oven Roasted White Turkey
Turkey Smoked White 95% Fat Free
White Oven Roasted 95% Fat Free Turkey
White Smoked 95% Fat Free Turkey

Perdue

Carving - Turkey Breast, Hickory Smoked

Carving - Turkey Breast, Honey Smoked

Carving - Turkey Breast, Mesquite Smoked

Carving - Turkey Breast, Oven Roasted

Carving - Whole Turkey

Carving Classics - Pan Roasted Turkey Breast, Cracked Pepper

Carving Classics - Turkey Breast Pan Roasted

Carving Classics - Turkey Breast Pan Roasted, Honey Smoked

Deli Dark Turkey Pastrami - Hickory Smoked

Deli Pick Ups - Sliced Turkey Breast, Golden Browned

Deli Pick Ups - Sliced Turkey Breast, Honey Smoked

Deli Pick Ups - Sliced Turkey Breast, Mesquite Smoked

Deli Pick Ups - Sliced Turkey Breast, Oven Roasted

Deli Pick Ups - Sliced Turkey Breast, Smoked

Deli Turkey Breast - Oil Browned

Fresh Ground Breast of Turkey

Fresh Lean Ground Turkey

Ground Turkey Burgers

Healthsense - Turkey Breast, Oven Roasted (Fat Free, Reduced Sodium)

Rotisserie Turkey Breast

Short Cuts Carved Turkey Breast - Oven Roasted

Whole Turkeys Seasoned with Broth

Plainville Farms

Turkey Products (All BUT Gravy/Relish and Dressing)

Publix ()

Extra Thin Sliced Oven Roasted Turkey Breast (Pre-Packed Sliced Deli Lunch Meats)

Extra Thin Sliced Smoked Turkey Breast (Pre-Packed Sliced Deli Lunch Meats)

Fresh Young Turkey Breast

Fresh Young Turkey, Whole

Fully Cooked Smoked Turkey Breast

Fully Cooked Smoked Turkey, Whole

Ground Turkey

Ground Turkey Breast

Smoked Turkey (Pre-Packed Sliced Deli Lunch Meats)

Turkey Breast (Pre-Packed Sliced Deli Lunch Meats)

Saag's

Saag's (All BUT British Bangers)

Shady Brook Farms

Shady Brook Farms (All BUT Beer Smoked Turkey Bratwurst Fully Cooked, Italian Style Meatballs, Appetizer Sized Meatballs, Cajun Fried Turkey, and Teriyaki Turkey Breast Tenderloins)

Sugardale ⓘ

Ultra Thin Sliced Deli Meat - Turkey

Thin 'n Trim

Thin 'n Trim (All)

Thumann's ✓

Meat (All BUT Deep Fry Hot Dogs)

Symbols Summary   gf = gluten-free

 GF Lines or Facility; or
No chance of cross-contamination

 Gluten Testing is performed

 Gluten-Free based on review of ingredient label
(as no GF list was provided)

 Procedures to Mitigate Cross-Contamination are in place,
although there are shared facilities or equipment

 Cross-Contamination is possible; or, Made with "gluten-free in-gredients" (with no mention of overall status by the company)

No Icon. The company reported that the product is gluten-free but provided no further context.

For the full key, see page 21 >>

ALWAYS READ LABELS

THE GLUTEN-FREE DIET:
AN EASY REFERENCE INGREDIENTS TABLE

Need a refresher on the gluten-free diet? These grains are safe: rice, soy, corn, potatoes, tapioca, buckwheat, arrowroot, amaranth, millet, quinoa, sorghum and teff. When plain, you can also eat: fruits, vegetables, milk, meat, eggs, beans, oil, wine, and distilled alcohols like vodka and gin.

As for what's off limits, "no wheat, rye, barley and oats*" in practice means, no (wheat) flour, pasta, croutons, bread, cookies, and "hidden" gluten sources like soy sauce, beer, and licorice. (But don't despair, there ARE specialty GF versions of these products in this guide!) Beyond these basics, even the most experienced shopper can stumped by mysterious ingredients like "guar gum."

We hope this ingredient list will make label-reading easier than ever, for both new and experienced GF shoppers!

Ingredient	Status
Mono and Diglycerides	✓
Monosodium Glutamate (MSG)	✓
Mustard Flour	?
Natural Colors	✓
Natural Flavors	✓
Polysorbates	✓
Psyllium	✓
Rennet	✓
Rice Malt	✓
Rice Syrup	?
Rum	✓
Saccharin	✓
Seitan	✗
Semolina	✗
Silicon Dioxide	✓
Sodium Benzoate	✓
Sodium Nitrate	✓
Sodium Nitrite	✓
Sodium Sulphite	✓
Sorbate	✓
Sorbic Acid	✓
Sorbitol	✓
Soy Sauce	✗
Spelt	✗
Starch (on labels, this refers to cornstarch)	✓
Stevia	✓
Sucralose	✓
Sucrose	✓
Sulfites	✓
Tabbouleh	✗
Tartaric Acid	✓
Triticale	✗
Vanilla Extract	✓
Vanilla Flavoring	✓
Vanillin	✓
Vinegar (All EXCEPT malt)	✓
Vodka	✓
Wheat Bran	✗
Wheat Germ	✗
Whey	✓
Wine	✓
Xanthan Gum	✓
Xylitol	✓
Yeast (All EXCEPT brewer's yeast)	✓

Ingredient	Status	Ingredient	Status
Agar-Agar	✓	Durum	✗
Alcohol, Distilled	✓	Einkorn	✗
Algin	✓	Farina	✗
Annatto	✓	Flax	✓
Arabic Gum	✓	Fructose	✓
Artificial Colors	✓	Fumaric Acid	✓
Artificial Flavoring	✓	Gelatin	✓
Ascorbic Acid	✓	Glucose	✓
Aspartame	✓	Glucose Syrup	✓
Baking Powder	?	Glutamic Acid	✓
Beer	✗	Glutinous Rice	✓
Beta Carotene	✓	Glycerides	✓
BHA	✓	Glycol	✓
BHT	✓	Graham Flour	✗
Bulgur	✗	Guar Gum	✓
Calcium Disodium EDTA	✓	Gum Arabic	✓
Caprylic Acid	✓	Hydrolyzed Corn Protein	✓
Caramel Color	✓	Hydrolyzed Soy Protein	✓
Carboxymethylcellulose	✓	Hydrolyzed Wheat Protein	✗
Carnauba Wax	✓	Inulin	✓
Carob Bean	✓	Invert Sugar	✓
Carrageenan	✓	Kamut	✗
Casein	✓	Lactic Acid	✓
Cellulose Gum	✓	Lactose	✓
Citric Acid	✓	Lecithin	✓
Corn Gluten	✓	Malic Acid	✓
Corn Syrup	✓	Malt (e.g., malt extract, malt flavoring, malt vinegar)	✗
Corn Syrup Solids	✓	Maltitol	✓
Cornstarch	✓	Maltodextrin	✓
Couscous	✗	Maltose	✓
Cream of Tartar	✓	Mannitol	✓
Dextrimaltose	✗	Matzo (matzoh)	✗
Dextrins	?	Molasses	✓
Dextrose	✓		

*See page 14 for a profile on "gluten-free" oats

This ingredient table was created in collaboration with Shelley Case, B.Sc., RD, registered dietitian and author of Gluten-Free Diet: A Comprehensive Resource Guide. She is a member of the medical advisory board of the Celiac Disease Foundation and Gluten Intolerance Group. For more in-depth information about the gluten-free diet, ingredients, labeling laws and healthy eating, please visit www.glutenfreediet.ca.